IARC Handbooks of Cancer Prevention

## Volume 7

# Breast Cancer Screening

**IARC Handbooks of Cancer Prevention**
**Programme Head: Harri Vainio**

**Volume 7: Breast Cancer Screening**

| | |
|---|---|
| Editors: | Harri Vainio, M.D., Ph.D.<br>Franca Bianchini, Ph.D |
| Technical editor: | Elisabeth Heseltine, M.Sc. |
| Bibliographic assistance: | Agnès Meneghel<br>Brigitte Kajo |
| Photographic assistance: | Georges Mollon/Pascale Rousson |
| Layout: | Josephine Thévenoux |
| Printed by: | LIPS, Lyon, France |
| Publisher: | IARCPress<br>International Agency for Research on Cancer<br>150 cours Albert Thomas, 69372 Lyon, France<br>Tel. +33 4 72 73 84 85<br>Fax. +33 4 72 73 83 19 |

WORLD HEALTH ORGANIZATION

INTERNATIONAL AGENCY FOR RESEARCH ON CANCER

# IARC Handbooks of Cancer Prevention

## Volume 7

# Breast Cancer Screening

**IARC**Press

Lyon, 2002

Published by the International Agency for Research on Cancer,
150 cours Albert Thomas, F-69372 Lyon cedex 08, France

Distributed by Oxford University Press, Walton Street, Oxford, OX2 6DP, UK (Fax: +44 1865 267782) and in the USA by
Oxford University Press, 2001 Evans Road, Carey, NC 27513, USA  (Fax: +1 919 677 1303).
All IARC publications can also be ordered directly from IARCPress
(Fax: +33 4 72 73 83 02; E-mail: press@iarc.fr)
and in the USA from IARCPress, WHO Office, Suite 480, 1775 K Street, Washington DC, 20006

**IARC Library Cataloguing in Publication Data**

Breast Cancer Screening/
    IARC Working Group on the Evaluation of
    Cancer-Preventive Strategies  (2002 : Lyon, France)

(IARC handbooks of cancer prevention ; 7)

1.  Breast Neoplasms - prevention & control 2. Mass Screening I, IARC Working
    Group on the Evaluation of Cancer-Preventive Strategies II. Series

ISBN  92 832 3007 8                                        (NLM Classification: W1)
ISSN  1027-5622

Printed in France

# International Agency For Research On Cancer

The International Agency for Research on Cancer (IARC) was established in 1965 by the World Health Assembly, as an independently financed organization within the framework of the World Health Organization. The headquarters of the Agency are in Lyon, France.

The Agency conducts a programme of research concentrating particularly on the epidemiology of cancer and the study of potential carcinogens in the human environment. Its field studies are supplemented by biological and chemical research carried out in the Agency's laboratories in Lyon and, through collaborative research agreements, in national research institutions in many countries. The Agency also conducts a programme for the education and training of personnel for cancer research.

The publications of the Agency contribute to the dissemination of authoritative information on different aspects of cancer research. Information about IARC publications, and how to order them, is available via the Internet at: **http://www.iarc.fr/**

---

This publication represents the views and opinions of an IARC Working Group on the Evaluation of Cancer-Preventive Strategies which met in Lyon, France, 5–12 March 2002

---

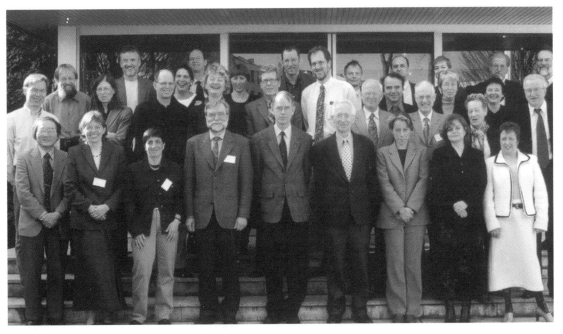

**Participants and members of the secretariat:**
*First row from left:* T. Kuroishi, M. Blettner, F. Bianchini, M. Hakama, P. Dean, B. Armstrong, P. Pisani, S. Robles, J. Thévenoux. *Middle row:* E. Suonio, K. Straif, C. Partensky, S. Taplin, E. Heseltine, C. Baines, J. Hall, I. Andersson, G. Welsch, D. Thomas, N. Segnan, A. B. Miller, A. Kricker, H. Sancho-Garnier, S. Redman, L. Nyström. *Back row:* H. Vainio, S. Narod, H. de Koning, A. Ullrich, J. Tyczynski, E. Weiderpass-Vainio, N. Day, L. Irwig. (Participants missing from photo: V. Beral, I. Ellis and R. Blanks)

## Note to the Reader

Anyone who is aware of published data that may influence any consideration in these *Handbooks* is encouraged to make the information available to the Unit of Chemoprevention, International Agency for Research on Cancer, 150 Cours Albert Thomas, 69372 Lyon Cedex 08, France

Although all efforts are made to prepare the *Handbooks* as accurately as possible, mistakes may occur. Readers are requested to communicate any errors to the Unit of Chemoprevention, so that corrections can be reported in future volumes.

## Acknowledgements

We would like to acknowledge generous support from the Foundation for Promotion of Cancer Research, Japan (2nd Term Comprehensive 10-Year Strategy for Cancer Control), and from the German Federal Ministry for Health.

# Contents

# List of participants

**I. Andersson**
Department of Diagnostic Radiology
Malmö University Hospital
Malmö
Sweden

**B. Armstrong (Chairman)**
Edward Ford Building A27
University of Sydney
Sydney
NSW 2006
Australia

**C. Baines**
Department of Public Health Sciences
University of Toronto
Toronto
Ontario M5S 1A8
Canada

**V. Beral**
Imperial Cancer Research Fund
Cancer Epidemiology Unit
University of Oxford
Gibson Building
Radcliffe Infirmary
Oxford OX2 6HE
United Kingdom

**R. Blanks**
Institute of Cancer Research
Royal Cancer Hospital
Cancer Screening Evaluation Unit
Sutton
Surrey SM2 5NG
United Kingdom

**M. Blettner**
Department of Epidemiology and
Medical Statistics
School of Public Health
33501 Bielefeld
Germany

**N. Day**
Strangeways Research Laboratory
University of Cambridge
Cambridge CB1 8RN
United Kingdom

**P. Dean**
Department of Diagnostic Radiology
University of Turku
20521 Turku
Finland

**H.J. de Koning**
Department of Public Health
Erasmus University Rotterdam
3000 DR Rotterdam
Netherlands

**I. Ellis**
Faculty of Medicine and Health
Sciences
Division of Histopathology
Nottingham City Hospital
NHS Trust
Nottingham NG5 1PB
United Kingdom

**S. Fletcher***
Harvard Medical School
Harvard Pilgrim Health Care
Boston
Massachusetts 02115
USA

**M. Hakama (Vice-Chairman)**
University of Tampere
School of Public Health
33014 Tampere
Finland

**L. Irwig**
Screening and Test Evaluation
Program (STEP)
Department of Public Health and
Community Medicine
University of Sydney
Sydney
NSW 2006
Australia

**A. Kricker**
NHMRC
National Breast Cancer Centre
Kings Cross
Sydney
NSW
Australia

**T. Kuroishi**
Division of Epidemiology &
Prevention
Aichi Cancer Center Research
Institute
464-8681 Nagoya
Japan

**A.B. Miller**
Division of Clinical Epidemiology
German Cancer Research Center
69120 Heidelberg
Germany

*Unable to attend

**S. Narod**
The Centre for Research in Women's
Health
Toronto M5G 1N8
Canada

**C. Nichols***
Office of Science Planning and
Assessment
National Cancer Institute
Bethesda
Maryland 20892
USA

**L. Nyström**
Department of Public Health and
Clinical Medicine
Unit of Epidemiology
Umeå University
901-85 Umeå
Sweden

**S. Redman**
NHMRC
National Breast Cancer Centre
Kings Cross
NSW
Australia

**S. Robles**
Pan American Health Organization
Regional Office of the World Health
Organization
HCP/HCN
Washington DC 20037
USA

**H. Sancho-Garnier**
EPIDAURE
Centre Val d'Aurelle
Parc Euromédicine
34298 Montpellier
France

**N. Segnan**
CPO Piemonte
Cancer Prevention Centre
Unit of Epidemiology
10123 Torino
Italy

**S. Taplin**
Group Health Cooperative
Center for Health Studies
Seattle
Washington 98101-1448
USA

**D.B. Thomas**
Fred Hutchinson Cancer Research
Center
Seattle
Washington 98109-1024
USA

**H.G. Welch**
Department of Medicine and
Community and Family Medicine
Dartmouth Medical School
Hanover
New Hampshire 03755
USA

**Observer**

A. Ullrich
WHO
Geneva
Switzerland

**Secretariat**

F. Bianchini
J. Cheney
J. Hall
E. Heseltine (Lajarthe, 24290 St
Léon-sur-Vézère, France)
C. Partensky
D.M. Parkin
P. Pisani
A. Sasco
K. Straif
L. Stayner
E. Suonio
J. Tyczynski
H. Vainio
E. Weiderpass-Vainio

**Technical assistance**

B. Kajo
J. Mitchell
C. Mogenet
J. Thévenoux

* Unable to attend

# Preface

# Why a Handbook on breast cancer screening ?

The scientific process of acquiring information about the efficacy of breast cancer screening was initiated in 1963, when Sam Shapiro and coworkers introduced the Health Insurance Plan study (Shapiro *et al.*, 1988a) in New York, USA, the first randomized controlled trial of the effect of mammography and clinical breast examination in reducing mortality from breast cancer. This study opened the era of randomized controlled trials for evaluation of screening techniques. Cancer screening techniques used before that, such as the Papanicolau (Pap) smear, never underwent proper evaluation in randomized trials before their introduction as a means for population screening.

Randomized controlled trials have been criticized many times as expensive and slow to provide results. The Breast Cancer Detection Demonstration Project (Baker, 1982) in the USA was initiated to provide data on the efficacy of breast cancer screening rapidly, and the first results appeared in 1979, 3 years before publication of the results of the Health Insurance Plan study. Three more studies — in Malmö, Sweden (Andersson *et al.*, 1988), Edinburgh, Scotland (Roberts *et al.*, 1990) and in two Swedish counties (Tabár *et al.*, 1985) — were initiated 13–14 years after the beginning of the Health Insurance Plan study, and another three studies were initiated in 1980–82, in Canada (Miller *et al.*, 1992a,b) and in Stockholm (Frisell *et al.*,

1986) and Göteborg, Sweden (Bjurstam *et al.*, 1997). Thus, a number of randomized controlled trials, initiated in five different countries over a 20-year period, provide the basis for evidence in the field of mammographic screening.

Mammography was first officially introduced in a population-wide, organized screening programme in Iceland and in several districts in Sweden in 1987. The Netherlands and several regions of Canada followed in 1988, and Finland in 1989. In 1988, the American Cancer Society and the Preventive Services Task Force established policies in favour of screening for breast cancer in the USA (US Preventive Task Force, 1996). In contrast to the policies in other countries, that in the USA emphasized a triple approach, involving breast self-examination, clinical breast examination and mammography. The Europe Against Cancer programme simultaneously initiated a series of pilot screening programmes in several countries in Europe (Commission of the European Communities, 1996) in order to develop expertise in planning and running high-quality population-based screening programmes before their incorporation into national policy. In the early 1990s, national screening programmes were initiated in Australia and the United Kingdom, and these were followed by organized programmes in several states of the USA, in Israel and, later, in France. Germany and

Switzerland were among the last western countries to join the international trend, with plans to introduce national screening at the beginning of the twenty-first century.

Experience in large-scale mammographic screening by the mid-1990s, and the availability of data on more recent follow-up from the trials, led to discussion about the value of mammographic screening for women under the age of 50. Even on the basis of the same scientific evidence, few countries have established the same breast cancer screening policy. The policies differ with respect to the target age group to be screened, the frequency of screening, the number of mammographic views to be taken and the screening modalities. In Japan, the policy was based on clinical breast examination until recently, when it was decided to add mammography.

In spite of the vast amount of information available from several randomized trials, some doubt has recently been cast on the value of breast cancer screening in reducing mortality from breast cancer (Gotzsche & Olsen, 2000; Olsen & Gotzsche, 2001). In this volume, the relevant published studies are thoroughly reassessed, together with the newest data, either recently published or in press, according to the procedures and guidelines followed in the Handbooks (see pp. 223)

# Chapter 1

# Breast Cancer and Screening

## The world-wide burden of breast cancer

Of the 10 million new cases of invasive cancer world-wide each year in males and females combined, 10% arise in the breast, which makes it the second most common site of malignant neoplasms after the lung (Parkin, 2001). In 2000, breast cancer accounted for 22% of all new cancers in women, making it by far the most common cancer in females (Figure 1). In high-income countries, the proportion rises to 27%, more than twice as common as any other cancer in women. In 2000, cancer of the breast was also the commonest tumour among women in low-income regions, with 470 000 new cases per year, whereas invasive cervical cancer had been the leading cancer during the previous two decades. More than half of the 1.05 million cases occur in high-income countries in North America and western Europe and in Australia and New Zealand (Figure 2), where an average of 6% of women develop invasive breast cancer before the age of 75. Incidence rates of a similar magnitude are observed in Argentina and Uruguay. The risk for breast cancer is low in the low-income regions of sub-Saharan Africa and Southern and Eastern Asia, including Japan, where the probability of developing breast cancer by the age of 75 is one-third that of other high-income countries. The rates are intermediate elsewhere. Japan is the only affluent country where in 2000 the incidence rate was low.

Clear increases in the incidence of and mortality from breast cancer were

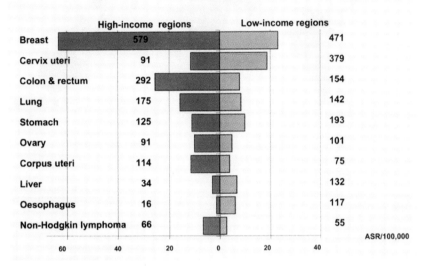

**Figure 1** The 10 commonest sites of cancer in women world-wide, with incidence rates for 2000. World age-standardized rates per 100 000 population and total numbers of cases (thousands)
From Ferlay *et al.* (2001)

### Breast cancer incidence

- Breast cancers accounted for 22% of all cancers in women worldwide (1 million new cases) in 2000.

- The incidence of breast cancer in women in high-income countries in 2000 was at least twice that of any other cancer in women, and was similar to the incidence of cancer of the cervix in low-income countries (see Figure 1).

- More than half the breast cancers that occurred throughout the world in 2000 were estimated to have been in high-income countries (see Figure 2).

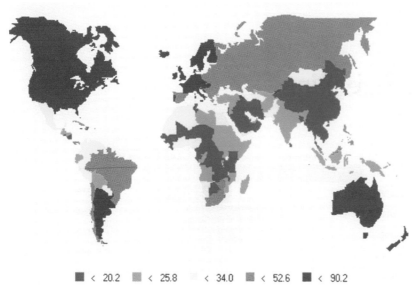

■ < 20.2  ■ < 25.8    < 34.0  ■ < 52.6  ■ < 90.2

**Figure 2** Estimated age-standardized incidence rates of breast cancer world-wide in 2000.
From Ferlay *et al.* (2001).

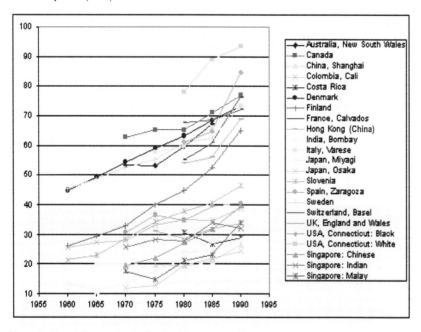

**Figure 3** Trends in age-standardized incidence rates of breast cancer among women in selected populations.
From Doll *et al.* (1966, 1970); Waterhouse *et al.* (1976, 1982, 1987), Parkin *et al.* (1992, 1997); http://www.depdb.iarc.fr/who/menu.htm

observed until the early 1980s in both high- and low-income countries (Figure 3). The subsequent advent of mammo-graphy and improvements in prognosis in high-income countries altered the reported rates of both incidence and

mortality, masking trends in the underlying risk for the disease. The risk continues to increase in eastern Europe and Latin America (Figure 3), as seen mainly from trends in mortality, and in some urban populations of Asia, as indicated by population-based incidence rates in, e.g., Japan, Singapore, Shanghai and Hong Kong (China) and Mumbai (India).

Around 1990, the incidence of breast cancer varied eightfold world-wide, indicating large differences in the distribution of the underlying causes (Parkin *et al.*, 1997). Studies of geographical variation, time trends and populations migrating from low- to high-risk areas (Geddes *et al.*, 1993; Ziegler *et al.*, 1993; Kliewer & Smith, 1995) suggest an important role of environmental factors in the etiology of the disease. Low parity, late age at first pregnancy, early menarche and late menopause are all factors that are consistently associated with an increased risk for breast cancer. Trends towards lower reproductive rates in western populations therefore explain part of the observed increase and may predict similar increases in populations where the reproduction rates are declining (Lopez-Carrillo *et al.*, 1997; dos Santos Silva & Beral, 1997; Gao *et al.*, 2000). As for most epithelial tumours, the risk for the disease increases steadily with age (Figure 4A).

Substantial improvements in survival have been recorded in western countries since the late 1970s (Adami *et al.*, 1989; Chu *et al.*, 1996; Quinn *et al.*, 1998), and an increasing number of women live with the consequences of the disease and its treatment. In the USA, survivors of breast cancer were estimated to constitute 1.5% of the female population (Hewitt *et al.*, 1999), which is about 10 times the annual incidence. The mortality rate, which had been increasing until the 1980s, levelled off or declined in several high-risk countries (Hermon & Beral, 1996; La Vecchia *et al.*, 1998; Howe *et al.*, 2001; Figures 4B, 4C, 4D). Despite these positive achievements,

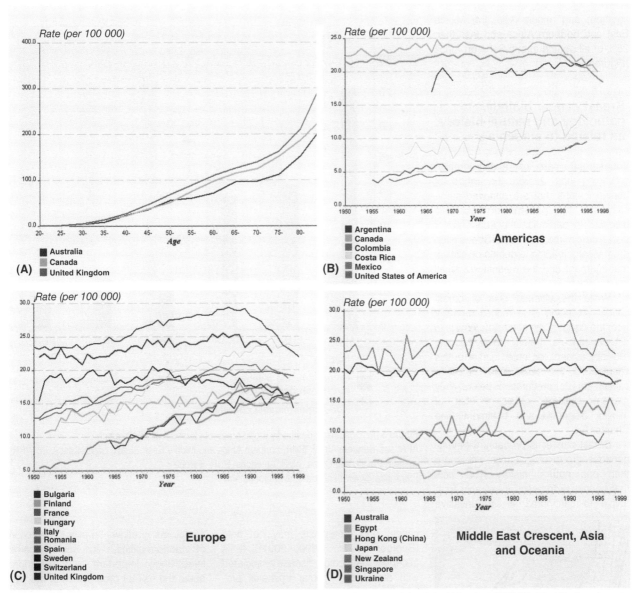

**Figure 4** Age-specific mortality rates from breast cancer in women in Australia, Canada and the United Kingdom, 1990 (A). Mortality from breast cancer, time trends of age-standardized rates per 100 000 female population in the Americas (B), Europe (C), Middle East Crescent, Asia and Oceania (D)

From http://www-depdb.iarc.fr/who/menu.htm

breast cancer remains the malignancy that causes the most deaths from cancer among women in high-income countries. The only exceptions are Canada and the USA, where mortality from lung cancer is still rising and is characterized by a poor prognosis (http://www-depdb.iarc.fr/who/menu.htm).

Survival from breast cancer in low-income countries is generally poorer than that in high-income regions, reflecting late presentation of cases (Sankar-

anarayanan et al., 1998). According to WHO, in 2000, noncommunicable diseases, including cancer, accounted for 75% of all deaths in the Americas, Europe and the Western Pacific region including China, half of all deaths in southern and middle Asia, the Middle East and northern Africa and less than 25% of all deaths in sub-Saharan Africa (Figure 5).

## Breast cancer biology, pathology and natural history as related to screening

Widespread use of mammographic screening has altered the range of benign lesions that are removed surgically and the patterns of neoplastic disease. In particular, the frequency of ductal carcinoma *in situ* (DCIS) has risen dramatically, leading to debate on clinical management and the meaning of small in-situ lesions.

While the ultimate goal of breast cancer screening is to reduce mortality from the disease, the immediate goal is to detect cancers before they become clinically evident, as noted earlier in this chapter. At the same time, detecting cancer (or its precursors) before they present clinically raises a risk of excess diagnosis and treatment (see Chapter 5).

Breast cancer is probably a heterogeneous group of diseases with more than one natural history. The view that cancer progresses inexorably from atypia to carcinoma *in situ*, invasive

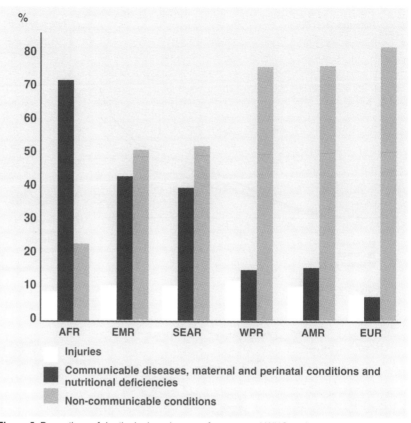

**Figure 5** Proportions of deaths by broad group of causes and WHO region.
AFR, sub-Saharan Africa; EMR, northern Africa and Middle East; SEAR, South-East Asia; WPR, western Pacific and China; AMR, Americas; EUR, Europe
From http://www-depdb.iarc.fr/who/menu.htm

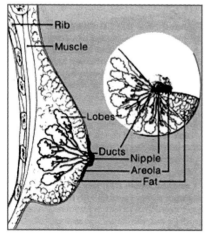

Normal breast structure

cancer and metastasis may not hold (Buerger *et al.*, 1999, 2001). It is accepted that benign disease associated with ductal and lobular epithelial proliferation and hyperplasia, especially with atypia, confers an increased risk for developing breast cancer, and these lesions may form part of a spectrum of neoplastic breast disease or an interface between some benign and malignant breast conditions. However, these lesions may not be the explanation or the basis for development of all forms of breast cancer.

As screening mammography and other techniques, in contrast to symptoms, allow earlier detection of abnormalities, it has become increasingly important to know more about the risk for progression of the various lesions identified. Understanding the progression rates is crucial for answering questions relevant to screening programmes, including how such abnormalities should be treated and how intensively they should be sought.

This section reviews what is known about the progression of breast cancer at three points in the disease course: benign disease, in-situ cancer and invasive cancer.

## Barriers to understanding of early cancers

At the outset, it is important to emphasize that there are two barriers to better understanding of progression. First, the nomenclature used for the microscopic appearance of lesions has been inconsistent, making comparisons across studies and time difficult. Secondly, there is concern about the reproducibility of pathological observations in early forms of breast cancer, some of which may reflect the problem of nomenclature and some the diagnostic threshold of a pathologist. In both cases, variation in diagnosis can confuse assessment of the risks for progression.

Most of the long-term data on progression of in-situ cancers and their precursors refer to lesions that presented clinically (e.g. a mass or nipple discharge) and not to those currently detected mammographically. Because disease detected at screening is asymptomatic and the tumours are generally smaller than those detected clinically, early detection could influence natural history. Thus, the progression rates reported here may be overestimates of the natural history of those detected by mammography.

## Benign breast disease
### Significance in breast screening

Many benign conditions can be seen mammographically, but those that lead to surgical biopsy are of particular concern. Woman may be recalled for assessment after primary mammographic screening because of benign disease or involutional changes, which can be seen mammographically as ill-defined masses (fibroadenoma and cysts), parenchymal deformity (radial scar, sclerosing adenosis) and calcification. A variety of benign calcified lesions are seen (Table 1; Spencer et al., 1994). The commonest abnormalities leading to benign surgical biopsy are non-comedo-type suspect calcification (29%) (Figure 6), a poorly defined mass (21%), architectural distortion (19%) and a well-defined mass (18%) (Spencer et al., 1994) (Figure 7) (American College of Radiology, 1995; Liberman et al., 1997).

The positive predictive value for malignancy by type of mammographic abnormality is shown in Table 2 (Burrell et al., 1996). The sensitivity of mammography in cancer detection must be high, but it is also important to achieve high diagnostic specificity to avoid morbidity associated with unnecessary surgical biopsy. The aim of assessments after screening should be both accurate diagnosis of breast cancer with prompt referral for treatment and accurate diagnosis of benign and involutional changes, if possible without surgical biopsy.

### Association with an increased risk for breast cancer

Many studies have shown an increased risk for cancer among patients with usual epithelial hyperplasia, which is 1.5–2.0 times greater than that of a reference population, and a 2.5–4-fold increase in risk for patients with atypical ductal hyperplasia (Dupont & Page, 1985; Dupont et al., 1993; Marshall et al., 1997) (Figure 8). Atypical lobular hyperplasia increases the relative risk by four to five times (Page et al., 1991; Marshall et al., 1997). Other forms of benign breast disease, such as sclerosing adenosis, fibroadenoma and papillary apocrine change, appear not to alter the risk or to be associated with a 1.5–2-fold increase (Jensen et al., 1989; Dupont et al., 1994). The invasive cancers occurring after diagnosis of these types of epithelial proliferation occur at roughly equal frequency in the ipsilateral and contralateral breast. All these epithelial proliferative lesions may be found coincidentally in a lesion found as a result of breast screening.

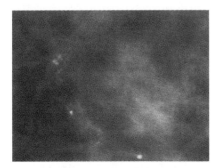

**Figure 6** Punctate calcification identified at mammographic screening. The resulting biopsy revealed benign stromal calcification

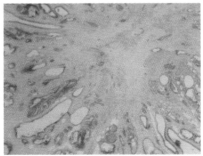

**Figure 7** A benign radial scar which has a stellate configuration similar to some forms of breast carcinoma and can produce a parenchymal deformity mimicking carcinoma mammographically

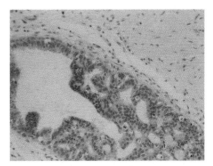

**Figure 8** An example of atypical ductal hyperplasia with a single duct space, part of which contains uniform, small-cell epithelial proliferation

## Table 1. Causes of indeterminate calcification diagnosed by core biopsy alone in 151 samples

| Lesion | (%) |
| --- | --- |
| Fibrocystic change | 33 |
| Fibroadenoma | 18 |
| Stromal calcification | 15 |
| Fibroadenomatoid hyperplasia | 15 |
| Involutional change | 11 |
| Sclerosing adenosis | 7 |
| Duct ectasia | 4 |
| Apocrine change | 4 |
| Blunt duct adenosis | 3 |
| Mucocoele | 2 |
| Vascular | 1 |
| Fat necrosis | 1 |
| Radiation change | 0.6 |
| Foreign body reaction | 0.6 |

From Spencer et al. (1994)

## Table 2. Positive predictive value (PPV) for malignancy of various mammographic abnormalities

| Abnormality | PPV (%) |
| --- | --- |
| Microcalcifications | |
| All | 45 |
| Comedo | 83 |
| Non-comedo | 35 |
| Masses | |
| Spiculate | 94 |
| Ill defined | 54 |
| Well defined | 4 |
| Parenchymal deformity | 37 |
| Density with calcification | 44 |

From Burrell et al. (1996)

## Carcinoma in situ

### Definition

Two non-invasive forms of breast carcinoma in situ are recognized: DCIS and lobular carcinoma in situ (LCIS). Each arises from its respective epithelial cell population in the lobule or duct of the normal breast. However, the neoplastic cell population is confined within the parenchymal site of origin, and the cells do not infiltrate beyond the limiting basement membrane. DCIS may harbour calcifications that make it mammographically apparent, but LCIS rarely gives rise to mammographic abnormalities (Goldschmidt & Victor, 1996).

### Association of LCIS with invasive carcinoma

Lobular neoplasia includes LCIS and atypical lobular hyperplasia and is typically found incidentally in other benign and malignant breast lesions on histological examination (Figure 9). The relative risk for subsequent development of invasive carcinoma among patients with lobular neoplasia ranges from 4- (atypical lobular hyperplasia) to about 10-fold in women with LCIS (Page et al., 1991; Dupont et al., 1993; Marshall et al., 1997), higher risks being associated with more extensive lesions (Page et al., 1991; Fisher et al., 1996). The invasive cancers seen after diagnosis of lobular neoplasia occur at roughly equal frequency in the ipsilateral and contralateral breast. Management of lobular neoplasia has evolved (Gump, 1993; Schnitt & Morrow, 1999) with better understanding of the disease. The current consensus is that both LCIS and atypical lobular hyperplasia are risk factors for subsequent development of invasive carcinoma in either breast. The value of routine mastectomy with or without contralateral breast biopsy has been questioned, and the majority of patients are managed by careful follow-up (Gump et al., 1998).

### Pathological classification of ductal carcinoma in situ (DCIS)

The classification of DCIS is evolving, and several groups have described systems for subdividing the lesions. The traditional classification, which is based on both architectural growth pattern and cytological features, is poorly reproducible, with up to 30% of cases in multicentre trials requiring reclassification (van Dongen et al., 1992a). The lack of agreement among pathologists may be due largely to the architectural heterogeneity of DCIS. There is less heterogeneity in nuclear grade characteristics, and most of the contemporary histological classification systems are based on a three-tier grading or differentiation system with nuclear grade (National Coordinating Group for Breast Screening Pathology, 1995; Sneige et al., 1998), grade and polarity (Holland et al., 1994) or grade in the presence or absence of necrosis (Poller et al., 1994: Silverstein et al., 1995). Silverstein and colleagues have been particularly innovative in using histological grade, lesion size and distance of the excision margin in making a prognostic index (Silverstein et al., 1996), and this has shown significant predictive power for local recurrence.

Although many of the histological classification systems appear to have

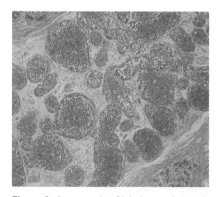

**Figure 9** An example of lobular carcinoma in situ, showing filling of a distention of the acini of a breast lobule by a uniform population of epithelial cells. There are no associated features, such as calcification, inflammation or fibrosis, which would allow mammographic detection, and LCIS is typically a chance finding in breast biopsies resulting from breast screening.

been predictive, questions remain about diagnostic reproducibility among pathologists (Douglas-Jones *et al*., 1996; Scott *et al*., 1997; Badve *et al*., 1998; Sneige *et al*., 1998). Pathologists appear to have little difficulty in separating the entities at either end of the spectrum: problems of concordance of classification are generally found in the middle group and its boundaries and also at the boundary between low-grade DCIS and atypical ductal hyperplasia (Rosai, 1991; Schnitt *et al*., 1992; Sloane *et al*., 1994, 1999). Three recent consensus meetings came to similar conclusions and recommended that, until better data on clinical relevance and agreement among pathologists emerge, the morphological features present in DCIS and their nuclear grade should be recorded (Recht *et al*., 1994, Australia–New Zealand Breast Cancer Trials Group, 1996; Consensus Conference Committee, 1997). Nuclear grade should be assigned according to internationally accepted guidelines (Commission of the European Communities, 1996; Tavassoli & Stratton, 2002).

Calcification can be seen in both high- and low-grade DCIS (Figure 10) (Elston & Ellis, 1998; Evans *et al.,* 1994a; Tavassoli & Stratton, 2002). The mammographic calcification found in high-grade DCIS is more predictive of malignancy and generally more obvious, often showing coarse rod and branching shapes (Burrell *et al.*, 1996). This profile of subtypes of screen-detected DCIS suggests that radiologists might be able to distinguish subtypes of DCIS with different risks of progression to high-grade invasive disease (Evans *et al.*, 1994a).

### Association of DCIS with invasive carcinoma

For ethical reasons, there are limited data on the natural history of untreated DCIS. The available studies are from the 1930s to 1950s and relate to symptomatic, extensive, high-grade comedo DCIS. At that time, DCIS was rare in

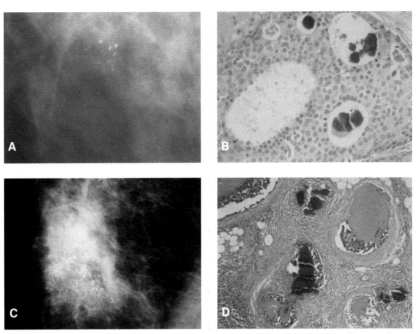

**Figure 10** Mammograms and histological photomicrographs of typical examples of low- and high-grade DCIS. **A** Mammogram showing fine punctate calcification corresponding to the calcifications seen in secondary luminal spaces in the example of low-grade DCIS seen in **B**. The mammogram in **C** shows an extensive area of coarse calcification arising in luminal necrotic debris formed in the centre of ducts involved by high-grade DCIS, illustrated in **D**.

clinical practice, and patients typically presented with a mass lesion, nipple discharge or Paget disease of the nipple. This form of DCIS was defined at the time as aggressive. One very small but widely quoted series showed a 75% rate of progression to invasive disease, with a mean time to progression of 4 years (Dean & Geshchicter, 1938). This type of experience led to the prevailing effective use of mastectomy as the treatment of choice for symptomatic DCIS.

More recent studies reflect the opposite end of the spectrum of DCIS and are based on lesions originally classified as benign. Virtually all are examples of low-grade DCIS. In the studies with the longest follow-up, about 40% progressed to invasive disease after 30 years. In contrast to epithelial hyperplasia, atypical hyperplasia and LCIS, invasive

tumours tend to occur in the same quadrant of the breast as the intitial lesion (Page *et al*., 1995).

Evidence from studies of recurrence after breast-conserving surgery for DCIS indicates that about 50% of recurrences are as invasive cancer and that high-grade DCIS and DCIS with necrosis represent a biologically aggressive subset of DCIS with higher rates of invasive and in-situ recurrence than low-grade DCIS lesions without necrosis (Solin *et al*., 1993; Silverstein *et al*., 1995, 1996; Fisher *et al*., 1999). One large randomized trial (Bijker *et al*., 2001a) showed that margin status is the most important factor in the success of breast-conserving therapy for DCIS. In this trial, the risk for subsequent development of distant metastasis after invasive local recurrence was significantly higher in patients with poorly differentiated DCIS than in those with well-differentiated DCIS. Analysis of recurrences in this trial also showed that most primary DCIS lesions and their local recurrences were similar histologically or in marker expression, suggesting that local recurrence usually reflects outgrowth of residual DCIS; progression of well-differentiated DCIS to poorly differentiated DCIS or grade III invasive carcinoma is unusual (Bijker et al., 2001b).

Invasive lesions with an extensive intraductal component also show a predisposition to local recurrence after breast-conserving therapy (van Dongen et al., 1989). The grade of DCIS associated with invasive cancers has been shown to correlate with both disease-free interval and survival (Lampejo et al., 1994). Strong associations also exist between the grade of invasive cancer and the grade of coexisting DCIS. High-grade DCIS is associated with high-grade invasive cancer and low-grade DCIS with low-grade invasive cancer (Lampejo et al., 1994; Douglas-Jones et al., 1996; Cadman et al., 1997). An association between grade 3 invasive cancer and poorly differentiated DCIS is seen whatever the grading system used (Douglas-Jones et al., 1996).

### Genetic changes seen in in-situ carcinoma and atypical ductal and lobular hyperplasia

Molecular genetic studies of low-grade DCIS and atypical ductal hyperplasia with loss of heterozygosity techniques have demonstrated similar genetic lesions, providing, in informative cases, confirmatory evidence that these lesions are clonal and therefore fulfil the basic criterion of neoplastic transformation (Lakhani et al., 1995). In addition, it has been shown that in-situ and invasive elements of breast cancers have identical molecular alterations, implying that they are stages in the same pathway (Stratton et al., 1995). These findings are consistent with the observation that the two components have similar morpho-

logical characteristics (Lampejo et al., 1994) and are also consistent with the hypothesis that low-grade in-situ cancer gives rise to low-grade invasive carcinoma and high-grade in-situ cancer to high-grade invasive carcinoma. Evidence from a study in two counties in Sweden (see Chapter 4) gave rise to an alternative hypothesis: that tumours progress from low to high grade, as the proportion of high-grade tumours increases with tumour size (Tabár et al., 1992).

Recent studies, and particularly those in which comparative genomic hybridization was used to investigate DCIS, prompted the proposal of a hypothetical model for the pathogenesis of DCIS in which genetic lesions are associated with particular morphological subtypes (Buerger et al., 1999). Different morphological classes of DCIS have specific genetic changes that are not shared by other types. In particular, low-grade and high-grade DCIS appear to be distinct, separate entities, on the basis of morphology, phenotype and molecular genetics. Well-differentiated DCIS is associated with loss of 16q and 17p, while tumours of intermediate and high grades often have losses of significantly more allelic chromosomal arms, frequently including 1p, 1q, 6q, 9p, 11p, 11q, 13q and 17q (Fujii et al., 1996). High-grade DCIS in particular is associated with gains at 17q but also at 11q and 13q (Chuaqui et al., 1997). Intermediate-grade DCIS appears to have a combination of lesions, which show 16q loss but gains at other chromosomes, particularly 1q; some cases show gain at 11q13q but lack the gain at 17q12 which is a feature of high-grade DCIS (Buerger et al., 1999). Similarly, atypical lobular hyperplasia and LCIS show the same genetic mutations, with loss of material from 16p, 16q, 17p and 22q and gain at 6q (Lu et al., 1998). Interestingly, although low-grade DCIS and atypical ductal hyperplasia have no molecular genetic similarity to high-

grade DCIS, they have similarities to LCIS and atypical lobular hyperplasia. These observations challenge the existing assumptions that lobular and ductal lesions are distinct and that DCIS is a homogeneous disease. They also raise the possibility that future molecular markers will provide better discrimination among morphologically similar cells.

### Implications for screening

Breast screening detects a wide spectrum of breast cancer, ranging from microfocal low-grade DCIS to large high-grade invasive cancer (Cowan et al., 1991; Klemi et al., 1992; Rajakariar & Walker, 1995). It has been proposed that detecting in-situ cancer, particularly high-grade DCIS, would prevent the development of high-grade invasive cancer (Lampejo et al., 1994; Evans et al., 1997, 2001a,b). It is well recognized that many low-grade, special invasive cancers are identified at screening (Cowan et al., 1991; Klemi et al., 1992; Porter et al., 1999) (Figure 11). Such tumours have an excellent prognosis but may be so indolent that they would never have presented clinically or have threatened the

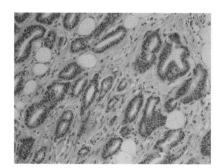

**Figure 11** A well-differentiated invasive adenocarcinoma of the breast of tubular type. The tumour cells are arranged in rounded or elongated glandular or tubular structures with a central luminal space which closely mimics the normal breast terminal duct or lobule. An associated stromal fibrous reaction produces the typical stellate mammographic appearance that allows detection of these tumours by screening.

life of the patients. It has been proposed alternatively that a proportion of these low-grade invasive tumours might de-differentiate over time into more aggressive, less well-differentiated tumours (Tabár et al., 1999), although this was not found in another screening programme (Hakama et al., 1995). Identification and removal of such cancers when they are at a low grade would avoid such progression. Detection of high-grade invasive cancers when they are small is clearly a means by which screening could reduce breast cancer mortality. In support of this possibility, it was shown in the two-county trial in Sweden that histological grade 3 invasive cancers detected when less than 10 mm have an excellent prognosis (Tabár et al., 1999), while it is widely recognized that large high-grade invasive cancers have a poor prognosis.

Ductal carcinomas of no specific type have time-dependent prognostic factors (i.e. size and lymph node stage) that are, in general, moderately good, suggesting that their detection at screening is effective. However, lobular cancers and lobular mixed cancers are larger and more frequently extended to lymph nodes at the time of mammographic detection; thus, identification of cancers with a lobular component by breast screening is not likely to be beneficial. This appears to be a consequence of the subtle mammographic features of lobular carcinoma, which are more commonly seen on only one mammographic view and less frequently contain calcification than ductal carcinomas not otherwise specified (NOS) (Cornford et al., 1995).

The same group examined the value of detecting DCIS at mammographic screening and showed that identification of high-risk types of calcification allows diagnosis of otherwise occult, co-existing, small grade 3 invasive carcinomas associated with calcific high-grade DCIS (Evans et al., 1997). In addition, comparison in their series of the biological characteristics of DCIS detected at screening with symptomatic DCIS lesions showed a higher proportion of adverse characteristics in those detected at screening. The most likely explanation for these findings is suggested by a comparison of the radiological findings of different DCIS sub-types. High-grade DCIS more frequently showed abnormal mammographic features than low-grade DCIS. The granular and punctate calcifications seen in low-grade DCIS (Evans et al., 1994b) are more subtle, less specific and often not picked up at mammographic screening, as they are similar to those seen in common benign conditions (Holland et al., 1990; Evans et al., 1994a).

## Invasive carcinoma
### Definition
Invasive carcinoma of the breast is defined as a malignant tumour, part or all of which penetrates the basement membrane of the epithelial site of origin (i.e. the duct or lobule). The vast majority of these tumours are adenocarcinomas and are believed to be derived from the mammary parenchymal epithelial cell population, particularly cells of the terminal duct lobular unit. The morphological appearance of these tumours varies widely, and many of the recognized morphological types have particular prognostic or clinical characteristics. More recently, specific genetic lesions have been identified in some types.

### Pathological classification of breast cancer
The prognosis of a patient with breast cancer is dependent on two distinct groups of variables. The first are those time-dependant variables that influence tumour stage, particularly the histological size of the tumour, the presence and extent of lymph node metastatic disease and the presence of systemic metastatic disease. The second group of variables, sometimes referred to as intrinsic characteristics, are related to the inherent biology of the individual tumour. This group includes the histological grade, tumour type, growth fraction, hormone and growth factor receptor status and an ever-lengthening list of molecular characteristics.

Of these features, tumour size, histological type, histological grade, vascular invasion status and lymph node status have been shown to be related to clinical outcome (Elston & Ellis, 1998). These features can be used:

- to decide on the most appropriate treatment for a particular patient, including the extent of surgery and the use and choice of adjuvant therapy;
- to monitor breast screening programmes, the success of which is reflected by more favourable prognostic features of the cancer detected; and
- to monitor changing patterns of disease incidence, particularly by cancer registries.

For these reasons, there is increasing international recognition that pathological classification of breast cancer should conform to a minimum dataset, which includes these key variables (Royal College of Pathologists, http). One common approach is based on a combination of invasive tumour size, nodal involvement and metastases (TNM). As it has three dimensions, it is commonly collapsed into one summary number from 0 to IV, where 0 is in-situ disease (UICC, 2002; American Joint Committee on Cancer, 2002)

### Morphological features of invasive breast carcinoma relevant to prognosis and screening
The factors described below have been shown to provide clinically relevant prognostic information and are valuable in evaluating breast screening programmes.

*Tumour size*

Ideally, the size of tumours should be assessed on resected pathological specimens. In situations in which pathological size cannot be determined, such as in patients receiving primary systemic or neoadjuvant therapy or when several estimates of size have been made, alternative means should be used, including magnetic resonance imaging, ultrasound and clinical examination (UICC, 2002; American Joint Committee on Cancer, 2002).

As tumour size is a time-dependent factor, it has been shown consistently in many studies to influence prognosis (Cutler *et al.*, 1969; Elston *et al.*, 1982; Fisher *et al.*, 1984; Carter *et al.*, 1989; Neville *et al.*, 1992). Patients with smaller tumours have better long-term survival rates than those with larger tumours (Figure 12).

Estimation of tumour size has assumed particular importance in breast screening. The term 'minimal breast cancer' was originally introduced to identify forms of breast cancer for which there was an exceedingly good prognosis (Gallager & Martin, 1971); these included all cases of in-situ carcinoma (ductal and lobular) and invasive carcinomas measuring 5 mm or less. Subsequently, for no clearly defined reason, the invasive component was re-defined by various groups. The Breast Cancer Detection Demonstration Projects (Beahrs *et al.*, 1979) and the American Cancer Society (Hartmann, 1984) used 9 mm or less as the maximum diameter, while the American College of Surgeons (Bedwani *et al.*, 1981) favoured up to and including 10 mm. This lack of uniformity in definition causes problems in the interpretation of data from different studies.

Tumour size is also an important quality assurance measure for breast screening programmes (Hartmann, 1984; Tabár *et al.*, 1987a; Royal College of Radiologists, 1997) and can be used in part to judge the ability of radiologists to detect small, impalpable invasive carcinomas on mammography. For example, the National Health Service Breast Screening Programme in the United Kingdom requires that 50% of the invasive cancers detected must measure less than 15 mm (Royal College of Radiologists, 1997). It is therefore incumbent on pathologists to measure tumour diameter as accurately as possible. As size decreases, so the risk for errors in measurement increases, and inconsistencies have been reported (Beahrs *et al.*, 1979; Sloane *et al.*, 1994).

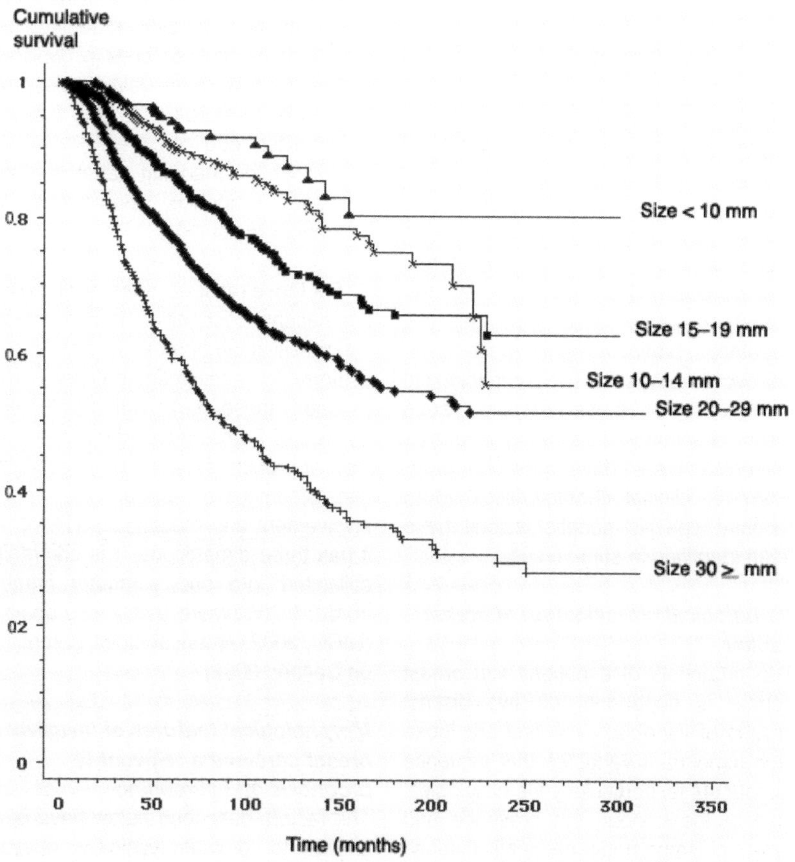

*Histological type*

A wide range of morphological patterns can be seen in invasive carcinoma of the breast (Fisher, E.R. *et al.*, 1975; Azzopardi *et al.*, 1979; Page *et al.*, 1987; Ellis & Fidler, 1995), and many types have distinct prognostic characteristics (Page *et al.*, 1987; Ellis *et al.*, 1992). The diagnostic criteria are described in detail elsewhere (Page *et al.*, 1987; Ellis *et al.*, 1992; National Coordinating Group for Breast Screening Pathology, 1995; Rosen, 1997; Elston & Ellis, 1998; Tavassoli & Stratton, 2002) and will not be repeated here. It must be appreciated that a considerable subjective element remains, and there is not yet universal agreement on the criteria for all types. This is reflected in the relative

**Figure 12** Relationship between tumour size and survival rate of patients with primary unoperable breast cancer. Kaplan-Meier plot of cumulative survival by size of invasive cancer.

## Prognostic characteristics of different tumour types

**Group 1:** **Excellent prognosis**
Tubular, tubulolobular, invasive cribriform, mucinous

**Group 2:** **Good prognosis**
Tubular variant or mixed, alveolar lobular, mixed ductal not otherwise specified and other special types

**Group 3:** **Average prognosis**
Medullary, atypical medullary, classicular lobular, lobular mixed

**Group 4:** **Poor prognosis**
Ductal not otherwise specified, solid lobular, mixed ductal not otherwise specified and lobular

From Pereira *et al.* (1995)

proportions of different types in published series (Elston & Ellis, 1998) and the observation that the consistency of diagnosis of histological type was disappointingly low in pathology quality assurance schemes (Sloane *et al.*, 1994, 1999), implying that pathologists should work to the same diagnostic protocols.

The favourable prognosis of certain histological types of invasive carcinoma of the breast is well established (see box; Pereira *et al.*, 1995). Thus, tubular carcinoma (Cooper *et al.*, 1978; McDivitt *et al.*, 1982; Carstens *et al.*, 1985), mucinous carcinoma (Lee *et al.*, 1934; Clayton, 1986), invasive cribriform carcinoma (Page *et al.*, 1983), medullary carcinoma (Bloom *et al.*, 1970; Ridolfi *et al.*, 1977), infiltrating lobular carcinoma (Haagensen *et al.*, 1978) and tubulolobular carcinoma (Fisher *et al.*, 1977) have all been reported to have a more favourable prognosis than invasive ductal carcinomas NOS, but few comprehensive long-term follow-up studies of histological type in relation to survival have been carried out. Dawson and colleagues (1982) found a higher proportion of tubular, mucinous, medullary and infiltrating lobular carcinomas in patients who had survived at least 25 years after mastectomy than among those who had survived for less than 10 years. These findings were confirmed in a similar study from Edinburgh (Dixon *et al.*, 1985), with the addition of papillary and invasive cribriform carcinomas among the cancers in long-term survivors. These 'special' or 'specific' forms of invasive carcinoma have also been found at higher frequency in the prevalence round of mammographic breast screening programmes (Anderson *et al.*, 1991; Ellis *et al.*, 1993) and more frequently in carcinomas detected at screening than in cancers found between screening rounds (interval cancers) (Porter *et al.*, 1999).

A study of one series comprising over 1500 patients with primary operable invasive carcinoma who were followed up for a minimum of 10 years confirmed the excellent prognosis of pure tubular, invasive cribriform and mucinous carcinomas (Ellis *et al.*, 1992). This study also showed that the categories of carcinoma with special characteristics, tubular mixed carcinoma and mixed ductal NOS and special type, are worth recording, as they carry a considerably better prognosis than ductal carcinoma NOS and form a significant proportion of all invasive cancers (15%). In previous studies, such mixed types were rarely recognized and the tumours were included in the general category of ductal carcinomas NOS.

It has become accepted dogma that medullary carcinoma (Figure 13) has an excellent or good prognosis (Moore & Foote, 1949; Richardson, 1956; Bloom *et al.*, 1970; Ridolfi *et al.*, 1977; Rapin *et al.*, 1988). It is interesting that this view has persisted, despite the fact that other studies have been unable to confirm better survival after medullary carcinoma than after ductal carcinoma NOS (Cutler *et al.*, 1966; Pedersen *et al.*, 1988; Fisher *et al.*, 1990; Ellis *et al.*, 1992). However, some of the latter studies showed that medullary carcinoma does have a better prognosis than ductal carcinoma NOS of grade 3 (Pedersen *et al.*, 1988; Fisher *et al.*, 1990; Ellis *et al.*, 1992). Some authors (Ellis *et al.*, 1992) therefore concluded that medullary carcinoma should be regarded as having a moderate rather than a good prognosis.

Overall, patients with infiltrating lobular carcinoma (Figure 14) have a slightly better prognosis than those with ductal carcinoma NOS (Haagensen *et al.*, 1978; Ellis *et al.*, 1992), although the 10-year survival rate of 54% in the latter study clearly implies no more than a moderate prognostic outcome. However, Dixon and colleagues (1982) found significant differences in the survival of patients with different morphological subtypes of lobular carcinoma, and this has been confirmed (Ellis *et al.*, 1992). Thus, the classical type has a good prognosis

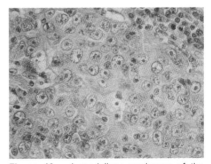

**Figure 13** A medullary carcinoma of the breast composed of syncytial sheets of large pleomorphic tumour cells surrounded by stroma rich in lymphocytes and plasma cells

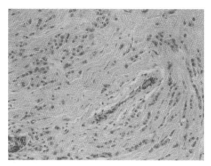

**Figure 14** Classical invasive lobular carcinoma of the breast is composed of narrow files of small, regular tumour cells, which typically infiltrate the breast, surrounding existing parenchymal structures and causing little disturbance to the tissue architecture. This infiltrative patterns produce few mammographic signs, and lobular carcinoma is a cause of false-negative results in mammographic examinations, due to occult disease.

(60% 10-year survival rate), the mixed lobular type an average prognosis (55% at 10 years) and the solid lobular type a poor prognosis (40% at 10 years). Tubulolobular carcinoma, which has an excellent prognosis (over 90% 10-year survival rate), is currently considered a separate, distinct type because of lack of agreement about its assignment as a tubular or lobular variant.

The detection by breast screening of carcinomas with tubular features is facilitated by the high frequency of spiculation seen at mammography (Elson et al., 1993). It is well recognized that pure tubular carcinomas detected at screening have a good prognosis. This is confirmed by the finding of Evans et al. (2001a) of a very low incidence of pure tubular cancers among women who subsequently developed metastatic disease (three of 173 patients (2%), three of the 16 grade 1 lesions (20%)). This suggests that these tumours may be overdiagnosed. The value of detecting pure tubular cancer at screening is therefore likely to be of benefit only if a proportion of tubular cancers de-differentiate if left in the breast. Overdiagnosis of

tumours with some tubular features (tubular variant or mixed carcinoma) is less clear, as 10% of cancers that metastasize are of the tubular mixed type and these tumours do not have the exceptionally good prognosis of pure tubular carcinoma.

*Grading of invasive carcinoma*
Despite the diversity of methods used, many studies have demonstrated a significant association between histological grade and survival from invasive breast carcinoma. Grade is now recognized as a powerful prognostic factor that represents a simple method for classifying differentiation in all invasive breast cancers (Figure 15). Grade should be included as a component of the minimum data set for histological reporting of breast cancer (Henson et al., 1991; Elston & Ellis, 1998; Royal College of Pathologists, http).

Various grading systems have been described, which are based on assessment of multiple cellular and architectural variables (Greenhough, 1925; Patey, 1928; Bloom, 1950a,b; Bloom & Richardson, 1957; Fisher et al., 1984; Contesso et al., 1987; Elston & Ellis, 1991) or nuclear variables (Hartveit, 1971; Black et al., 1975; Le Doussal et al., 1989). The absence of uniform defintion makes comparison of findings difficult.

Given the nature of the methods, assessment of histological differentiation will always carry an underlying subjective element; however, one of the fundamental problems with many of the early systems was the lack of strictly defined written criteria. Bloom and Richardson (1957) made a useful contribution by adding numerical scoring to the method described by Patey (1928) but did not provide clear criteria for their cut-off points. Elston and Ellis (1991) added further modifications to the above method and to their system and achieved greater objectivity and acceptable concordance. This method has been shown to be highly reproducible (Dalton et al., 1994; Frierson et al., 1995; Robbins et al., 1995) and has been adopted internationally as the method of choice (National Coordinating Group for Breast Screening Pathology, 1995; Connolly et al., 1996; Commission of the European Communities, 1996; American Joint Committee on Cancer, 2002; Tavassoli & Stratton, 2002; UICC, 2002). In this system, three characteristics of the tumour are evaluated: tubule formation as an expression of glandular differentiation, nuclear pleomorphism and mitotic counts (Table 3). A numerical scoring system on a scale of 1–3 is used to ensure that each factor is assessed individually, and an overall grade is assigned as follows:

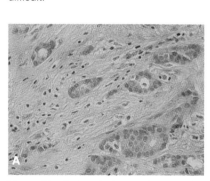 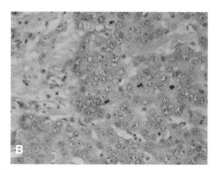

**Figure 15** **A** A grade 3 or poorly differentiated invasive breast carcinoma. The tumour cells are arranged in sheets with no apparent gland formation. The cells are large and vary in size, and obvious mitotic figures are present. **B** Vascular invasion seen as a group of tumour cells present in a peritumoral lymphatic vascular channel

**Table 3. Summary of semi-quantitative method for assessing histological grade of breast carcinoma**

| Feature | Score |
|---|---|
| **Tubule and gland formation** | |
| Majority of tumour (> 75%) | 1 |
| Moderate degree (10–75%) | 2 |
| Little or none (< 10%) | 3 |
| **Nuclear pleomorphism** | |
| Small, regular, uniform cells | 1 |
| Moderate increase in size and variation | 2 |
| Marked variation | 3 |
| **Mitotic counts** | |
| Dependent on microscope field area | 1–3 |

Reproduced from Elston and Ellis (1991)

- Grade 1: well differentiated; 3–5 points
- Grade 2: moderately differentiated; 6–7 points
- Grade 3: poorly differentiated; 8–9 points

*Lymph node stage*
Involvement of loco-regional lymph nodes in breast cancer has long been recognized as one of the most important prognostic factors. Clinical assessment of lymph node status is not sufficiently accurate for therapeutic use, and evaluation of lymph node stage should be based on histological examination of excised nodes (Barr & Baum, 1992). Patients who have histologically confirmed loco-regional lymph node involvement have a significantly poorer prognosis than those without nodal involvement (Cutler et al., 1969; Fisher, E.R. et al., 1975; Elston et al., 1982; Ferguson et al., 1982; Haybittle et al., 1982; Galea et al., 1992; Veronesi et al., 1993a). The overall 10-year survival rate is reduced

from 75% for patients without nodal involvement to 25–30% for those with involved nodes. Prognosis is also related to the number and level of loco-regional lymph nodes involved: the greater the number of nodes involved, the poorer the patient survival (Nemoto et al., 1980; Fisher et al., 1984). Most groups stratify patients into two groups for therapeutic purposes: those with one to three positive nodes and those with four or more (American Joint Committee on Cancer, 2002; UICC, 2002). Similarly, involvement of nodes in the 'higher' levels of the axilla, and specifically the apex, carries a worse prognosis (Handley, 1972; Haagensen, 1986; Veronesi et al., 1993a), as does involvement of the internal mammary nodes (Handley, 1972).

The frequency of disease with involved lymph nodes is significantly lower in women in whom disease is detected at screening. Approximately 40–50% of symptomatic patients have iinvolved nodes, in contrast to approximately 10–20% of patients with disease detected at screening (Cowan et al., 1991; Klemi et al., 1992; Rajakariar & Walker, 1995). This finding has raised concern that routine axillary lymph node dissection is over-treatment for many women with breast cancer detected at screening and has led to interest in use of sentinel lymph node biopsy for effective staging of the axilla (Krag et al., 1998; Bundred et al., 2000).

Vascular invasion (Figure 16) is defined as the presence of tumour cells in vascular spaces (lymphatic or blood) in tissues surrounding an invasive tumour (Örbo et al., 1990; Pinder et al., 1994). Vascular invasion correlates very closely with survival and loco-regional lymph node involvement (Rosen, 1983; Davis et al., 1985; Örbo et al., 1990; Pinder et al., 1994). Possibly because of this association, it has been claimed that the prognostic information it provides is as powerful as lymph node stage (Bettelheim et al., 1984). There is certainly a correlation between the pres-

ence of vascular invasion and early recurrence in patients with no lymph node involvement (Rosen et al., 1981; Roses et al., 1982; Bettelheim et al., 1984), and some (Roses et al., 1982; Pinder et al., 1994) have shown that adverse prognostic effects are also independent of occult axillary node involvement. In addition, vascular invasion is a predictor of local recurrence after conserving therapy (Roses et al., 1982; Locker et al., 1989a; Rosen, 1991; Pinder et al., 1994) and of flap recurrence after mastectomy (O'Rourke et al., 1994).

As stated above both nodal and vascular invasion status are powerful independent prognostic factors in patients with invasive breast carcinoma (Bettelheim et al., 1984; Todd et al., 1987; Pinder et al., 1994; Seidman et al., 1995; Tabár et al., 1999). In a study of the features associated with the development of metastatic disease after a previous breast cancer (Evans et al., 2001a), 72% of 173 women who developed metastatic disease had nodal metastases and 59% had definite vascular invasion; 84% had either lymph node metastases or vascular invasion, or both. This finding was consistent, whatever the histological grade of the primary tumour. The absence of vascular invasion and nodal involvement in invasive breast cancer indicated a low risk for subsequent development of metastatic disease. Trends in the frequency of

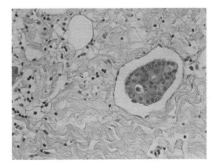

**Figure 16** Vascular invasion seen as a group of tumour cells present in a peritumoral lymphatic vascular channel

nodal involvement and vascular invasion status according to histological grade, invasive size and tumour type were then examined in a group of 573 women with invasive cancers detected at screening, in order to predict the likelihood of development of systemic disease. Grade 1 invasive cancers less than 20 mm in diameter and grade 2 and 3 cancers less than 10 mm were associated with low rates of nodal involvement and vascular invasion. The criteria for selecting groups for analysis were the intrinsic morphological features of the invasive tumour (i.e. histological grade and tumour type) at different sizes. Of the well-differentiated, less intrinsically aggressive (grade 1) carcinomas, only those over 20 mm were associated with a high rate of lymph node involvement. Nevertheless, 9% of the primary breast cancers that metastasized were grade 1 lesions. Thus, large grade 1 invasive cancers can, and do, spread. Detection of these lesions when they are small might be seen as overdiagnosis but could prevent progression to a size associated with metastasis. Some types of low-grade invasive breast carcinoma have, however, an exceptionally good prognosis even when metastatic disease is present (Diab et al., 1999). The detection of low-grade invasive and in-situ breast carcinoma therefore remains of questionable value.

The low rates of nodal positivity and vascular invasion of grade 2 invasive cancers less than 10 mm in diameter identified by screening indicate the value of detecting them at this size. Grade 2 cancers of 10–15 mm were associated with moderately high rates of nodal involvement but low rates of vascular invasion. The benefit of detecting grade 2 cancers 10–15 mm in size is therefore less clear. Larger grade 2 cancers (over 15 mm) were already associated with high rates of nodal involvement and vascular invasion at the time of diagnosis. Their detection by mammographic screening may therefore be of limited benefit.

Low rates of both nodal positivity and vascular invasion were seen in grade 3 invasive cancers less than 10 mm in diameter detected at screening, suggesting that detection of these small high-grade tumours is valuable, especially as larger grade 3 invasive cancers have such a poor prognosis. Women with grade 3 cancers over 20 mm in this series had high rates of affected lymph nodes and vascular invasion; therefore, detection at this stage is unlikely to influence survival. The moderate rates of nodal involvement and vascular invasion in grade 3 cancers of intermediate size (10–20 mm) suggest that their detection is less likely to be beneficial than when they are small. Similar views have been developed from reviews of other mammographic screening populations (Tabár et al., 1999).

*Molecular markers*
Many molecular alterations have been identified which reflect the biological characteristics of invasive breast carcinomas. Some are related to survival, but, more importantly, these changes indicate which molecular pathways affect a tumour and could therefore predict benefit from specific forms of molecular therapy.

One such marker is steroid hormone receptors (the estrogen receptor (ER) and the progesterone receptor (PR).

Estrogen is an important mitogen, which expresses its activation by binding to its nuclear receptor (ER) (Figure 17). ER is expressed in 60–80% of invasive breast tumours, and ER-positive tumours have a better initial prognosis than ER-negative tumours. The presence of nuclear hormone receptors is useful for predicting response to hormone therapy, such as adjuvant tamoxifen (Osborne, 1998; Bundred, 2001; Isaacs et al., 2001). ER- and PR-positive tumours have a 60–70% response rate, while that of ER- and PR-negative tumours is less than 10%. ER-positive, PR-negative tumours have an intermediate response of approximately 40%.

The *ERBB2/HER2* oncogene, located on 17q21, is amplified in approximately 20% of invasive breast cancers, leading to overexpression of the coded HER2 protein, a transmembrane receptor with tyrosine kinase activity (Figure 18). The prognostic value of *HER2* overexpression, first reported in 1987 (Slamon et al., 1987), has been studied extensively (Tsuda et al., 2001; Yamauchi et al., 2001). *HER2* overexpression is a weak to moderate independent predictor of survival, at least for patients with node involvement. Amplification or overexpression can be measured by Southern blot analysis, fluorescent in-situ hybridization (FISH) or differential polymerase chain reaction to detect

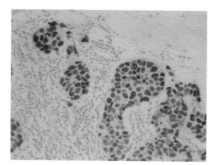

**Figure 17** An invasive breast cancer stained immunocytochemically for estrogen receptors. The estrogen receptor protein is seen as a brown pigment in the tumour cell nuclei.

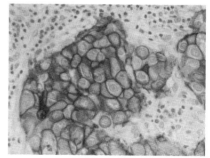

**Figure 18** An invasive carcinoma stained immunocytochemically for HER 2 protein. The protein, seen as a brown pigment, is overexpressed on the tumour cell membranes.

gene amplification and immunohisto-chemistry or enzyme-linked immuno-sorbent assay to detect protein expression (Tsongalis & Ried, 2001). The results of studies of the predictive value of HER2 status have not been consistent. A review by Yamauchi et al. (2001) concluded that HER2 is a weak-to-moderate negative predictor of response to alkylating agents and a moderate positive predictor of response to anthracyclines and that the data are insufficient to draw conclusions on the response to taxanes or radiotherapy. A humanized anti-HER2 monoclonal antibody, trastuzumab (Herceptin), has been developed as an anti-cancer drug targeting amplified and overexpressed HER2 (Cobleigh et al., 1999).

Markers of proliferation have been investigated extensively in relation to prognosis (Fitzgibbons et al., 2000; Isaacs et al., 2001). Mitotic count is part of histological grading (see above). Other methods include DNA flow cytometry measurement of the S-phase fraction and immunohistochemistry with antibodies directed against antigens present in proliferating cells like Ki-67. Several hundred studies on the S-phase fraction, with various techniques, indicated that a high S-phase fraction is associated with inferior outcome. Ki-67 is a labile, non-histone nuclear protein that is not expressed in resting cells but is detected in the G1 through M phases of the cell cycle. The percentage of Ki-67-positive cells can be used to stratify patients into good and poor survivors.

*Genetics and invasive cancers*
In the past decade, the ability to measure both molecular markers of cancer activity and the genes that control cell growth has increased tremendously. In future, this information may complement (and even supplant) the histological categorization described above. The basic approach is to relate the pattern of expression of multiple genes to the rate of growth of the tumour. This process may help clinicians to predict which cancers will grow fast and which will not.

*Genetic changes in specific types of invasive breast cancer.* Specific genetic lesions or regions of alteration are associated with specific histological types of cancer and are related to grade in large ductal carcinoma NOS. The latter group appear morphologically similar but include a number of tumours with unrelated genetic evolutionary pathways (Buerger et al., 2001). They also show fundamental differences from some special type tumours, including lobular (Gunther et al., 2001) and tubular carcinoma (Roylance et al., 1999). Furthermore, recent cDNA microarray analyses have shown that ductal tumours NOS can be classified into subtypes on the basis of expression patterns (Perou et al., 2000; Sorlie et al., 2001) .

Genetic changes have also been found in invasive lobular carcinoma (Frixen et al., 1991; Vleminckx et al., 1991; Gamallo et al., 1993; Rasbridge et al., 1993; Berx et al., 1995; Nishizaki et al., 1997; Flagiello et al., 1998), but they are identified less frequently than in ductal cancers (Nishizaki et al., 1997; Flagiello et al., 1998).

Tubular carcinomas of the breast have a lower frequency of genetic alterations than other types of breast carcinoma (Man et al., 1996; Roylance et al., 1999; Waldman et al., 2001). Of particular interest is the observation that sites of chromosomal alteration frequently affected in other types of breast cancer are not seen, implying that tubular carcinoma of the breast is a genetically distinct group of breast cancers.

Up to 13% of carcinomas arising in carriers of the *BRCA1* gene are of the medullary type (Marcus et al., 1996; Breast Cancer Linkage Consortium, 1997), and 35–60% exhibit medullary-like features (Marcus et al., 1996; Armes et al., 1998). Reciprocally, in a group of medullary cancers, germ-line mutations of *BRCA1* were observed in 11% of cases (Eisinger et al., 1998). There is thus a large overlap between medullary features and the phenotype of *BRCA1* germ-line-associated tumours, but not all *BRCA1* mutations lead to the medullary phenotype. Medullary carcinomas are also characterized by a high rate of *P53* alterations (de Cremoux et al., 1999)

*Gene expression.* Gene expression profiles may offer more information than morphology and provide an alternative to morphology-based tumour classification systems. The recent development of laser capture microdissection and high-density cDNA arrays provides a unique opportunity to generate such profiles of cells from tumours in various stages of progression (Kitahara et al., 2001). Although this field is still in its infancy, it has already been shown that variations in gene expression can be used to classify breast cancers into a basal epithelial-like group, a luminal epithelial/ER-positive group, an HER2-overexpressing group and a normal breast-like group (Perou et al., 2000; Sorlie et al., 2001). The luminal group has since been divided into at least two subgroups, each with a distinctive expression profile. It is expected that gene sets will be identified that correlate with patient outcome or predict patient response to treatment.

Expression profiles based on micro-arrays will make it possible to analyse the expression of thousands of genes simultaneously and will allow the classification of tumours into new groups according to gene expression patterns (Alizadeh et al., 2001; Gruvberger et al., 2001; Hedenfalk et al., 2001; Perou et al., 2000; Sorlie et al., 2001; West et al., 2001). Expression patterns have shown biological differences between tumours: hereditary breast cancers with *BRCA1* mutations could be distinguished from those in *BRCA2* carriers (Hedenfalk et al., 2001), and ER-positive and ER-negative cancers had different expression profiles (Gruvberger et al., 2001; West et al., 2001). Analysis of a number of breast cancer series has resulted in identification of at least five different subtypes with different prognostic outcomes (Perou et al., 2000; Sorlie et al., 2001; van't Veer et al., 2002).

*Familial risk.* Breast cancer has been recognized for over 100 years as having a familial component (Brocca, 1866). Its genetic basis is discussed in Chapter 4.

## Can a patient be 'cured' of breast cancer?

The concept of cure in breast cancer has been problematic, as deaths occurred at all intervals in short-, medium- and long-term follow-up studies. Three concepts of cure have been defined — statistical, clinical and personal — and the evidence for the curability of female breast cancer according to each of these concepts has been examined (Haybittle, 1991). The author concluded that there was no convincing evidence of statistical or clinical cure in series of treated patients, but that one-fourth of such patients had experienced individual cure, in that they died from some other cause without overt signs of breast cancer. This view was based on the few large studies with long-term follow-up, which showed persistently worse survival up to 30 years after diagnosis when compared with aged-matched controls, some of the later deaths being attributed to treatment rather than metastatic disease (Haybittle et al., 1989). The level of individual cure in series of patients treated more recently should be higher, due mainly to better stage distribution. It has been shown that deaths rarely occur 20 years after diagnosis (Joensuu & Toikkanen, 1995), indicating that cure may be achieved. Analysis of one large, long-term follow-up study showed that the time to death of patients dying of breast cancer is influenced not by the time-dependent factors of tumour size and lymph node status (which appear to pre-dict the risk for death) but by the intrinsic factor, histological grade (Blamey et al., 2000). Of women who died, 90% of the deaths occurred within 8 years of diagnosis in patients with grade 3 tumours and within 13 years in patients with grade 2 tumours and were projected to occur within 30 years in patients with grade 1 tumours. The survival curves of patients with grades 2 and 3 tumours mirrored that of the general population after 90% of deaths had occurred. Patients with grade 1 tumours had a low overall risk of dying. These results suggest that not all patients with invasive breast carcinoma have systemic disease at diagnosis, and that patients could be offered advice on their risk of death depending on the grade of their tumour. Those patients who live for defined times after diagnosis could be reassured that their risk for death from breast cancer is the same as if they had not had breast cancer and is equivalent to cure.

## Diagnosis and treatment

Diagnostic and treatment approaches have changed throughout the history of breast screening. In the early 1960s, when the first evaluation of mammography began, radical mastectomy was the predominant form of therapy, and this did not vary with tumour or patient characteristics. At present, breast conserving techniques with radiation therapy, adjuvant chemotherapy and hormonal treatments are used in a variety of ways, depending on age and tumour size and stage. Diagnostic approaches have also evolved over the past 40 years to accommodate the need to find smaller and smaller tumours. European guidelines for quality assurance in diagnosis and treatment provide a reference for implementing present practice (Commission of the European Communities, 2001). This section gives a summary of diagnosis and treatment strategies, reflecting current evidence-based practices in high-income regions.

### *Current diagnostic strategy*

Diagnosis of breast cancer depends on whether or not a lesion can be felt (whether it is palpable). When there is a palpable lesion, a diagnosis is made on the basis of the results of three techniques: inspection and palpation, mammography and core-cutting needle biopsy or fine-needle aspiration biopsy. If there is a suspicion of malignancy, operative excision is recommended.

Non-palpable lesions pose a greater diagnostic challenge. In this circumstance, a suspect area on a mammogram is localized by further magnification, stereotactic mammography and/or ultrasound. Biopsy is performed by core cutting or fine-needle aspiration, usually with guidance by imaging techniques, such as ultrasound or mammography. Operative excision of the area is again undertaken for any suggestion of malignant change.

### *Evolution of treatment guidelines*
#### *Operative treatment*
*Breast-conserving surgery.* Breast cancer treatment was based for a long time on the Halsted hypothesis, according to which breast cancer spreads only by direct infiltration or via the lymphatic vessels into the lymph nodes. Halsted radical mastectomy was the predominant method of operation until the 1970s, when two prospective randomized trials confirmed that the prognosis was similar with less extensive operation (Turner et al., 1981; Maddox et al., 1983). It was thus concluded that breast cancer can send distant metastases at an early stage, and lymph node metastases are not necessarily a result of cancer spread along the lymphatic vessels but rather an indicator of systemic disease. Consequently, the extent of local treatment will not affect survival. This hypothesis has since been replaced by the view that breast cancer is a heterogeneous disease, some forms remaining local for a long time and others becoming systemic relatively early. According to this third hypothesis, the role of local treatment is

often crucial (Hellman, 1994). Prospective randomized studies conducted since the 1970s showed that survival after breast-conserving surgery combined with radiotherapy was similar to that after mastectomy (Sarrazin et al., 1989; Fisher et al., 1989; Veronesi et al., 1990; Blichert-Toft et al., 1992; van Dongen et al., 1992b; Fisher et al., 1995; Jacobson et al., 1995; van Dongen et al., 2000).

Although breast-conserving surgery has become more popular since the 1980s, there is wide variation in the proportion of breast-conserving operations, due to differences in patient populations, hospital resources and surgeons' abilities and attitudes (Kotwall et al., 1996; Margolese, 1999). Breast-conserving surgery was first shown to be safe for patients with tumours less than 2 cm in diameter. Initially, the local relapse rate was higher after breast-conserving surgery for patients with tumours 2–5 cm in diameter and for those with axillary node involvement (van Dongen et al., 1992b). Later, breast-conserving surgery combined with various adjuvant treatments was shown to give results similar to those of mastectomy (van Dongen et al., 2000). Currently, breast-conserving surgery is preferred whenever possible, i.e. for invasive tumours less than 3 cm in diameter and for DCIS with tumour-free margins.

*Axillary lymph nodes.* Axillary lymph nodes are removed primarily for staging, but the operation also has therapeutic significance, preventing axillary recurrence. The number of metastatic lymph nodes among all the lymph nodes removed is reported. At least 10 nodes should be removed (Grabau et al., 1998; Orr, 1999). The number of metastatic lymph nodes is an important prognostic factor. Thus, if more than 10 lymph nodes are removed from I and II axillary levels and they are all free of metastasis, there will be no local recurrence in the subsequent 5 years (Axelsson et al.,

1992). If no involvement of axillary lymph nodes is detectable by palpation and ultrasound examination and the nodes are not excised, survival will be reduced by 5% (Orr, 1999). All I and II level axillary lymph nodes are removed from patients with invasive breast carcinoma. If, during the operation, lymph nodes suspected of containing metastasis are detected, III level axillary lymph nodes are also removed.

*Post-operative radiotherapy*
Post-operative radiotherapy with approximately 50 Gy for 5 weeks reduces local recurrence after breast-conserving surgery (Fisher et al., 1989; Clark et al., 1992; Veronesi et al., 1993b) and after mastectomy (Overgaard et al., 1997). Post-operative radiotherapy is given after breast-conserving surgery. For patients with lymph node metastases or tumours in stage 3 or 4, post-operative radiotherapy is also given after mastectomy.

*Adjuvant cytostatic chemotherapy*
For most of the past century, breast cancer was considered to require mainly local treatment. In the 1970s, it was shown in controlled trials that adjuvant cytostatic chemotherapy reduced local recurrence in patients with lymph node involvement (Fisher, B. et al., 1975; Bonadonna et al., 1977) and improved the disease-free and overall survival rates by 15–20% (Bonadonna et al., 1995). The standard regimen until the late 1990s was 4–6 months of cytoxan, methotrexate and 5-fluorouracil. This has been replaced gradually by anthracycline-based combinations, especially for younger patients.

Adjuvant therapy is recommended when the risk for recurrence is intermediate or high, i.e. more than 10% over 10 years (Fisher et al., 1992). Adjuvant treatment is given to all women under 35 years of age. Currently, a growing number of patients with no node involvement receive adjuvant cytostatics,

according to their tumour characteristics (Fisher et al., 1997; Kroman et al., 2000).

*Adjuvant hormonal therapy*
Adjuvant hormonal treatment with the anti-estrogen tamoxifen improves the disease-free and overall survival rates of patients who have undergone radical surgery (Nolvadex Adjuvant Trial Organisation, 1985, 1988). The current standard treatment for post-menopausal, ER- and/or PR-positive patients is 20 mg/day for 5 years. This treatment increases the 5-year survival rate by 15% (Veronesi et al., 1998). Newer selective ER modifiers and/or aromatase inhibitors may improve the survival of patients who would otherwise have received tamoxifen (Bonneterre et al.; 2001).

## Screening for breast cancer: Conceptual considerations

The core concept of screening is that detection of early disease offers the opportunity to change its prognosis. Earlier diagnosis may improve prospects for survival because early intervention permits treatment at a more tractable stage (Morrison, 1992). However, as experience with screening has accumulated and understanding of cancer biology has evolved, it is apparent that there is substantial heterogeneity among cancers at particular sites, and this heterogeneity may well influence the impact of screening. Models of screening should incorporate this heterogeneity.

The epidemiological model discussed in this section is an operational one for screening and incorporates heterogeneitiy among cancers. It makes no assumption about the biological nature of the process of cancer progression. The model applies principally to mammographic screening for breast cancer, in which the great majority of detected lesions are invasive cancer, and it is assumed that these will not progress.

## General definitions

Several definitions are needed to understand this simplified screening model, and these are shown in Figure 19. First, the model assumes that there is a period in which there is no detectable disease, but early malignant changes may have taken place and a clone of cells is dividing and de-differentiating until it attains a size that could be detected by screening. The point at which a tumour could be found by screening begins the sojourn time (Zelen & Feinleib, 1969) or 'detectable preclinical phase'. 'Lead time' refers to the period between when a cancer is found by screening and when it would appear through clinical signs and symptoms (Morrison, 1992). Sojourn time is a characteristic jointly of the lesions and the screening test. Lead time will in addition be affected by the frequency of screening. Neither the sojourn time nor the lead time is directly observable for an individual, unless a screening test is repeated at frequent intervals, the results of a positive screening test are ignored and the person is observed until she becomes sympto-matic. Such a situation is clearly not tenable. However, in a population that has undergone screening, the distribution of lead time and sojourn time can be estimated (see below).

Sojourn time is a characteristic of a particular lesion. It is expected to vary widely for different lesions, reflecting the wide biological heterogeneity of breast cancer. Sojourn time notably depends for example on histological grade.

In addition to sojourn time and lead time, two parameters of traditional importance in screening are sensitivity and specificity. For a condition which either exists or does not, such as Tay Sachs disease, these two parameters are defined in terms of a 2 x 2 table:

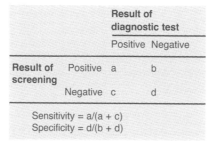

|  |  | Result of diagnostic test | |
|---|---|---|---|
|  |  | Positive | Negative |
| Result of screening | Positive | a | b |
|  | Negative | c | d |

Sensitivity = a/(a + c)
Specificity = d/(b + d)

The situation is more complex for screening for breast cancer, because it is a progressive condition. At the time at which screening is performed, there is no 'gold standard' diagnostic test for the disease: the condition being screened for is a future clinical disease. The 'true' disease state at the time of screening is a lesion that will progress into a clinically invasive cancer. This state can be determined for an individual only by following her forward in time. Since, however, a positive result at screening should lead to an intervention to prevent the development of a clinical cancer, much of the information required for direct estimates of sensitivity and specificity will be missing. There is no direct measure of 'a' in the table. The quantity 'c', however, can be estimated directly, since, if one follows forward in time a group of individuals who showed no lesion on the screening test, some will develop clinical invasive disease. The length of time after screening that is used to define this group of 'screen-negative' and 'disease-positive' individuals is commonly 1 year, but that is a somewhat arbitrary interval. The women presenting with clinical disease in the year after a negative result thus constitute the cell entry 'c' in the above table.

In a number of programmes, a 2-year interval is used to define sensitivity. This has the advantage that it is less subject to statistical variation due to small numbers and less dependent on the exact date of diagnosis, although more affected by new cancers. Clearly, the longer the interval used to define sensitivity, the lower will be the resulting estimate (as follows from the discussions below and Figure 20).

Attention should also be paid to the definition of the screening test. Mammographic screening is essentially a multiple-step process, with the initial screening mammogram leading, if positive, to a series of more detailed

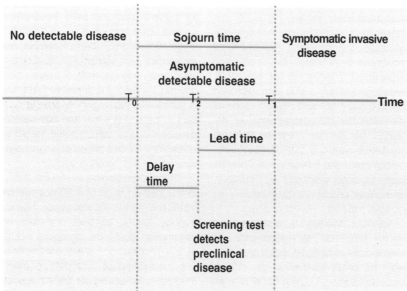

**Figure 19** Scheme of progression of a chronic disease, with the intervention of an early-detection screening test

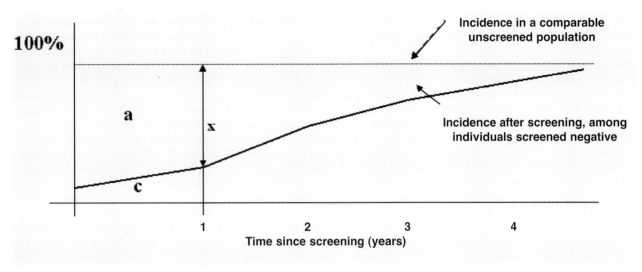

**Figure 20** Sensitivity defined in terms of 1-year proportionate incidence: incidence of interval cancers as a proportion of the incidence in comparable unscreened population
c = interval cancers in first year; a = deficit of cancers in first year by comparison with an unscreened population; x = deficit of incidence at 1 year

investigations, culminating in a biopsy for a definitive diagnosis of malignancy. The definitions of sensitivity and specificity discussed in this section refer to the complete screening episode, the final assessment of positivity or negativity being based on the results of the mammogram and all further assessment. It is a common experience that women with a positive mammogram but classified as negative, i.e. disease free, on further assessment are at higher risk of subsequent disease than the general population. The implication is that if only the screening mammogram is considered as the screening test, it will be more sensitive than the overall screening episode, although of course with less specificity. The sensitivity of screening mammograms could be estimated in analogous fashion to the sensitivity of the complete screening episode, but in practice such estimation is rarely attempted. It would refer strictly to the sensitivity of the test itself.

To estimate sensitivity, one then must identify the individuals, or indirectly estimate their number, who constitute the cell entry 'a'. As the 'true' disease state is agreed to be clinical cancer appearing within 1 year of a screening test, to estimate 'a' one needs to estimate the number of true cancers that were detected at screening and treated, and thus prevented from presenting clinically in this period of 1 year after screening. This group forms the screen-positive, disease-positive group. The quantity 'a + c' is the number of cancers that would have presented clinically in the group that was screened if no screening had taken place. Thus, if one has a directly comparable unscreened population, e.g. as in a randomized trial, the quantity 'a + c' is observable. In the absence of a comparison group strictly defined by randomization, other approaches would be needed, but for any general population sample, estimates based on age-adjusted cancer incidence data from a comparable population or time when screening was not practised should provide a good approximation if used judiciously. The quantity 'a' is then obtained by subtraction, and the sensitivity estimate is given as before (Day, 1985):

$a/(a + c)$.

For the test sensitivity, the same expression, $a/(a + c)$, applies, except one moves from 'c' to 'a' the interval cancers that were positive on the mammography test but negative on follow-up. This approach to the estimation of sensitivity, called the 'incidence method', can be expressed graphically as in Figure 20 and can be used to estimate sensitivity as the 1-year proportionate incidence of interval cancers (see below). In a definition of sensitivity that was sometimes used in the past, the 'gold standard positive' tumours were considered to be all those diagnosed at screening or within 1 year after screening, so that, in the above terminology, sensitivity was given by (a + b)/(a + b + c). This quantity has no clear interpretation, since the cancers diagnosed at screening could have surfaced at any (including infinite) time in the future or never (overdiagnosis), whereas the false-negative results at screening surfaced in the first year after screening. The two groups are clearly not comparable.

## Positive predictive value, specificity and the issue of over-diagnosis

A similar approach can be taken to the definition of specificity and positive predictive value, as, if one has estimates of the values of 'a' and 'c', and 'a + b' and 'c + d' are known from the results of screening, then clearly one has estimates of 'b' and 'd'. However, for determining specificity and positive predictive value, an interval of 1 year after screening may not be appropriate. For positive predictive value, for example, it would be of more interest to estimate the proportion of lesions detected at screening that would have progressed to clinical cancers (i.e. a/(a + b)) by the next round in a periodic screening programme. This parameter is of direct relevance to the question of overdiagnosis, which relates to invasive cancers detected at screening that will not progress to a clinical cancer within some defined time interval.

For specificity, or rather its complement, one might be interested in the proportion of individuals who had a positive screen among those who would not have developed a clinical cancer in the interval between screening tests (i.e. b/(b + d)). For the test specificity, the false-positive results should be included. The test validity indicators correspond to each other like those of episode validity. In particular, it is deficient to report (only) episode specificity and only test sensitivity.

In screening for a progressive disease, such as breast cancer, it is important to define the interval over which sensitivity and the other parameters are being defined and to ensure that they are comparable across populations. As demonstrated by Rosenberg et al. (2000), lengthening the observation period after a screening mammogram will decrease the sensitivity. Conversely, the shorter the interval the more important it is to remove the time assumed by episode from the woman–years of interval cancer incidence.

## Cancers detected at screening, interval cancers and distribution of lead time and sojourn time

When a population of women undergoes screening, a certain number of breast cancers will be detected at the initial screening test, and further cancers will be diagnosed clinically in the post-screening period among those with negative results at screening (so-called 'interval cancers'). This process is represented graphically in Figure 20. The probability of a cancer being detected at screening clearly depends on the length of time the lesion is detectable preclinically, i.e. on the sojourn time: the longer the sojourn time, the greater the chance that the lesion will be detected. Cancers detected at screening thus represent a biased sample of preclinical lesions, with an undue proportion of cancers with a long sojourn time and probably a good prognosis. This bias is known as length bias.

In Figure 21, the incidence rate of breast cancer after screening is expressed as a proportion of the incidence rate in an equivalent unscreened population. The deficit in incidence in comparison with the unscreened represents those cancers detected at screening, as described in the definition of sensitivity. The curve of incidence after screening not only gives the proportion of cancers that are detected at screening (sensitivity), but also the time at which after screening the cancers detected would have presented clinically. Thus, in Figure 21, there is an incidence deficit of 'x' 1 year after screening. According to the definition of lead time, this deficit of 'x' corresponds to cancers detected at screening with a lead time of 1 year. The complete distribution of lead time among the cancers diagnosed at screening that would have presented clinically is there-fore given by the difference between the unscreened incidence rate and the post-screening incidence rate, from time zero through to the maximum time for which observations are available.

The curve of the proportionate incidence after screening will increase monotonically from time zero until it approaches unity, at which time the effect of screening essentially disappears. Shortly after screening, the curve will represent largely the cancers missed at screening. The increase with time then represents cancers that were not in the preclinical detectable phase at the time of screening. So, 1 year after screening, the interval cancers will consist of all those with a sojourn time less than 1 year, and hence not detectable 1 year previously, plus those with a sojourn time greater than 1 year but missed at screening. The curve of proportionate incidence after screening thus represents a combination of sensitivity and the cumulative distribution of sojourn time among cancers diagnosed at screening that would have presented clinically. Separation of the two is difficult (Walter & Day, 1983; Day & Walter, 1984), but broad areas of acceptable (and correlated) values can be identified.

## Periodic screening: Length bias and the unbiased set

Population screening programmes usually aim at screening each woman at regular intervals, normally between 1 and 3 years. In this situation, cancers would be detected at each screening test, and clinically detected cancers would present in each of the intervals between screening rounds. Figure 21 shows the process graphically. One can define a screening cycle as the period between the ends of two screening rounds.

A useful extension of the concept of sensitivity can be derived from programme sensitivity. This refers to the cumulative incidence of interval cancers during the screening cycle, as a proportion of the cumulative incidence

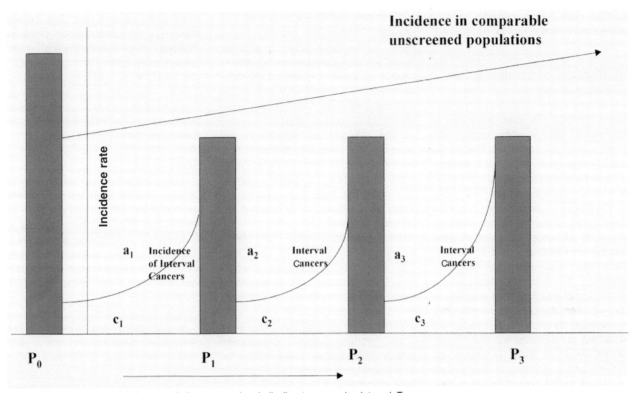

**Figure 21** Cancers occurring in a population screened periodically, at a screening interval, T
$P_0$, cancers detected at prevalence screen; $P_i$, cancers detected at the 'i'th incident screen; $c_i$, interval cancers diagnosed in the 'i'th inter-screening interval; $a_i$, incidence gap in the 'i'th inter-screening interval

during this interval that would have occurred in the absence of screening, programme sensitivity being 1 minus this proportion. Programme sensitivity thus gives a measure of the proportion of incident cases that would be diagnosed by screening among women who are screened according to the programme schedule. The denominators can be woman–years among the screened, invited or the target population. The last results in a measure that is relevant to organized programmes and is comparable with overall mortality reduction in the target population.

As described in the previous section, cancers detected at screening represent a biased sample of cancers in the population. Those detected at the first screening test, the prevalence screen, will be the most biased, as lesions with a sojourn time that is long in comparison with the inter-screening interval will be more strongly overrepresented. After the prevalence screen, the successive screening cycles soon approach a steady state. The cancers diagnosed in one screening cycle, i.e. from immediately after one screening test to immediately after the next, thus approximate the incident cancers during that period, although with a threshold of detection lower than for incident clinical cancers. They thus form a set of cancers from which length bias has been removed and have been termed the 'unbiased set' (Tabár et al., 1992). Their prognostic characteristics can be compared with those of clinically incident cancers, a comparison from which length bias has been approximately removed. Unbiased sets should include nonresponders as well.

## A more complex view of cancer
The model shown in Figure 19 describes the operational process of screening, incorporating no information on the biology of the carcinogenic process. Current knowledge of the neoplastic process allows us to distinguish a number of steps, which may begin with mutation at specific genetic loci and other cellular events and continue until cells divide and disseminate throughout the organism. Cancer development is a long process, and not all the steps are necessarily irreversible. In the future, screening modalities may be developed to target these early molecular changes.

In that case, more complex models of the screening process will be required.

## Evaluation of screening for breast cancer

Mammography has been evaluated in randomized trials in which women with breast cancer were excluded. These trials are fully discussed in Chapter 4, where it is shown that the effect of early detection of invasive disease can take 5–7 years to emerge. The emergence may take even longer when the women who are screened are under 50 years at entry into the trial (Tabár et al., 1997). With the introduction of population screening programmes, the methods developed for evaluation of trials must be adapted to the more complex public health situation. In contrast to trials, population-based screening programmes will take considerably longer to have an impact on breast cancer mortality in the general population. Unlike the participants in trials, the general population have staggered entry into a programme, and women with a pre-exisiting diagnosis of breast cancer are not easily excluded from the overall mortality estimate (Blanks et al., 2000b; Jonsson et al., 2001). The conditions for estimating refined mortality rates imply the existence of a cancer register and linkage to it of screening data which is not prevented by data protection legislation. Therefore, predictive measures of the process of cancer screening based on short-term outcomes are useful for evaluating the potential of a programme to make long-term reductions in mortality that are quantitatively comparable to those seen in randomized trials. Short-term parameters for this purpose that have been partially validated as accurate predictors of long-term reductions in breast cancer mortality include sensitivity and sojourn time distribution, both expressible in terms of the post-screening incidence of interval cancer (Day & Duffy, 1996).

Estimates of benefit based on predicted breast cancer mortality may be useful in the initial stage of a public health screening programme but cannot replace analysis of observed mortality, as discussed at length in Chapter 5 (see also Hakama et al., 1999; Blanks et al., 2000b; Jonsson et al., 2001).

The efficacy of screening programmes for reducing mortality from breast cancer, particularly by mammography, has been analysed in a number of randomized trials (see Chapter 4), which are referred to throughout the following sections.

In December 1963, the Health Insurance Plan of Greater New York, USA, had 490 000 members, of whom 80 000 were women aged 40–64. About two-thirds were employees of local, state or Federal agencies and their family members. The next largest group were union groups outside Government service (Shapiro et al., 1966). In 23 of the 31 medical groups, about 62 000 women were randomized to annual mammography screening and clinical breast examination for 4 consecutive years. Randomization was done by pair-matching by age, size of insured family and employment group through which the family had joined the Plan. Sixty-seven per cent attended the first round. There were no differences between attenders, a 10% sample of non-attenders and a 10% sample of controls with respect to age, socioeconomic status and histories of pregnancy and breastfeeding (Shapiro et al., 1988a). This study is referred to as the 'Health Insurance Plan study'.

In Edinburgh, Scotland, between 1978 and 1981, 87 general practitioners' practices covering 44 268 women aged 45–64 years, were randomized for a breast cancer screening trial (Alexander et al., 1999). The 22 926 women in the intervention group practices were invited to participate in a screening programme, which included clinical breast examination every year and two-view mammog-

raphy every second year. The 21 342 women in the control group practices received only usual medical care. Subsequently, additional eligible women who joined these practices and existing patients who reached 45 years of age were recruited into two further cohorts: 4867 women in 1982–83 and 5499 women in 1984–85 (Alexander et al., 1999). This study is referred to as 'the Edinburgh trial'.

Two trials were conducted in Canada, one with women aged 40–49 and the other with women aged 50–59 (Miller et al., 1981). Women randomized to screening in both age groups were offered annual clinical breast examination and mammography and were taught how to practise breast self-examination. Control women aged 40–49 were given a single clinical examination, taught how to practise breast self-examination and received a questionnaire every year. Control women aged 50–59 were offered only annual clinical breast examinations and were taught how to practise breast self-examination, as the objective was to evaluate the contribution of mammography over and above that of clinical breast examination and breast self-examination. Women were eligible for the trials if they had not had breast cancer, had had no mammogram in the previous 12 months, were currently not pregnant and completed a questionnaire giving full identification and data on risk factors for breast cancer (Miller et al., 1981). Before randomization, all participants gave written informed consent and were told that they had a 50% chance of having a mammogram. They then received a screening clinical breast examination (and instruction in breast self-examination), and the findings were recorded. While the participant remained in the examining room, the examiner went to receive the results of randomization from the centre coordinator and then told the participant whether she would receive mammography. A total of 50 430 women aged 40–49 and 39 405 women aged 50–59 were enrolled (Miller et al., 1992a,b).

Several trials have been conducted in Sweden, and these are summarized below. The trials have been the subject of two overview analyses (Nyström et al., 1993, 2002).

In the first of two trials in Malmö, Sweden, all women born between 1908 and 1932 were identified from the population register and randomized by a computer program within each birth year cohort. The lists were divided, the 21 088 women on the first half being invited and the 21 195 on the second serving as controls (Andersson et al., 1988). Women were invited to screen–film mammography alone in the first two rounds, with two views (cranio-caudal and medio-lateral oblique), and either both views or only the oblique view, depending on the parenchymal pattern, in the subsequent rounds, every 18–24 months. A single medio-lateral oblique view was taken for women whose breasts were mainly fatty on mammography, and both views were taken for women with dense breasts. After August 1978, the investigators aimed to continue to recruit women who attained the age of 45 years and to randomize them to either receive or not receive an invitation to mammography. In this second trial, 17 786 women born in 1933–45 were ultimately recruited, with 9574 in the invited group and 8212 in the control group. Owing to financial restraints, it was not possible to include one birth-year cohort every year. The randomization and screening procedures were the same as in the first trial, and recruitment continued up to 1990 (Andersson & Janzon, 1997). These trials are referred to in this handbook as the first and second Malmö trials.

In 1975, the Swedish National Board of Health and Welfare invited five county councils to start mammography screening. Two counties, Kopparberg and Östergötland, accepted the invitation. Women in this trial were randomized by cluster within geographical areas (municipalities, parishes, tax districts). The sparsely populated municipalities in the county of Östergötland were grouped pairwise with respect to the size of the population and geographical characteristics, adjacent municipalities being constituted into pairs, as they were considered to be similar in most respects. The more populated municipalities of Linköping, Norrköping and Motala were split into six, eight and two clusters, respectively, of similar size, creating three, four and one pairs, respectively, in order to increase the number of clusters. The clusters were allocated to invitation or a control group at a meeting of the county council by tossing a coin. A total of 76 617 women aged 40–74 were randomized to mammography or usual care (Nyström et al., 2002). In the County of Kopparberg, the invited group was planned to be twice as large as the control group. Thus, triplets of geographical areas were identified by dividing each block into three units of roughly equal size, two of which were randomized to receive screening and one to the control group. A total of 56 782 women aged 40–74 were randomized (Tabár et al., 1985). In this handbook, this trial is referred to as 'the Two-county study'.

A trial was performed in the south-eastern part of Greater Stockholm, Sweden, in which about 60 000 women aged 40–64 years in March 1981 were randomized by day of birth to be invited for mammography or to a control group (Frisell et al., 1986). Women born on days 1–10 and 21–31 of the month were invited for screening (total, 40 318), and women born on days 11–20 to the control group (about 20 000). In the overview of Nyström et al. (2002), women born on day 31 were not included, and the totals analysed were 39 139 in the intervention group and 20 978 in the control group. In this handbook, this study is referred to as 'the Stockholm trial'.

Between December 1982 and April 1984, all 51 611 women born between 1923 and 1944 and living in the city of Göteborg, Sweden, were randomized to mammographic screening or a control group, of whom 25 941 were aged 39–49. Randomization was by cluster on the basis of date of birth for the cohorts born in 1929–35 and by individual birth date for those born in 1936–44 (Bjurstam et al., 1997). In order to be able to re-screen women every eighteenth month, despite a fixed capacity for mammography, the ratio of women randomized to the invited and the control group was 1:1.2 in the age group 39–49 years and 1:1.6 in the age group 50–59 years. In this handbook, this study is referred to as 'the Göteborg trial'.

In addition to the randomized trials described above, the Finnish national programme was evaluated after randomization. The programme was begun in 1987, when the Finnish National Board of Health recommended identification of women aged 50–59 years and invitation to screening every second year. The Finnish Cancer Society established 11 mammography centres, and local municipalities, responsible in Finland for public health services, were entitled to establish an arrangement with one of these screening centres. In 1987, 84% of the municipalities made arrangements with the Cancer Society and followed the guidelines of the National Board of Health. The programme was introduced gradually, and decisions about adding cohorts were taken at random. Thus, in 1987, women born in 1928, 1932 and 1936 were invited to be screened by mammography; in 1988, women born in 1930, 1934 and 1938 were invited, and in 1989 women born in 1931 and 1937 were invited. This facilitated comparison of these birth cohorts, considered to be the study cohorts, with the birth cohorts invited after 1990, considered to be the control cohorts (Hakama et al., 1997).

# Chapter 2
# Screening techniques

## Screening mammography

Mammography is an X-ray technique that was developed specifically for soft tissue radiography of the breast. It is based on the differential absorption of X-rays between the various tissue components of the breast such as fat, fibroglandular tissue, tumour tissue and calcifications. Mammography is used both as a clinical tool to examine symptomatic patients and as a screening examination. The goal of screening mammography is to detect breast cancer early (Figure 22). To reach this goal, mammographs of consistently high quality must be produced with minimal exposure of the women to radiation.

### X-ray equipment
The physics of modern screen–film mammography techniques have been reviewed elsewhere (Säbel & Aichinger, 1996; Barnes, 1999; Haus, 1999; Hendrick & Berns, 1999; Haus & Yaffe, 2000).

Image contrast and spatial resolution are important determinants of image quality in mammography. The contrast depends on many factors, such as beam quality, screen–film combination, film processing and scattering of radiation.

### *Beam quality*
The image contrast depends on the energy distribution of the radiation used. The attenuation coefficients of fat, fibroglandular tissue and tumour tissue differ more at lower energy (below 20 keV) than at higher energy. However, compromises have to be made to keep the exposure within acceptable limits. This is accomplished by using various target–filter combinations. Most current mammography systems have molybdenum targets combined with molybdenum filtration; many also have rhodium filtration. Dual-target tubes, such as molybdenum–wolfram or molybdenum–rhodium, are also available.

The combination of a molybdenum target with molybdenum filtration results in an energy distribution that is ideal for imaging small-to-medium-sized breasts (energy, 15–20 keV) at tube voltages of 25–30 kVp. Increasing the voltage increases the penetration of the beam and thus decreases the dose; however, it also decreases the image contrast by decreasing the attenuation differences.

Switching to rhodium filtration and rhodium or wolfram targets has the same effect (Thilander-Klang, 1997; Thilander-Klang *et al.*, 1997; Figures 23 and 24). Many modern mammography units have programmes that choose automatically, on the basis of breast thickness and composition, a target–filter combination, that represents a reasonable compromise between image contrast and dose.

### *Tube current*
The tube current must be high enough to produce adequate film density with short exposure. Exposure times longer than about 1 s imply a risk of added dose and also lack of sharpness due to motion. Rhodium targets cannot be operated at

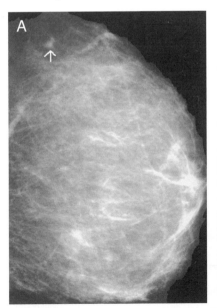
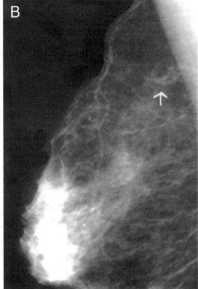

**Figure 22** Screening mammograms of early breast lesions
**A**, slightly spiculated tumour measuring 0.5 cm (arrow); a 0.6-cm invasive ductal carcinoma grade 2 was found on microscopy; **B**, cluster of calcifications (arrow); a ductal carcinoma *in situ* grade 2 measuring 1.4 cm was found on microscopy

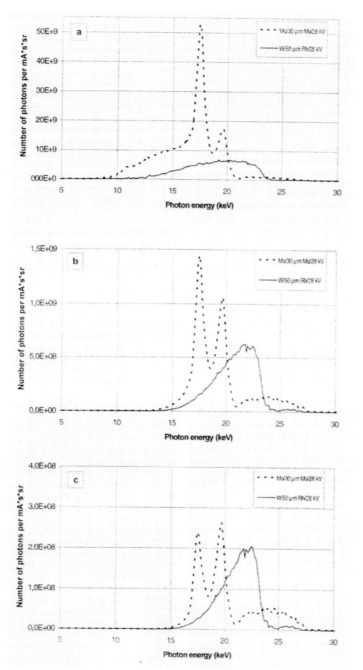

**Figure 23** Absolute X-ray spectra, with (a) measured entrance, (b) calculated transmitted energy with 40-mm polymethyl methylacrylate phantom and (c) calculated transmitted energy with 60-mm polymethyl methylacrylate phantom, obtained with various anode–filter combinations and a tube voltage of 28 kV

Dotted lines, molybdenum–molybdenum; solid lines, wolfram–rhodium

as high a tube current as molybdenum and wolfram targets because of a lower melting-point.

### Scatter control

One important factor that degrades image contrast is scattering of radiation (Friedrich, 1975; Barnes & Brezovich, 1978). The amount of scatter depends heavily on breast thickness and to some extent also on breast area. This is one of the reasons why breast compression is necessary to obtain a good mammogram. Further control of scatter can be obtained locally by spot compression, which can be combined with magnification.

The most important means of scatter reduction is the anti-scatter grid, which consists of thin lead lamellae separated by a radiolucent spacer. The grid ratio (height of lead lamellae divided by inter-space thickness) is usually 4:1 or 5:1. The grid usually starts moving during exposure and acts to absorb most of the scattered radiation (75–85%) while transmitting most of the primary radiation (60–75%) (Yester et al., 1981). As a result, image contrast is improved at the price of increased dose. Improvement in contrast is related to breast thickness, being greater with increasing thickness. The grid technique was introduced in the late 1970s. It was not used in most of the mammography screening trials, the exception being that in Göteberg, where it was used throughout (Bjurstam et al., 1997).

An even more efficient way of reducing scatter is the slot scanning technique (Barnes et al., 1989a,b), in which the X-ray beam is collimated to a thin fan beam which is scanned across the breast. Conventional linear grids reduce scatter only perpendicular to the grid septa, and there is little reduction in the direction parallel to the grid lines. Another solution is the cellular grid (Rezentes et al., 1999), which has a square pattern and therefore controls scatter in two dimensions. These grids have been shown to reduce scattered radiation further and

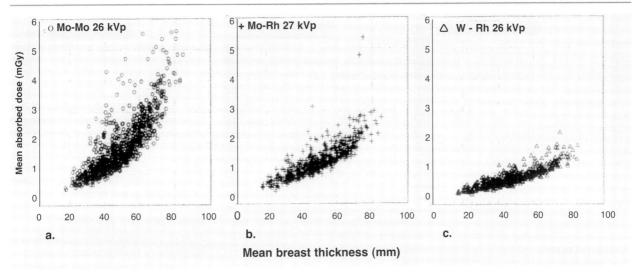

**Figure 24** Mean absorbed dose to glandular tissue versus mean breast thickness with (a) molybdenum–molybdenum, (b) molybdenum–rhodium and (c) wolfram–rhodium target–filter combinations

thus to improve image contrast over conventional grids.

Still another way of reducing scatter is geometric magnification with an air gap. The magnification factor is usually 1.7–2.0. For magnification work, a focus of 0.10–0.15 is necessary. Modern mammography machines are equipped with magnification capabilities.

### Automatic exposure control

Adequate automatic exposure control makes it possible to achieve optimal, reproducible density of images, independently of breast thickness and the beam quality used. Automatic exposure control devices have been refined substantially over the past few years. Most can be operated either manually or automatically. In the automatic mode, the instrument can choose both voltage and filter and, in some cases, also the target, depending on the thickness and density of the breast. The sensor should be of sufficient size and location to cover various components of breast tissue, and it should be moveable away from the chest wall, as the exposure should be determined by the densest part of the breast.

An automatic exposure control device should meet certain standards. A minimum requirement is that it should maintain a uniform film density to ± 0.10 or 0.15 optical density unit when the thickness of the phantom varies from 2 to 7 cm, for all techniques used (Social-styrelsen, 1998). Optical density is one determinant of the sensitivity of mammography (Young *et al.*, 1997). According to the European guidelines (Commission of the European Communities, 2001), the optical density should be between 1.4 and 1.8 (National Health Service Breast Screening Programme, 1998).

### Compression

Optimal compression is an important part of the mammography procedure. Compression improves contrast by reducing scatter and hardening the X-ray beam and also reduces the dose to the breast. Furthermore, patient motion is reduced, and the density of the image becomes more uniform. With proper compression, the structures of the breast are spread apart, facilitating image interpretation.

### Screen film, processing and viewing

The introduction of rare-earth intensifying screens in the mid-1970s represented a major step forward, as these screens could be combined with fast-speed films, thereby reducing the dose. The screens are virtually always used as back-screens combined with a single emulsion film in order to achieve optimal spatial resolution. Various phosphors have been used; one that is commonly used is gadolinium oxysulfide ($Gd_2O_2S$:Tb), which emits visible light in the green spectral region (wavelength, about 500 nm).

Film processing is critical for obtaining a high-quality mammogram, and suboptimal image quality is frequently due to suboptimal processing. Processing is one of the key determinants of film contrast, as reflected in the so-called characteristic curve of the film. Critical factors in processing are temperature, processing time and replenishment rate.

Extended cycle processing is sometimes used for single-emulsion films (Kimme-Smith *et al.*, 1989), thereby increasing film contrast and speed. Today, a 90-s processing cycle is recommended by almost all film manufacturers.

Once the key processing parameters have been set, a quality control programme should be implemented. Base parameters like film speed, contrast and base plus fog can be determined easily by sensitometry, either by manual measurement or by running a sensitometry strip through an automatic reader.

Light boxes of adequate luminance and a low level of ambient light are important for viewing, as well as masking of films to reduce stray light (Commission of the European Communities, 2001).

## Radiation dose

The mammographic imaging system must be optimized in order to keep the radiation dose as low as possible. Such a requirement has been included in national legislation in some countries and in international guidelines.

The mean absorbed dose in the breast gland per mammographic film is in the order of 1.0–1.5 mGy for the average breast examined with modern equipment. Surveys have shown considerable variation in dose among centres. In southern Sweden, the dose varied by a factor of 4.3, depending on the radiologists' preference in terms of optical density of the films, variation in film processing parameters and other factors (Socialstyrelsen, 1997). In Sweden, the mean absorbed dose to the breast gland per film must not exceed 1.5 mGy at the optical density setting used and should not exceed 1.0 mGy at net density 1.0 as measured with a 4.5-cm polymethyl methylacrylate phantom according to the European protocol (Zoetelief et al., 1996). According to the European guidelines (Commission of the European Communities, 2001), the dose should be < 2.0 mGy. A woman being screened every 2 years between the ages of 40 and 70, with two views of each breast, would thus receive an absorbed dose of 64 mGy or less from the screening. For a discussion of the possible hazard of mammographic radiation, see Chapter 5.

## Quality control

Guidelines for quality assurance have been issued by several bodies, such as the Commission of the European Communities (2001). Many factors affect the accuracy of mammography, including those related to the X-ray machine and film processing, the examination technique including positioning and compression (Taplin et al., 2002) and the radiologist's performance. It has been shown that radiologists vary, sometimes substantially, in their interpretation of mammograms (Elmore et al., 1994; Beam et al., 1996a,b). One determinant may be the volume read per day (Esserman et al., 2002). Recommendations vary regarding the minimum number of mammograms that should be read yearly, from 480 to 5000 (Food & Drug Administration, 1997; National Health Service Breast Screening Programme, 1998). Another factor is training, which has been shown to improve sensitivity with no change in specificity (Linver et al., 1992).

Continuous correlation of radiographic findings with cytology and pathology is another essential component, with training and continuing education. Furthermore, a database should be established that contains basic information such as patient identification, date of mammographic examination, mammographic diagnosis, results of needle biopsy and surgical procedures, including microscopic diagnosis. If cancer is present, the tumour size, lymph node status, malignancy grading and the presence or absence of distant metastasis should be recorded.

High, consistent image quality is mandatory to achieve the objectives of mammography. To maintain the image quality at an acceptable level, regular tests must be carried out. The day-to-day consistency of the procedure should be based on sensitometry and phantom exposure. While sensitometry specifically monitors the performance of the processor, phantom exposure provides an overall check of the imaging system. If the process is stable, as shown by sensitometry, the phantom film will indicate the status of the X-ray machine. Sensitometry and phantom exposure can be performed by radiographers, whereas several parameters relating to mammography machines should be checked by a medical physicist semi-annually or at least annually. An example of a quality control programme for mammography is shown in Table 4.

## Sensitivity and specificity

Several estimates of the sensitivity and specificity of mammography have been published. In most of them, the cancers detected at screening, expressed as the proportion of all these cancers and those occurring during the first 12 months after screening ('interval cancers') were used as a proxy for sensitivity. This was called the 'detection' method by Fletcher et al. (1993). The preferred expression for sensitivity is 1 minus the incidence of interval cancers expressed as a proportion of the estimated underlying incidence of breast cancer in the population. This was called the 'incidence' method by Fletcher et al. (1993; see Chapter 1).

Table 5 summarizes estimates of the sensitivity, specificity and positive predictive value of mammography, with or without clinical breast examination, as reported in breast screening trials (described above in Chapter 1 and more fully in Chapter 4) and some population-based screening programmes, which covered screening from as early as 1963 to as late as 1997. In all instances in this table, the estimates of sensitivity are based on 1-year interval cancer rates and are calculated by the detection method, the incidence method or both (Fletcher et al., 1993). The estimates of specificity and predictive positive value take into consideration all women referred for further investigation after a positive result at screening. Unless otherwise specified, the estimates are based on invasive cancers only in the

## Table 4. Technical quality control programme for mammography used in southern Sweden

| Function to be checked | Method, test and/or responsibility | Frequency |
|---|---|---|
| Film processing | Sensitometry (technologist or radiologist) | Daily |
| Entire imaging process | Phantom exposure (technologist or radiologist) Visual comparison with reference | Daily |
| Phototimer | PMMA phantom exposure with recording of milliamperes (technologist or radiologist) | Daily if batch processing |
| Beam quality: filtration, tube potential, half-value layer | Service or physicist | Annually or semi-annually |
| Phototimer: reproducibility, dependence on object thickness and tube potential | Service or physicist | Annually or semi-annually |
| Output: millampere accuracy and linearity | Service or physicist | Annually or semi-annually |
| Beam geometry: radiation field extension | Service or physicist | Annually or semi-annually |
| Compression device | Service or physicist | Annually or semi-annually |
| Film cassettes: sensitivity, film screen contact, spatial resolution | Service or physicist | Annually or semi-annually |
| Anti-scatter grid | Service or physicist | Annually or semi-annually |
| Absorbed dose | Physicist | Annually or semi-annually |

Modified from Commission of the European Communities (2001)
Milliamperes are the product of tube current x length of exposure
PMMA, polymethyl methacrylate

first screening round or the combination of second and subsequent screening rounds.

The estimates of sensitivity derived with the detection method, available from almost all the programmes, varied from low values of 68% (Stockholm trial of one-view mammography) and 74% (Health Insurance Plan trial of early two-view mammography and clinical breast examination) to high values of over 90% in several populations. There is no strong evidence that the sensitivity of these programmes increased over time. As expected from differences in the way in which they are computed, the estimates of sensitivity derived with the preferred incidence method were generally smaller than those computed with the detection method and varied by 52–82%, again with little evidence of a trend over time. The estimates of sensitivity were generally higher by a small margin in first than in subsequent screening rounds.

The estimates of specificity were derived mainly from the screening trials and exceeded 90%, with few exceptions; many exceeded 95%. The corresponding values for positive predictive value ranged from 2% to 22%; most were 12% or less.

Estimates of sensitivity for women in different age groups have been reported from a number of studies, and some are shown in Table 5. In addition, Tabár et al. (1987b) reported estimates obtained by

**Table 5. Summary of estimates of sensitivity and specificity of breast cancer screening by mammography with or without clinical breast examination reported from screening trials and some population-based screening programmes**

| Trial or programme | Screening method, period, age group | Sensitivity (%) Detection method | Incidence method | Specificity (%) | PPV (%) |
|---|---|---|---|---|---|
| Health Insurance Plan (Fletcher et al., 1993; Shapiro, 1997) | Two-view mammmography and CBE 1963–66, 40–64 | 74 | 77 | 98.5 | 12 |
| Breast Cancer Detection Demonstration Project (Seidman et al., 1987) | Two-view mammography, CBE and thermography 1972–81, 40–59 | 88[1], 84[2] | | | |
| Utrecht, Netherlands (de Waard et al., 1984a) | Two-view mammography and CBE 1974–80, 50–67 | 91 | | | |
| Nijmegen, Netherlands (Verbeek et al., 1988) | One-view mammography 1975–85, 35–64 | 89 | 82 | | |
| Malmö, Sweden (Fletcher et al., 1993) | Two-view mammography 1976–90, 43–70 | 79 | 68 | 96[1], 97[2] | 10[1], 22[2] |
| Two-county trial, Sweden (Fletcher et al., 1993) | One-view mammography 1977–81, 40–75 | 76 | 60[1],70[2] | 95[1], 98[2] | 12 |
| Edinburgh, Scotland (Fletcher et al., 1993) | Two-view mammography and CBE 1979–86, 45–64 | 88 | 79 | 96[1], 97[2] | 15[1], 4[2] |
| Edinburgh, Scotland (Chamberlain et al., 1991) | Two-view mammography and CBE 1979–86, 45–64 | 92[1],93[2] | 73[1,3],78[1,3] | 96[1], 97[2] | 15[1], 4[2] |
| Guildford, England (Chamberlain et al., 1991) | Two-view mammography and CBE 1979–86, 45–64 | 94[1], 90[2] | 73[1,3],78[1,3] | 92[1], 94[2] | 6[1], 2[2] |
| Canada 1 (Fletcher et al., 1993) | Two-view mammography and CBE 1980–85, 40–49 | 81 | 58 | 82[1], 93[2] | 2 |
| Canada 2 (Fletcher et al., 1993) | Two-view mammography and CBE 1980–85, 50–59 | 88 | 72 | 83[1], 96[2] | 4[1],6[2] |
| Stockholm, Sweden (Fletcher et al., 1993) | One-view mammography 1981–83, 40–64 | 68[1] | 75 | 95[1], 97[2] | 8[1],10[2] |
| Stockholm, Sweden (Fletcher et al., 1993) | One-view mammography 1981–83, 40–49 | 53[1] | 39 | | |

## Table 5. (contd)

| Trial or programme | Screening method, period, age group | Sensitivity (%) | | Specificity (%) | PPV (%) |
|---|---|---|---|---|---|
| | | Detection method | Incidence method | | |
| Göteberg, Sweden (Bjurstam et al., 1997) | Two-view mammography 1982–84, 39–49 | | 82 | | |
| Sydney, Australia (Rickard et al., 1998) | Two-view, double reader film–screen mammography 1988–92, 40–69 | | 71 | | |
| Ontario, Canada (Libstug et al., 1998) | Two-view mammography and CBE 1990–95, 50–69 | 90[1], 81[2] | | 87[1], 92[2] | 6.7[1], 6.2[2] |
| British Columbia, Canada (Olivotto et al., 2000) | Two-view mammography 1988–97, ≥ 40 | 86 <br> 86 | | 94 | 6 |
| East Anglia, England (Day et al., 1995) | One- and two-view mammography 1990–93, 52–64 | | 76[4] | | |
| Netherlands (Fracheboud et al., 1999) | One- and two-view mammography 1990–93, 50–69 | 92[1], 85[2] | 73[1], 74[2] | | |
| Victoria, Australia (BreastScreen Victoria, 2001) | Two-view, double reader film–screen mammography 1996, 50–69 | 91[1], 82[2] | | | |

PPV, positive predictive value; CBE, clinical breast examination

[1] First round

[2] Subsequent rounds

[3] Edinburgh and Guildford combined

the incidence method for the Two-county trial of 62%, 88% and 85% for women aged 40–49, 50–59 and 60–69, respectively. In a study in Utrecht, the Netherlands, in which mammography and clinical breast examination were used, Day et al. (1988) reported a sensitivity of screening of 83% for women aged 50–59 and 86% for women aged 60–64. In a study in Nijmegen, in which mammography alone was used, Verbeek et al. (1988) reported a sensitivity of 44% for women aged 35–49 and 75% for women aged 50–64. Peer et al. (1996) later replicated this age difference in screening rounds four through eight, with an estimate of 64% for women under 50 and 85% for those above 50. Chamberlain et al. (1991) evaluated sensitivity by age for all screenings in the combined programmes in Edinburgh and Guildford (United Kingdom); the sensitivity was 70% for women aged 45–54 at entry and 84% for those aged 55–64 at entry. In the screening programme in British Columbia, Canada, the sensitivity (with the detection method) was 76% for women aged 40–49, 85% for those aged 50–59, 90% for those aged 60–69, 91% for those aged 70–79 and 91% for those aged 80 or more (Olivotto et al., 2000). Thus, there was a consistent trend for increasing sensitivity with increasing age.

In the Canadian trials, review by the reference radiologist allowed identification of the cancers missed by the radiologists in the screening centre and suspected by the reference radiologist. This process included both the interval cancers and the cancers detected at the second screening (Baines et al., 1986a). These, together with the cancers identified by physical examination but missed on mammography, allowed identification

## Mammographic density

- Breast parenchymal 'density' as seen on a mammogram is a determinant of the sensitivity of mammography.

- Breast parenchymal density decreases with age.

- Hormone replacement therapy of the combination type may result in increased breast density.

- Tamoxifen may decrease breast density.

of the false-negative findings. This is in practice a refinement of the detection method. On this basis, two reports of the sensitivity of mammography were made for the first screening for both components of the trial together (i.e. for women aged 40–59 on entry). The first related to the first five centres in the trial, which were entered in 1980 and 1981 (Baines *et al.*, 1986b), with an overall sensitivity of 69%, a specificity of 94%, and a positive predictive value of 8.6%. Baines *et al.* (1988a) subsequently reported the sensitivity of the first screening in all 15 centres to be 75%, a specificity of 94% and a positive predictive value of 7%. The authors postulated that the differences in sensitivity between the first and second reports were a consequence of a general improvement in mammography with time since the trial was initiated, and the benefit the later centres derived from entering the trial with mammography quality control procedures fully in place.

Chamberlain *et al.* (1991) determined what they called the 'relative' sensitivities of mammography and clinical breast examination as the proportion detected by each of all cancers found at each round in the Trial of Early Detection of Breast Cancer in the United Kingdom. The relative sensitivity of mammography was 94% at the prevalence screen and 90% at the incidence screens. For comparison, the relative sensitivities were 72% and 45% for clinical breast examination.

### Host factors that affect sensitivity

Mammography is based on the principle of differential absorption of X-rays between fat, fibroglandular tissue, tumour tissue and calcifications, fat being more radiolucent (blacker on the film) than the other tissues (which are 'denser' or whiter on the film). Thus, the density of a mammogram is determined by the relationship between fat and fibroglandular tissue or tumour tissue, the mammogram being 'denser' the more of the latter tissue components are present. The mammographic pattern of the breast thus varies between individuals (Figure 25). Furthermore, breast cancer is more readily detected in a fatty breast than in a dense breast (Mandelson *et al.*, 2000).

In addition to age, several other factors seem to be related to the amount of fibroglandular tissue in the breast,

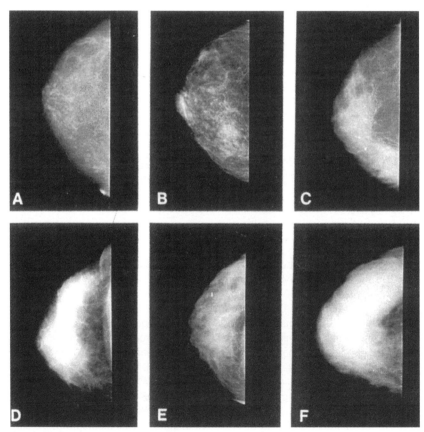

**Figure 25** Six categories of mammographic density. A = 0%; B = 0 < 10%; C = 10 < 25%; D = 25 < 50%; E = 50 < 75%; F = > 75%
From Boyd *et al.* (2001)

including parity and age at birth of first child (Andersson *et al.*, 1981; de Waard *et al.*, 1984b); greater age at birth of first child and nulliparity are associated with denser breasts. There is also suggestive evidence that density may vary with the phase in the menstrual cycle, being on average greater in the luteal phase (White *et al.*, 1998). This might explain the lower sensitivity and specificity of mammography in women in the luteal phase than in the follicular phase seen in one study (Baines *et al.*, 1997).

It has been demonstrated fairly consistently that breast density increases in a certain proportion of women undergoing hormone replacement therapy, especially if they are treated with combinations of estrogen and progestin (Figure 26; Sala *et al.*, 2000). In one study, greater density was seen in 3.5–23.5% of women, depending on the preparation used (Greendale *et al.*, 1999). The increase in density

usually appears within months after the start of treatment and appears to subside within a few months of termination of treatment.

Increased density after hormone replacement therapy can be assumed to decrease the sensitivity of mammography, and this has been demonstrated (Laya *et al.*, 1996). Kavanagh *et al.* (2000) reported a sensitivity of 80% for non-users of hormone replacement therapy and 64% for users in a large screening programme. Furthermore, the specificity was marginally lower for users. However, Thurfjell *et al.*, (1997) found no decrease in sensitivity of mammography in women on hormone replacement therapy.

Tamoxifen, which has mainly antiestrogenic effects, has been reported to decrease the density of the breast parenchyma in some women (Atkinson *et al.*, 1999; Chow *et al.*, 2000).

## One *versus* two views

Screening with a single view (the medio-lateral oblique) was suggested by a pioneer of mammographic screening, Lundgren (1977), on the presumption that virtually all breast cancers could be detected with one view. However, it was soon demonstrated that addition of a second view (the cranio-caudal) could improve sensitivity. The results of the Malmö mammographic screening trial suggested that 10–20% of invasive carcinomas < 10 mm in diameter would have been overlooked if only one projection had been used at screening. This applied mainly to mass lesions, while calcifications were consistently observed in both projections (Andersson, 1981).

Ample evidence in the same direction came from the screening programme in the United Kingdom (Wald *et al.*, 1995), which changed from using one to two views in the mid-1990s. A 25–42% increase in detection of invasive cancers < 15 mm in diameter was seen in incidence screens (Blanks *et al.*, 1997). Furthermore, the increase in sensitivity with two views was greatest for small cancers and cancers of low grade (Given-Wilson & Blanks, 1999).

The results of studies of the effect of two views on specificity varied. No significant change was noted in several, while a decrease was found in one study (Thurfjell *et al.*, 1994a). The results also indicated that the rate of false-positive findings was higher with one view only (Andersson, 1981).

The strategy used in several Swedish programmes is to classify the parenchyma as either 'dense' or 'not dense' at baseline, representing breasts with more than and less than approximately 25% fibroglandular tissue, respectively, as assessed visually. In subsequent screening rounds, 'not dense' breasts are examined with the oblique view only and at a 2-year interval. Women with 'dense' breasts are examined with two views, the cranio-caudal and oblique, at intervals of 18 months (Socialstyrelsen, 1998).

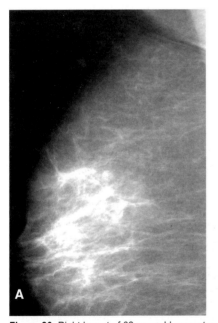 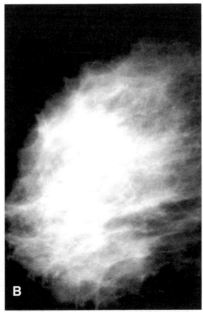

**Figure 26** Right breast of 62-year-old asymptomatic woman
**A**, before hormone replacement therapy: the breast is predominantly fatty; **B**, after hormone replacement therapy (combined estrogen–progestin preparation): the density of the breast parenchyma has increased substantially

There are currently no published comparisons of this strategy with two-view mammography.

## Double reading

An increase in sensitivity of 10–15% has been reported as the result of double reading compared with single reading (Anttinen et al., 1993; Anderson et al., 1994; Thurfjell et al., 1994b). However, Ciatto and collaborators (1995) found only a 5% increase. Most authors report decreased specificity with independent double reading, although consensus decisions or arbitration on selected cases improves specificity (Anttinen et al., 1993; Brown et al., 1996). There are two main reasons for not detecting a significant lesion at screening: overlooking it or misinterpreting it. Of all interval cancers, 15–30% were found retrospectively to have been overlooked and about 15% misinterpreted (Ikeda et al., 1992). Double reading can reduce these proportions and can detect some of the cancers that pass unnoticed until a subsequent screening. Furthermore, the wide variability in radiologists' interpretations of screening mammograms (Beam et al., 1996a) can be partly offset by double reading (Beam et al., 1996b).

Most authors recommend double reading, although Ciatto et al. (1995) questioned the cost–effectiveness of the procedure. In a Finnish programme, the incremental cost per cancer with double reading was not drastically higher than with single reading (39%) (Leivo et al., 1999). Several factors have to be taken into consideration, such as the experience of readers (Warren & Duffy, 1995). With very experienced readers, the advantage of double reading is probably smaller (Ciatto et al., 1995). In the European guidelines (Commission of the European Communities, 2001), double reading is mandatory in decentralized programmes and in programmes in which the radiologists are not yet sufficiently experienced. In centralized programmes with radiologists experienced in screening and diagnosis, double reading is not mandatory. Double reading practically doubles the resources required in terms of radiologists in a screening programme. Good results have been reported with suitably trained radiographers as second readers (Pauli et al., 1996). Computer-aided detection systems may replace a second reader in the future (Warren Burhenne et al., 2000).

## Other and emerging imaging techniques

X-ray mammography is the only imaging method for breast cancer screening that has received serious evaluation. More recently, alternatives and adjuncts have begun to be evaluated, primarily for their potential in breast cancer diagnosis. This section deals with their potential application to breast cancer screening. An overview of the techniques described below is given in Table 6.

The evidence for the accuracy of recently proposed methods of screening is reviewed below. To avoid bias, the literature was reviewed systematically to ensure that all relevant studies had been located, and their quality and applicability were examined before their results were assessed (Glasziou et al., 1999). To ensure the applicability of the results to screening, the studies had to have been done on women eligible for screening. Studies on women presenting clinically cannot be used to infer the accuracy of a new technique for screening, because the objective of testing is different. In clinical settings, the objective is to determine whether a previously detected abnormality is cancer. In screening, it is to identify abnormalities that may be found on further testing to be early cancers. Furthermore, the spectrum of disease is different, as the clinical abnormalities are larger and more advanced. Papers were therefore included only if they referred to new tests done in asymptomatic women, including populations at higher risk for breast cancer because of genetic predisposition or those in whom mammography is less accurate because they are younger or have radiologically dense breast tissue. Very few studies fulfilled these criteria. The remainder of the papers were review articles, were concerned with the development of tests or referred to use of tests in individual cases or as a diagnostic tool in women with a clinically or mammographically detected breast abnormality. Papers on screening were excluded if important technological changes made them no longer relevant. On these grounds, articles on thermography before 1988 were excluded, as were papers on ultrasonography with water baths or frequency probes with a resolution < 7.5 mHz.

No eligible papers were found for computed tomography scanning, magnetic resonance spectroscopy, scintimammography, electrical impedance or infrared spectroscopy. Light scanning and thermography have been suggested for screening but hold little promise. Light scanning was evaluated in two studies conducted over a decade ago (Alveryd et al., 1990; Braddick, 1991), and thermography was evaluated in one study (Williams et al., 1990); all suggested that these techniques are of insufficient accuracy, and no further eligible studies were identified. The results for the remaining techniques are described below. The relative sensitivities are presented for those studies in which interval cancers were not counted. Relative sensitivities allow comparison of tests but overestimate true sensitivity.

### Digital mammography

In digital mammography, the image receptor (screen–film) used in conventional mammography is replaced by a digital receptor; in all other respects, the imaging techniques are the same. From the woman's point of view, receiving a digital mammogram is similar to having a conventional mammogram, as breast

| Table 6. Other and emerging imaging techniques. Description and potential strenghts and limitations | | | |
|---|---|---|---|
| Screening technique | Description | Potential strengths | Current limitations |
| Digital mammography | Electronic detectors capture X-rays in a matrix of square picture elements. Computer generates image. | Image processing Easy display, transmission and storage Lower radiation dose Computer-aided detection | Higher cost than mammography for low-volume operations |
| Ultrasonography | High-frequency ultrasound waves generate images based on the acoustic–mechanical properties of breast tissue | Increased sensitivity for mammographically dense breasts. No X-irradiation | Operator-dependent More expensive than mammography Less specific than mammography |
| Magnetic resonance imaging | Based on radiofrequency signals generated by exciting hydrogen nuclei (protons) in a strong magnetic field. Dynamic study of spatial and temporal distribution of intravenous contrast medium | More sensitive than mammography No X-irradiation | Less specific than mammography More expensive than mammography Claustrophobic |
| Positron emission tomography (PET) | Tomographic nuclear imaging procedure with positron-emitting tracers (usually fluorodeoxyglucose) | Staging of breast cancer | Expensive Limited access Low sensitivity |
| Scintimammography | Nuclear imaging technique usually technetium-99m isonitrile (Sestamibi) | May be more sensitive for detection of certain histological types of breast cancer e.g. lobular invasive carcinoma | Poor spatial resolution Expensive |
| Electrical impedance imaging | Technique involving low-level bio-electric currents to map electrical impedance properties of the breast | No harmful radiation | |
| Infrared thermography | Measurement of heat emissions | No harmful radiation | Less sensitive and specific than mammography |
| Transillumination (near-infrared spectroscopy, light scanning) | Technique for scanning the breast with red or near-infrared light and recording the light image on infrared-sensitive film or with a television camera | No harmful radiation | Less sensitive and specific than mammography |
| Laser transillumination | Refinement of the above with extremely short laser pulses and time-resolved detection | Better resolution than infra-red transillumination | Still experimental |

compression and positioning are unchanged.

The digital receptor consists of a matrix of square picture elements (pixels), usually measuring 50–100 mm. In most current receptors, the signal is created in a two-step procedure. In the first step, the X-ray energy is converted to light in a structure that is similar to a conventional intensifying screen. In a second step, the light is converted to an electrical signal, which is digitalized. In other detectors, the light step is omitted, and the X-rays interact directly with the detector, creating electrical charges that are digitalized. Still other detectors count the X-ray photos directly.

The signal value of pixels is usually digitalized into 12–16 bytes, which creates a grey scale of 4096–65 536 levels. This wide dynamic range is a major advantage over conventional techniques and represents the basis for higher contrast resolution and various image processing and display techniques. One practical advantage is that areas that are very dark or bright on screen–film mammograms can be displayed to better advantage. The images can be printed on paper, but, to obtain full advantage of the technique, a monitor is required.

For high-volume screening, special work stations have been developed in order to handle large data sets and to display the images in a rational, customized way. One digital image may comprise 8–32 megabytes. Other advantages of digital mammography are related to storage and communication. Digital images can be transmitted electronically for centralized reading or consultation.

Digital mammography has the potential to provide images with lower doses of radiation than screen–film mammography. This may apply even more to the photon counting detectors, but no data have so far been published to support this contention. The cost of acquiring a complete digital system is several times that of a conventional system; however, in a high-volume screening setting, this cost may be offset by more rational working procedures and the elimination of fibre and developing chemicals.

Full-field digital mammography has been evaluated as a screening modality in one study (Lewin et al., 2001), which showed it to have similar sensitivity to screen–film mammography and greater specificity.

Computer-aided detection can be incorporated into the work station and the results of the computer analysis added onto the image, thereby assisting the radiologist in detecting suspect lesions. Computer-aided detection has been assessed in several studies (te Brake et al., 1998; Warren Burhenne et al., 2000; Birdwell et al., 2001; Freer & Ulissey, 2001), which suggest an incremental value in terms of sensitivity. The

evidence on specificity is conflicting. Some data suggest that computer-aided detection could replace a second reader (Warren Burhenne et al., 2000).

## Ultrasonography

Ultrasound images are produced from reflected high-frequency sound waves, without exposure to ionizing radiation. The technique is currently used mainly as an adjunct to mammography to characterize suspected lesions further and to guide needle biopsy. Breast ultrasound examination of asymptomatic women has some potential limitations:

- The sensitivity is highly dependent on the operator (Teh & Wilson, 1998).
- The field of view is limited to a few centimeters, which makes a full breast examination difficult and time-consuming (Nass et al., 2001) as well as more expensive than mammography.
- Creation of hard copies of ultrasound images is costly; recording the entire examination is impractical (Teh & Wilson, 1998).
- It is relatively ineffective for detecting microcalcifications (Nass et al., 2001; National Alliance of Breast Cancer Organizations, 2001)

In a type of ultrasonography called elastography, the firmness of tissue is imaged. Softer tissues, such as fat, appear brighter on the images than do firmer tissues—including tumours. The

technique involves combining two ultrasound images of the same tissue: a compressed view and an uncompressed view. While elastography may become a useful adjunct for distinguishing between benign and malignant lesions, its potential has not yet been clarified.

Ultrasonography has been assessed in several studies, primarily in women who had mammographically dense breasts of who were at high risk for breast cancer (Kolb et al., 1998; Buchberger et al., 2000; Warner et al., 2001). The results suggest that ultrasonography may increase the sensitivity of screening if used as an adjunct to mammography for mammographically dense breasts. Combined testing is likely to decrease specificity. It is not clear whether ultrasonography on its own is better than mammography in an unselected population.

## Magnetic resonance imaging

Magnetic resonance imaging (MRI) involves use of rapidly fluctuating, high magnetic fields to excite the protons of the hydrogen atoms within the water molecule. Weak electromagnetic signals produced within the body are detected by antenna coils and used to generate planar and three-dimensional images of internal structures. Planar images can be created from virtually any viewing angle, at a resolution of approximately 1 mm$^3$, and without ionizing radiation. The magnetic field presents minimal hazards.

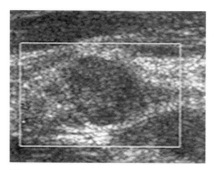

Ultrasonography image

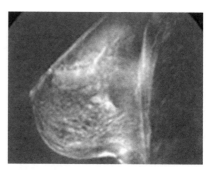

Magnetic resonance imaging

As used in breast cancer detection, MRI must be performed as a dynamic study of contrast enhancement of breast tissue after intravenous administration of contrast medium (Heywang-Köbrunner et al., 1988; Kaiser, 1989). The patho-physiological basis for the contrast enhancement of breast cancer is the presence of newly formed vascular structures, which have increased permeability and, furthermore, increased extravascular space. In typical cases, the rapid contrast enhancement is followed by an immediate decrease (so called wash-out). Benign lesions tend to enhance more slowly. Most invasive cancers show the typical enhancement pattern, but there are exceptions, especially lobular invasive carcinoma, which may resemble a benign lesion. This is also true for many uninvasive carcinomas. In contrast, some benign lesions, such as some fibroadenomas and papillomas, show rapid enhancement, similar to carcinomas.

MRI is considerably more expensive than ultrasound and mammography. Other drawbacks to MRI include the following:

- It is more time-consuming than mammography; an MRI examination takes approximately 30 min to complete, during which time the woman must remain motionless within the cramped quarters of the MRI device.
- The restricted MRI machinery conditions might discourage women with claustrophobic tendencies from undergoing the examination.
- The current technique requires an intravenous infusion of a contrast agent.
- The image obtained in MRI is affected by the phase of a woman's menstrual cycle. It is best done during the second or third week of the cycle, to minimize hormonal effects (Stoutjesdijk et al., 2001).

There are several well-established indications for use of MRI in the clinical setting, such as in investigation of possible multifocality or multicentricity of breast cancer in patients who cannot be fully evaluated with conventional techniques. Other indications are breast prostheses or extensive scarring, which may be difficult to evaluate with conventional techniques, and cases of axillary metastases and an unknown primary (Heywang-Köbrunner et al., 1988).

MRI has not been evaluated as a screening modality in unselected populations. Four studies on the sensitivity of MRI in high-risk women have been published within the past 2 years and are summarized in Table 7. The combined studies covered fewer than 40 cancers. The results suggest that MRI is more sensitive than mammography but may be less specific. A study is under way on a larger number of women (UK MRI Breast Cancer Screening Advisory Group, 2000).

## Positron emission tomography

Positron emission tomography (PET) scans create computerized cross-sectional images of metabolic changes within a tissue. A radiolabelled tracer (usually a glucose analogue) is used to highlight differences in metabolic activity. The usefulness of PET in screening for breast cancer has not been demonstrated. Small studies have indicated

| **Table 7. Sensitivity and specificity of magnetic resonance imaging** | | | | | | |
|---|---|---|---|---|---|---|
| Reference | Population | Age | No. of invasive cancers | Total sample size | Sensitivity (%) | Specificity (%) (% requiring biopsy) |
| Warner et al. (2001) | High risk (BRCA or several family members) | Mean, 43 Range 26–59 | 6 | 196 | M, 33 CBE, 33 Ultrasound, 60 MRI, 100 | M, 99.5 CBE, 99.5 Ultrasound, 93 MRI, 91 |
| Stoutjesdijik et al. (2001) | BRCA lifetime risk > 15% | 21–71 | 13 | 262 exams on 179 women | M, 42 MRI, 100 | M, 96 MRI, 93 |
| Tilanus-Linthorst et al. (2000a,b) | High risk (> 25%) and > 50% breast density | Mean, 41.5 | 3 | 109 | | MRI, 95 |
| Kuhl et al. (2000) | High familial risk | Mean, 39 Range, 18–65 | 9 | 105 | M, 33 Ultrasound, 33 MRI, 100 | M, 93 Ultrasound, 80 MRI, 95 |

M, mammography; CBE, clinical breast examination; MRI, magnetic resonance imaging

fairly good sensitivity and more limited specificity, with poor sensitivity for tumours smaller than 1 cm (Nass et al., 2001). PET might be useful in screening women with implants, scarring or dense breast tissue (Cole & Coleman, 1999; National Cancer Institute, 2001a). In addition, some lesions are seen on PET scans but not on mammograms, which makes biopsy difficult. Finally, the technique is costly, and PET scanners are relatively scarce because they must be located near particle accelerators that produce the short-lived radioisotopes used as tracers (National Cancer Institute, 2001a).

PET scanning is also time-consuming. After receiving the radioactive tracer, the woman must lie still for about 45 min while the tracer circulates, and the scanning takes another 45 min (National Cancer Institute, 2001a).

The National Cancer Institute (2001a) is sponsoring a clinical trial to evaluate PET and other imaging techniques in women with a diagnosis of breast cancer, but there is little likelihood of any use for PET in breast cancer screening in the near future.

PET has been evaluated as a screening tool in only one study of consecutive screenees (Yasuda et al., 2000). There were only five breast cancers, of which one was detectable with PET only.

## Scintimammography

In scintimammography—also called mammoscintigraphy—a radioactive tracer is introduced into the body and may accumulate at higher levels in tumour and some other tissues. A camera that detects γ-rays is then used to produce images. Newer cameras specifically designed for breast imaging are being evaluated clinically. The images can be two- or three-dimensional. One radioactive tracer (technetium-99m) has been approved by the Food and Drug Administration, and others are being studied (Nass et al., 2001).

The current role of scintimammography is as an adjunct to mammography to identify metastatic cells distant to the breast and to localize tumours. The technique does not appear to be affected by implants, scarring or dense breast tissue. The health risks are minimal and similar to those from mammography, although the entire body is exposed to radiation. Scintimammography is more expensive than mammography or ultrasound, but less expensive than MRI or PET.

## Electrical impedance imaging

Some cancerous tissue may conduct electricity much better than normal tissue does. Electrical impedance scanning is done with a hand-held probe connected to an electrode patch placed on a woman's arm. The probe measures the current passing through the skin covering the breast, and this information is used to reconstruct parametric images of the breast (National Cancer Institute, 2001a).

Electrical impedance imaging is painless and requires no exposure to ionizing radiation (Nass et al., 2001). The technique may give false-positive results because of problems such as poor contact of the device on the skin, air bubbles and superficial skin lesions. The images reflect the superficial tissues, limited to about 35 mm deep, and cancerous lesions directly behind the nipple were difficult to detect (Malich et al., 2001). At present, electrical impedance may have promise as an adjunct, but the high false-positive rates and other limitations compromise its use as a primary screening tool.

## Other techniques
### Radioactive antibodies
This technique involves radiolabelling antibodies to proteins that are selectively produced by cancer cells. Some have shown promise, but there have been no large-scale studies to determine a role for this technique in screening.

### Infrared thermography
Changes in blood flow cause temperature changes, and some breast tumours can raise skin temperature, which can be detected by thermography (Sudharsan et al., 1999). Infrared thermography was tested several decades ago, then essentially abandoned after the 1970s until recently. The technique is uninvasive and does not require compression of the breast or exposing women to radiation. The sensitivity and specificity of thermography are poor, and its application to screening is unlikely.

### Near-infrared spectroscopy
Near-infrared techniques involve use of light sources at 700–900 nm to image the breast. Some differences between oxygenated and unoxygenated haemoglobin can be detected, with imaging of excessive oxygen consumption in some tumours. As with all imaging methods based on sources prone to problems such as scatter and diffraction, the sensitivity of this method for imaging deep lesions will remain limited.

### Electrical potential measurement
As rapid cell proliferation disrupts the tissue's normal polarization, tools that measure electrical potential might allow identification of this disruption. Trials of the use of this technique in diagnosis, rather than screening, showed a specificity of only 55–60% (Fukuda et al., 1996; Cuzick et al., 1998).

### Electronic palpation
This technique, also called 'tactile imaging', is essentially an objective method for specifying the parameters of a clinical examination. A company in Massachusetts (USA) is seeking approval of their hand-held device containing a group of sensors which is pressed against the breast and moved around to image the tissue. It has undergone only limited evaluation (Wellman et al., 2001) and has not been assessed for screening.

### Other techniques at an early stage of development

Other techniques—including magnetic resonance spectroscopy, magnetomammography, Hall effect imaging, thermoacoustic computed tomography, microwaves and three-dimensional interactive visualization—are in early stages of development.

## Conclusions

None of the tests evaluated showed sufficient accuracy to support their use in general screening. However, the conduct and reporting of the studies were limited, and the populations were generally too small for adequate precision in critical measures, such as test sensitivity. Future studies should have adequate sample sizes, for example as is being done in a trial of digital mammographic imaging screening, which aims to enroll 49 500 asymptomatic women presenting for screening (http://www.acrin. org/protocols/6652/-6652abstract.html). Studies should conform to high standards of conduct and reporting (http://www.consort-statement.org/stardstatement.htm).

The design of cross-sectional studies to assess the accuracy of new techniques depends on how they are to be used. If a new technique is to replace an old one, the assessments (e.g. reading of images) should be performed independently and with similar information (e.g. clinical history) available to the readers of both tests. As the objective is usually to compare the accuracy of the tests under set conditions, procedures to deal with reader inaccuracy, e.g. selection of well-trained, experienced readers or the number of readers, should be similar for the two tests.

A new technique might be meant to complement an older one. For example, in a study by Lewin et al. (2001), the sensitivity of conventional mammography was 63% and that of full-field digital mammography was 60%. As the two modalities detected different cancers,

however, doing both tests increased the sensitivity of mammography by 26%.

Larger, better studies of new techniques should be started soon after their introduction. As new techniques often change rapidly, it might be argued that evaluation should be left until the new technique has become 'stable'. Unfortunately, evaluations are often problematic and a technique may come into common use before the evaluation is finalized. It is therefore wise to start evaluation early, using the technique in order to assess how changes and developments can be incorporated (Lilford et al., 2000).

# Clinical breast examination

Clinical breast examination long pre-dates imaging for evaluating mammary health and disease. While it depends on the eyes and fingers and subjective assessment of any abnormality found, it may still have a place in modern breast cancer screening programmes.

## Technique

### Procedure

No one technique for screening breasts for cancer has been shown to be better than any other in comparative studies against an assumed 'gold standard' or combination of methods. A systematic technique described by Pennypacker and Pilgrim (1993) was developed after extensive research with silicone breast models. This system illustrates the rigour that may be required to maximize the accuracy of clinical breast examination.

In the protocol of the Canadian National Breast Screening trials, described in Chapter 1, a 'spoke of the wheel' search pattern was used, with no explicit recognition of three levels of palpation (Bassett, 1985). In other respects, the technique was similar to that described by Pennypacker and

Pilgrim (1993). Use of a vertical strip pattern was subsequently shown to result in more complete coverage of breast tissue than either a 'spoke of the wheel' pattern or a search in concentric circles (Saunders et al., 1986).

The duration of a clinical breast examination depends on the skill of the examiner, the size and lumpiness of the breast and how many components of the examination are included. Visual examination is often cursory or omitted; applying three levels of pressure at each site is relatively uncommon. A study of periodic health examinations in an ambulatory care setting showed that the average duration of a complete clinical examination of both breasts and counselling on self-examination was 1.8 min (Kahn & Goldberg, 1984). Pennypacker et al. (1999) suggest a minimum of 5 min per breast for an experienced examiner using their programme.

### Sensitivity and specificity

No studies have been reported that document the sensitivity or specificity of clinical breast examination done fully in accordance with the recommendations of Pennypacker and Pilgrim (1993). The studies mentioned below include those described in Chapter 1.

In the Canadian National Breast Screening trials, the sensitivity, specificity and predictive values of a first screening were estimated for women who were randomized to receive only clinical breast examination. Three estimates were made: one for the examiner, a second for the surgeons involved in the study (who saw only participants who were deemed to have an abnormal result) and a third for the overall programme (which depended on implementation by community physicians of the diagnostic procedures recommended by the surgeons). For the examiners, a true positive result was an abnormality reported at the first screen by clinical breast examination, during the 12-month interval after the first screen or at the

## Clinical breast examination

- visual examination of the woman in three different standing positions: arms relaxed at her sides; hands pressed firmly on her waist and leaning forward; and arms over her head. The examiner seeks subtle asymmetries in the appearance of the breasts;

- palpation of the supraclavicular and axillary nodes with the woman seated and re-palpation of the axillary nodes with the woman supine;

- vertical-strip search of the breasts over an area extending from the mid-axillary line to the mid-sternum and from above the sub-costal margin (fifth rib) to the clavicle, including palpation of the nipple and areola;

- application in this search of three levels of pressure, superficial, medium and deep, at each palpation site. Palpation is done with the finger pads of the three middle fingers, and pressure is applied with circular motions at each site. For the lateral half of the breast, the torso is rotated in the medial direction; for the medial half of the breast, the torso is rotated laterally in order to spread out the breast tissue;

- when an abnormality is detected, the corresponding area of the other breast is examined. If the finding is not bilateral, further investigation is required.

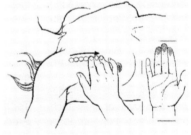

**Palpation technique**
Pads of the index, third, and fourth fingers (inset) make small circular motions.

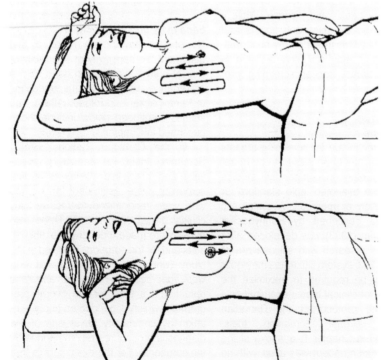

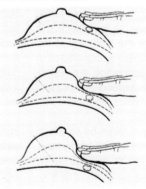

**Position of patient and direction of palpation for clinical breast examination**
*The figure shows the lateral portion of the breast and, bottom, the medial portion of the breast. Arrows indicate vertical strip pattern of examination.*

Levels of pressure for palpation of breast tissue shown in a cross-sectional view of the right breast

second screen. At the first screen, they achieved 71% sensitivity, 84% specificity and a positive predictive value of 1.5% in women aged 40–49 years at entry and 83%, 88% and 3%, respectively, in women aged 50–59 at entry. With repeated screening of the older women, the sensitivity of screening by the examiners decreased and the specificity increased. These estimates represent detection, in that cancers detected up to 12 months after screening were taken into account (Baines *et al.*, 1989).

Barton *et al.* (1999) pooled data from the study of the Health Insurance Plan of New York, USA, the trial in the United Kingdom, the Canadian national breast screening trials, the Breast Cancer Detection Demonstration Project in the USA and a study in West London, United Kingdom. Sensitivity was defined as the number of women with cancer detected by clinical breast examination divided by the sum of cancers detected at screening plus cancers detected within 12 months of screening. This yielded an overall estimate for the sensitivity of clinical breast examination of 54% (95% confidence interval [CI], 48–60%) and a specificity of 94% (95% CI, 90–97%). These estimates are remarkably close to similarly derived values reported by Bobo *et al.* (2000) in an analysis of 752 081 clinical breast examinations performed in the USA in the National Breast and Cervical Cancer Early Detection Program between 1995 and 1998. They found an overall sensitivity of 59%, a specificity of 93% and a predictive value of 4%; however, their ascertainment of interval cancers was limited to women who had undergone more than one screening. Ohuchi *et al.* (1995) reported 85% sensitivity and 97% specificity for clinical breast examination in Miyagi Prefecture, Japan, and Morimoto *et al.* (1997) reported 73% sensitivity in Tokushima Prefecture (see Chapter 4 for a description of these studies).

Studies with silicone models have shown that the sensitivity of clinical breast examination increases with increasing lump size and with increasing firmness of lumps, while greater depth is associated with decreased sensitivity (McDermott *et al.*, 1996). Barton *et al.* (1999) reported a sensitivity of 14% for 3-mm lumps and 79% for 1-cm lumps. Others have shown that the duration of the examination is positively correlated with sensitivity (Fletcher *et al.*, 1985; Campbell *et al.*, 1991). Comparisons of the results obtained with models with pre- and post-menopausal characteristics indicated that the sensitivity of clinical breast examination increases with age (McDermott *et al.*, 1996; Barton *et al.*, 1999).

Seven screening studies afford the opportunity to document whether offering clinical breast examination and mammography simultaneously in a screening programme increases sensitivity. There is clear variation among the studies in the mode of detection (by mammography alone, by clinical breast examination alone or by combined mammography and clinical breast examination) for cancers detected at screening. Some of the variation is due to study design; for example, in the Edinburgh trial, women were screened annually by clinical breast examination alone alternately with combined breast examination and mammography. Another explanation for the variation would lie with the adequacy of the protocol for clinical breast examination and its monitoring (Baines, 1992a). Only the Canadian national breast screening trials incorporated a protocol for clinical breast examination with evaluation and feedback (Baines *et al.*, 1989). As shown in Table 8, the detection rate with mammography alone is increasing over time and that with clinical breast examination decreasing. It has been shown in experimental situations that sensitivity decreases with lump size and with other factors such as duration of examination (Fletcher *et al.*, 1985).

More recently, Bobo *et al.* (2000) analysed the results of the National Breast and Cervical Cancer Early Detection Program in the United States for 1995–98 and found that at least 5.1% of breast cancers were not detected by mammography but were detected by clinical breast examination alone. A further 11% for which the mammography results were not reported were detected by breast examination. The procedure for clinical breast examination was not standardized.

## Training

Over the past two decades, training in clinical breast examination has been conducted increasingly with manufactured silicone models of the breast (Pennypacker & Pilgrim, 1993). Models can be designed to display the characteristics of pre- or postmenopausal breasts and lumps of varying size, depth and firmness. The models are placed horizontally for palpation, corresponding to a patient in the supine position. They have proved acceptable to health professionals for evaluation of their competence in clinical breast examination (Fletcher *et al.*, 1985). Furthermore, the rate of lump detection on such models correlated with that in in actual breast tissue (Hall *et al.*, 1980).

A randomized controlled trial was conducted with silicone breast models to evaluate the effect of training on the accuracy of lump detection by physicians and nurses (Campbell *et al.*, 1991). The mean sensitivity increased in the intervention group from 57 to 63% but decreased in the control group from 57 to 56%. Mean specificity declined in the experimental group from 56 to 41% and increased in the control group from 56 to 68%, indicating that the number of false-positive results increased with training. The recommended technique had six components: use of pads of the middle three fingers, circular motion, vertical-strip search pattern, three levels of pressure and total coverage. Four months after training, 80% of the intervention group were still using the correct tech-

## Table 8. Rates of cancer detection in programmes with combined mammography and clinical breast examination

| Study (date of start)[a] | Age (years) | Frequency | Percentage detected at screening | | |
|---|---|---|---|---|---|
| | | | Mammography only | Clinical breast examination only | Both |
| Health Insurance Plan, USA (1963) | 40–49 | Annual | 19 | 61 | 19 |
| Breast Cancer Detection Demonstration Project, USA (1972) | 40–49 | Annual | 45 | 8 | 46 |
| Canadian National Breast Screening Study-1 (1980) | 40–49 | Annual | 40 | 23 | 36 |
| Health Insurance Plan, USA (1963) | 50–59 | Annual | 41 | 41 | 18 |
| Breast Cancer Detection Demonstration Project USA (1972) | 50–59 | Annual | 47 | 7 | 45 |
| Utrecht, Netherlands (1975) | 50–64 | Variable | 56 | 10 | 35 |
| Canadian National Breast Screening Study-2 (1980) | 50–59 | Annual | 53 | 12 | 35 |

Adapted from Baines and Miller (1997)

[a] For descriptions of these studies, see Chapters 1 and 4.

nique. Training thus achieved increased sensitivity at the cost of decreased specificity.

Campbell *et al.* (1994) compared standardized with unstandardized training of medical students in clinical breast examination. The group with standardized teaching achieved improved accuracy of lump detection and technique, accompanied by decreased specificity. Interestingly, women with no previous medical experience were found to be able, after training, to teach a standardized technique as well as medical personnel. Another study showed that practice on silicone breast models and volunteers in medical schools was more effective than lectures alone for teaching clinical breast examination (Pilgrim *et al.*, 1993).

A recent controlled study (Lane *et al.*, 2001) showed that continuing medical education for community-based primary care physicians effectively improved their communication and counselling skills with respect to screening, clinical breast examination and administrative strategies to enhance routine screening. Of the two continuing medical education strategies used—face-to-face teaching and self-study—the former was more effective. However, use of such strategies on a national basis would be difficult. An alternative to physicians is nurse-examiners, as shown in the Canadian national breast screening trials (Miller *et al.*, 1991a). Acceptance of screening with clinical breast examination was increased by sending an invitation to women who were at high risk for breast cancer, although, again, nationwide implementation of such a strategy is unlikely (Richardson *et al.*, 1996).

### Maintainance of standards

No programme for evaluating clinical breast examination in large screening programmes has been published. However, the 15 centres of the Canadian national breast screening trials were provided with a protocol. Furthermore, at each centre, the examiners benefitted from regular feedback from study surgeons when participants with abnormal results from either clinical breast examination or mammography attended the review clinic. Annual (semi-annual when required) site visits allowed the deputy-director of the trial to observe examiner–participant interactions and to identify violations of the protocol for clinical breast examination; however, the consequences of these interventions were not evaluated (Baines *et al.*, 1989).

Detection of lumps in silicone breast models may be a useful way of evaluating performance of clinical breast examination and could be used to identify practical standards and to monitor and improve performance against them. This technique has been used in assessing physicians' performance in breast examination and in evaluating the effectiveness of standardized training in breast examination (Fletcher et al., 1985).

## Costs and potential harms

The costs of clinical breast examination include the cost of training, the cost of delivery, the cost of enhancing delivery and acceptance and the cost of diagnostic follow-up when abnormalities are found. Substantial costs are associated with training for the method of Pennypacker and Pilgrim (1993). The cost of delivery depends on the professional status of the examiner, being highest for physicians and lowest for 'supporting personnel'. The cost of enhancing implementation and acceptance of clinical breast examination depends on the intervention. Diagnostic follow-up may include fine-needle aspiration, fine-needle aspiration biopsy, core-needle biopsy, open biopsy, ultrasonography and diagnostic mammography. The procedures implemented, their frequency and the associated costs vary.

There are also direct and indirect costs to the women being examined. The palpation procedure itself is associated with no physical hazards other than minor discomfort. However, Elmore et al. (1998) calculated the 10-year risk associated with false-positive results in 10 905 clinical breast examinations among 2400 women in the Boston area (USA). After 10 annual examinations, the estimated cumulative risk for a false-positive result was 22%, and these all required further diagnostic follow-up, with the attendant expenses and anxiety. It is important that clinically suspect masses be evaluated even if a mammogram is normal (Pruthi, 2001).

## Other issues

One survey of 2800 participants in the Canadian national breast screening trials (82% response rate) revealed that women found clinical breast examination more acceptable than mammography, in that there was less associated discomfort. Furthermore, only 20% expressed a preference for clinical breast examination performed by physicians rather than nurses. Attendance at screening is enhanced by convenient site location, punctual appointments and courteous and supportive staff (Baines et al., 1990).

# Breast self-examination

Systematic breast self-examination has been recommended for almost 70 years (Adair, 1933), in the absence of compelling evidence of its efficacy. Initially, self-examination was justified because a substantial proportion of breast cancers were discovered by women themselves (Hislop et al., 1984; Joensuu et al., 1992); more recently, the practice has been seen to empower women, allowing them to take responsibility for their own health.

## Technique
### Procedure
Mamon and Zapka (1983) outlined one of many techniques that have been described for breast self-examination. Eight steps were to be performed lying down, first for the left and then for the right breast. They included: placing one hand behind the head and a prop under the shoulder; using the hand opposite to the breast being examined; pressing with the finger pads; covering the entire breast area; squeezing the nipple; examining the armpit; and using a circular or 'ladder' search pattern. Seven steps were outlined for a similar process in the upright position, including squeezing the nipple. Finally, there were four steps for conducting a visual examination in front of a mirror. Expecting women to comply

with 34 steps may be unrealistic, and such complexity may lead to lack of confidence (Eggertsen et al., 1983; Baines, 1988).

Thus, Baines (1992b) argued for a simplified technique based on the paedagogical principle that 'less is more' in terms of remembering what has been taught (Russell et al., 1984). Baines (1992b) also urged that the nipple squeeze, likely to be a deterrent to self-examination, be eliminated, because it is a spontaneous discharge, not a manually expressed discharge, that is pathognomic (Pilnik & Leis, 1978; Haagensen et al., 1981). Another disincentive to women may be the requirement that the practice be done in two positions, lying down and standing up. This led to a proposal that women with large breasts might choose to do self-examination lying down, while women with smaller breasts might prefer to do it while standing (Baines, 1992b). The proposal is consistent with a 21-step procedure in the upright position described by others (Carter et al., 1985).

The crucial components of breast self-examination appear to be visual examination and palpation of the entire breast with the finger pads in an effective search pattern. Hislop et al. (1984) showed that visual inspection was associated with smaller tumours and that careful palpation was associated with the absence of palpable nodes. Harvey et al. (1997), in a case–control study, identified three important components for the efficacy of breast self-examination, namely visual examination, palpation with the finger pads and using the three middle fingers. The proposed search patterns are of three types: concentric circles, radial spokes and vertical strips. The last has been shown to provide the of breast tissue (Saunders et al., 1986; Murali & Crabtree, 1992). Frequency of breast self-examination has been reported not to be a proxy for competence in practising it (Howe, 1980; Assaf et al., 1983; Fletcher et al., 1989; Janz et

## Breast self-examination

- Is any visual examination done ?

- Is most of the breast examined ?

- Are the armpits examined ?

- Is there a systematic search pattern?

- Are three fingers used?

- Are finger pads used ?

- Is a rotatory palpation applied?

- Is breast self-examination performed 12 times a year?

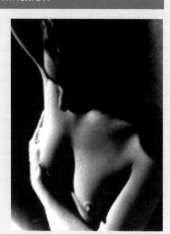

al., 1989), although contrary conclusions were drawn from the Canadian national breast screening trials (Baines & To, 1990).

### Sensitivity and specificity

Many published measures of the sensitivity of breast self-examination were based on detection of lumps in a silicone model of a breast or by a health professional in vivo. Assaf et al. (1983) concluded that the number of lumps that women detect in a silicone model is positively related to the number of components of breast self-examination that are performed correctly. Another study showed that increased accuracy (sensitivity) of detection of lumps in breast tissue, increased duration of examination and increased confidence were associated with training; however, training also increased the rate of false-positive findings and thus diminished specificity (Hall et al., 1980).

In the Canadian national breast screening trials, a proxy for the sensitivity of breast self-examination was estimated for 18 242 women who received five screening examinations (Baines, 1989). A report of a positive finding from breast self-examination was considered a 'true'

positive if it agreed with the subsequent findings of the examiner. On the basis of their self-examination scores, participants were divided into good, medium and poor performers. The scores improved over time. Higher scores were associated with higher sensitivity (never higher than 17%), and the positive predictive value improved from 39% at the third screen to 45% at the fifth. There was no difference between women who entered the programme when in their 40s and those who entered when in their 50s with regard to competence in breast self-examination (Baines et al., 1986c).

### Training

A frequently used system for training in breast self-examination is the MammaCare programme, which includes approximately 45 min of instruction from a nurse. The programme stresses tactile skills (lump detection and discrimination) and examination techniques. Silicone breast models are used both during teaching and in private sessions at home (Pennypacker et al., 1982).

A randomized controlled trial involving 300 women aged 40–68 was conducted to compare three methods for teaching breast self-examination:

MammaCare, traditional instruction from a nurse and no instruction, half of each group being encouraged by their physicians to do self-examination (Fletcher et al., 1990). The follow-up evaluation 1 year later was completed by 260 women. The group taught by MammaCare achieved more long-term improvement in lump detection in silicone models and in breast self-examination than those given traditional instruction or encouragement by a physician. Other investigators showed that female university students found significantly more lumps in breast models after MammaCare training than health professionals not taught with the MammaCare system, and the two groups had similar false-positive rates (Jacob et al., 1994).

The MammaCare system is not often used for training in breast self-examination. Other approaches have been shown to be most effective when done on a one-to-one basis, even though one study showed that competence in breast self-examination can be improved and the frequency increased after one session (Dorsay et al., 1988). In a study in which women were randomized to one of four approaches to training in self-examination, individual instruction was more successful in terms of proficiency and frequency than group teaching, and individual teaching plus reminders was even more successful (Bennett et al., 1990). Coleman et al. (1991) found that individual instruction resulted in greater proficiency than did group teaching. Ferro et al. (1996) concluded that instruction in breast self-examination based on theoretical and practical discussions significantly improved the quality of examination when compared with instruction based only on mailed material.

In a cohort of almost 90 000 women in the Canadian national breast screening trials, the scores for breast self-examination improved over time when it was taught annually and was reinforced on an individual basis in the context of a clinical breast examination (Baines & To, 1990).

## Maintenance of standards

### Reinforcement

Reinforcement was shown to be necessary in order to maintain skills in breast self-examination in a research setting involving 29 women trained in Mamma-Care (Pinto, 1993), in a programme involving almost 90 000 women in the Canadian national breast screening trials (Baines & To, 1990) and in four communities in Vermont, USA (Worden et al., 1990). Pinto (1993) showed that women whose skills were evaluated 2 months after MammaCare training and who had received re-training as needed had greater proficiency at 4 months and 1 year follow-up than women who were not evaluated or re-trained at 2 months. The results of the Canadian national breast screening trials showed that annual evaluation and re-training consistently improved breast self-examination scores over time (Baines & To, 1990), and Worden et al. (1990), comparing four communities, concluded that maintenance measures improved competence in breast self-examination over and above that achieved with training alone. The maintenance measures were designed to overcome barriers to self-examination: forgetfulness, by prompts and rewards; decreased confidence, by supportive messages in the media; and anxiety, by more media messages. Such interventions are unlikely to be widely generalizable.

Thomas et al. (2002) also reported improved performance on silicone breast implants in terms of technique and lump detection after reinforcement.

Regular observation (with feedback) of all examiners in the Canadian national breast screening trials to evaluate their performance with respect to instruction and evaluation of breast self-examination (Baines, 1987) may also have enhanced instruction in this practice.

### Performance indicators

A study with silicone breast models involving 126 women showed that three indicators were strongly associated with accurate detection of lumps: pressing firmly and deeply, examining all regions and adequate duration of examination (Haughey et al., 1984). The indicators used in another study were frequency, knowledge about when to do breast self-examination, technique and number of lumps detected in a silicone model (Carter et al., 1985). A more complex set of performance indicators was based on a combination of three scores: one for technique with four components, one for completeness based on nine components and one for lump detection based on the number of lumps detected in a silicone model (Dorsay et al., 1988). Such an approach is useful in a research setting.

In contrast, Baines (1988) proposed eight indicators appropriate for evaluation in a clinical setting (see box). The weakness of these indicators is that they are equally weighted, and it is extremely unlikely that they are equivalent.

The performance indicators used by Celentano and Holtzman (1983) were also equally weighted. They concluded that most women do not do breast self-examination correctly and that their competence can be evaluated from a self-report. The indicators they used were the components described by Mamon and Zapka (1983), listed above. However, when 81 women were asked to report their usual breast self-examination practice and were assigned a score on the basis of the number of components mentioned, the score was not associated with performance on a silicone model, indicating that what women say they do is not a reliable indicator of performance (Newcomb et al., 1995).

Researchers studying the MammaCare method developed a weighted scoring system for performance of breast self-examination that could be used in a clinical setting (Coleman & Pennypacker, 1991). The components, in descending order of weight, were: area examined, pressure used, motion while applying pressure, part of fingers used, search pattern, number of fingers used, number of motions and duration of examination.

## Mechanisms for improving breast self-examination

Encouragement or instruction by a physician is related to the frequency of breast self-examination (Senie et al., 1981; Bennett et al., 1983; Celentano & Holtzman, 1983; Amsel et al., 1984; Champion, 1987). However, achievement of both competence and adequate performance probably requires more than encouragement.

Cue enhancement was investigated by providing calendars with reminders and sending monthly reminders on postcards (Grady, 1984). These interventions were effective in achieving high rates of breast self-examination but only by menstruating women, and the frequency of practice declined after the experimental period. In contrast, distribution within the Canadian national breast screening trials of 1166 calendars on which women were asked to enter their findings from breast self-examination, analogous to the Finnish Mama Programme (Gästrin, 1981), had no effect on performance or the competence of breast self-examination when compared with that of 1027 women who did not receive the calendars (Baines et al., 1988b). Craun and Deffenbacher (1987) evaluated the efficacy of three approaches to increasing the frequency of breast self-examination and found that sending women monthly reminders was successful, while educational and demonstration programmes were not.

A 12-month public education campaign aimed at 40% of the Australian population was conducted through the mass media, with the support of local doctors, to teach women how to practise breast self-examination (Hill et al., 1982). Surveys of the general public, of patients in general practitioners' practices and of patients with newly diagnosed breast cancer before and after the campaign showed that 13% more of the general public and 6% more of breast cancer patients reported practising breast self-examination than at baseline. Performance was self-reported, and the competence of practice was not evaluated.

## Costs and potential harms

The costs associated with use of breast self-examination as a screening intervention are easy to conceptualize. The direct monetary costs include those for supportive health education and for training trainers, that to trainers in terms of professional time expended and that involved in evaluating the outcome. The indirect monetary costs include those for visits to health professionals triggered by findings at breast self-examination and any diagnostic and therapeutic procedures arising from such visits.

From the woman's perspective, the costs are the time it takes to acquire skill in breast self-examination, the associated monetary costs in terms of lost time from work and that of the instruction programme, the time it takes to do breast self-examination on a regular basis and the anxiety associated with lack of confidence or with problems in interpreting findings.

Only one well-designed study of the benefit of breast self-examination was identified (O'Malley, 1993). Benefit was defined as the increase in the number of women performing competent, frequent self-examination after training by nurses in MammaCare or traditional methods. Interestingly, the medical costs after teaching were not increased. Nevertheless, the costs associated with breast self-examination are considerable.

The potential for harm from the practice of breast self-examination resides in over-confidence, which might lead to delayed presentation with symptoms of cancer, false reassurance by health professionals when cancer is present and unnecessary investigation of benign lesions with subsequent morbidity and scarring. These harms may be most relevant to women under 30 who practise breast self-examination (Frank & Mai, 1985).

## Other issues

A study based on self-administered questionnaires of women's attitudes to screening after participation in the Canadian national breast screening trials achieved an 82% response rate (Baines et al., 1990). Analysis of 2299 questionnaires revealed a strong commitment to continuing breast self-examination. It also revealed that women found it difficult to do so, and almost 50% rated their competence in breast self-examination as only adequate or poor; only 7% considered it excellent. Self-reported impediments to breast self-examination were laziness, forgetfulness, being too busy and lack of confidence in both skills and interpretation. These attitudes are surprising, given that these women had annual instruction and reinforcement in breast self-examination. Janz et al. (1989) noted that, because breast self-examination is done in private, it excludes social approval and regular critical feedback. Also, breast self-examination does not alleviate symptoms or make women feel 'better' for doing it.

Some women practising breast self-examination may experience fear of cancer, pain and death (Moore, 1978). It has also been suggested that breast self-examination might arouse fear of mutilation and loss of desirability and be a threat to sexual identity (Bernay et al., 1982). Whatever the factors are that influence women's practice of breast self-examination, it is clear that, after years of research and encouragement, compliance with breast self-examination is less than impressive.

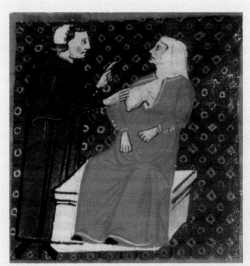

*Examination of the breast by the surgeon Teodorico Borgognoni (1275)*

Given the date of the painting (1275), breast cancer has probably been common in nuns for many centuries.
The painting is from Leiden University.

# Chapter 3
# Use of breast cancer screening

## Delivery and uptake of screening

This chapter describes breast cancer screening in the Americas, Asia, Europe and Oceania. Screening facilities are lacking in nearly all countries of sub-Saharan Africa (Anim, 1993). Published information from countries of the Middle Eastern crescent does not allow an appropriate description of breast cancer screening studies. Two countries in Oceania (Australia and New Zealand) have organized mammographic screening programmes; other countries have initiated breast cancer screening with varying degrees of organization.

Screening is done differently in countries according to their health care and financing systems and culture. Nevertheless, screening must be organized in such a way as to follow the process illustrated in Figure 27 and described below. The process includes specific types of care and the transitions between them. The types of care include identifying the target population, recruiting them for screening, delivering screening, diagnosing cancer among those with an abnormal screening result and treating those in whom breast cancer is diagnosed. The transitions between these types of care must also be considered, as they affect what services are delivered to whom. Use of letters of invitation to screening and use of media announcements have different effects on the transition to screening. A woman with a positive result in a screening mammogram must be evaluated, and her condition must be diagnosed and treated if necessary. Ensuring that the care is of high quality, that transitions

between types of care occur and that women have the best possible outcomes is the challenge in implementing screening.

As shown in the box, organized screening comprises six characteristics: a written policy specifying the target age categories, the method of screening (mammogram, clinical breast examination and/or breast self-examination) and interval; a defined target population, usually for the purpose of inviting women for screening; a management team that is responsible for overseeing facilities where screening occurs and for ensuring that the target population is screened; a clear decision structure and responsibility for health care management; a quality assurance structure, in which data relevant to the evaluation of the screening techniques, facilities and implementation are collected and validated; and a method for identifying whether breast cancer occurs in the target population.

Although organized screening programmes all have common characteristics, they can be defined in many different ways. For example, organized pro-

grammes may include policies set at a national or regional level; target populations specified by geographical region, voter registration, national population registries or health care insurance enrolment; management centralized in a national governmental structure, such as in the United Kingdom, spread throughout regional government structures, as in France, or concentrated in a committee of a health plan, such as sometimes occurs in the USA; management of health care by various combinations of physicians, nurses and other care providers, who operate independently or as part of a team; quality assurance by members of the programme management team or independent bodies, using a modified or selected set of measures such as clinical and technical image quality; and identification of cancer cases through national, regional or facility-based registries.

Screening is also conducted outside organized programmes, when it is known as 'opportunistic screening'. This form is the predominant one in the USA but also occurs in other countries outside of

---

### Organized screening programme

- an explicit policy, with specified age categories, method and interval for screening;

- a defined target population;

- a management team responsible for implementation;

- a health care team for decisions and care;

- a quality assurance structure; and

- a method for identifying cancer occurrence in the target population

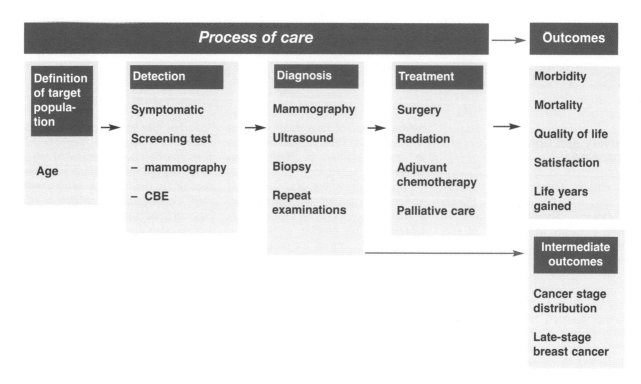

**Figure 27** Screening implementation and outcome

programmes. The effectiveness of screening in a country will differ, depending on whether it includes an organized programme targeted at the population at risk and an evaluation of abnormal results on screening mammograms or simply of delivery of high-quality mammography. An evaluation of the impact of screening on populations must therefore take into account the organizational structure through which it is delivered. As noted in Chapter 5, evaluation of the effect of screening in a population is much more complicated than is its evaluation in a randomized trial.

Use of the three screening techniques, mammography, clinical breast examination and breast self-examination, throughout the world is described below. The purpose of screening is to reduce mortality from breast cancer, but that can be acheived only if the techniques are used appropriately. In the

context of this chapter, 'use' of screening means the proportion of a population that has had a mammogram during a specified period. The period varies from country to country, depending on the data available, and it is different from 'participation'. 'Participation' is a prospective measure of the proportion of women who receive a mammogram within a specified period.

Table 9 summarizes the organized screening programmes in Australia, Canada, Europe, Israel, Japan and Uruguay. In the text that follows, the information in the table is discussed. For other countries and areas, information is summarized in the text or other tables, as comparable information was not available.

## Europe
Breast cancer screening in Europe varies widely. It can include organized

national programmes, opportunistic screening, both or neither. The programmes that exist are managed at national or regional level or are only pilot efforts. Mammography is the commonest screening test and may be associated with clinical breast examination. One or two views are offered every 1, 2 or 3 years. Double reading is generally done, and the age of the target population varies from 40 to 74 years, although most European countries emphasize the 50–69 age category. Mammography facilities can be centralized, as are quality control systems, the registration of data and evaluation.

### How screening is delivered
Table 10 includes 19 European countries (del Moral Aldaz *et al.,* 1994; Moss *et al.,* 1995; Giordano *et al.,* 1996; Shapiro *et al.,* 1998b; Mammography Screening Evaluation Group, 1998; Ballard-

## Table 9. Organized mammography screening programmes and services

| Screening | Country | Year implemented (year nationwide) | Number of programmes | System | Detection method | Cancer registry available |
|---|---|---|---|---|---|---|
| Nationwide | Australia | 1991 | 1 | PC | M | Yes |
| | Finland | 1986 (1989) | 1 | C | M | Yes |
| | France | 1989 (2002) | 32 (100) | PC | M ± CE | Yes[a] |
| | Iceland | 1987 (1989) | 1 | C | M + CE | Yes |
| | Israel | 1997 | 1 | C | M | Yes |
| | Luxembourg | 1992 | 1 | PC | M + CE | Yes |
| | Netherlands | 1989 (1997) | 1 | PC | M | Yes |
| | Sweden | 1986 (1997) | 27 | PC | M | Yes |
| | United Kingdom | 1988 (1996) | 1 | PC | M | Yes |
| Regional | Austria | 1999 | 2 | C | M | |
| | Belgium | 1989/1992 | 2 | D | M ± CE | No |
| | Canada | 1988 | 10 | PC | M+ CE + BSE | Yes[a] |
| | Denmark | 1991–1993 | 2 | C | M | Yes |
| | Ireland | 1989 | 1 | C | M | No |
| | Italy | 1985–93 | 15 | D | M± CE | Yes[a] |
| | Norway | 1996 | 1 | PC | M | Yes |
| | Portugal | 1990 | 1 | PC | M | Yes[a] |
| | Spain | 1990 | 4 | C | M | Yes[a] |
| | Switzerland | 1999 | 3 | D | M | Yes[a] |
| Pilot | Greece | 1989 | 2 | PC | M + CE +BSE | No |
| | Germany | 1999 | 3 | C | M | No |
| | Hungary | 1991 | 1 | C | M + CE | No |
| | Japan | 1999 | 1 | C | CE+ BSE | Yes |
| | Uruguay | 1996 | 1 | C | M+CE +BSE | Yes[a] |

From: Del Moral Aldaz *et al*. (1994); Moss *et al*. (1995); Giordano *et al*. (1996); Mammography Screening Evaluation Group (1998); Shapiro *et al*. (1998a); Ballard-Barbash *et al*. (1999); de Landtsheer *et al*. (2000); Klabunde *et al*. (2001a); de Wolf (2001); Autier *et al*. (2002)

PC, partly centralized: national policy, local implementation protocol; C, centralized: common policy and implementation protocol; D: decentralized: different policies

M, mammography; CE, clinical examination; BSE, breast self-examination

[a] Regional population-based cancer registry overlapping with breast screening programme.

Barbash *et al*., 1999; de Landtsheer *et al*., 2000; Klabunde *et al*., 2001a; de Wolf, 2001; Autier *et al.,* 2002). In nine countries, the scope of the programme is intended to be national, although complete implementation has not been achieved in all (Table 9).

The first organized programmes were begun in 1986–89 in the Nordic countries and the United Kingdom (Shapiro *et al.*, 1998a). Within the framework of the Europe Against Cancer programme, a European network of pilot projects for breast cancer screening was begun in

1986 (de Waard *et al.*, 1994). Pilot projects were established in France, Greece, Ireland, Portugal and Spain and later in Denmark, Germany, Italy and Luxembourg. These pilot projects were initially funded by the Commission of the European Communities, and most were

## Table 10. General characteristics of organized screening programmes

| Country | Age of screened population | Population access (%)[a] | Participation rate (1988) (%)[b] | Assessment of sensitivity[c] of programme | Interval (years) | No. of views (first, subsequent) | Financing |
|---|---|---|---|---|---|---|---|
| Australia | 40–69 | 75–100 | 54 | | 2 | 2, 2 | |
| Finland | 50–59 –(69)[d] | 100 | 89 | Yes | 2 | 2, 2 | GT + PT |
| Iceland | 40–69 | 100 | | Possible | 2 | 2, 1 | |
| Israel | 50–74 | 70 | | | 2 | | |
| Luxembourg | 50–65 | 98 | 56 | Possible | 2 | 2, 2 | PT |
| Netherlands | 50–69 –(74)[d] | 75–100 | 81 | Possible | 2 | 2, 1 | GT |
| Sweden | 40/50 –69/74 | 100 | 81 | | 1.5[e] /2 | 2, 1 | GT + S |
| United Kingdom | 50–64 | 100 | 76 | | 3 | 2, 1 | GT |
| France | 50–69 (74)[d] | 30 | 50 (17–60) | Yes | 2 | 2, 2 | GT + PT + C |
| Austria | | | | | | | Mixed |
| Belgium | 50–64/69 | < 25 | 28 | No | 2 | 1/2, 1/2 | PT |
| Canada | 50–69 | < 25 | | | 2 | | GT |
| Denmark | 50–69 | 18 | 71 | Yes | 2 | 2, 1 | GT |
| Ireland | 50–65 | < 25 | 62 | | | 2, 1 | GT, Pr |
| Italy | 50–69 | < 25 | 64 (46–72) | Yes | 2 | 2, 1 | GT + PT |
| Norway | 50–69 | 40 | 79 | Yes | 2 | 2, 2 | PT |
| Portugal | ≥ 40 | 25–50 | 34 | Possible | 2 | 2, 1 | GT + PT |
| Spain (Navarra) | 45–64 | < 25 | 85 | Yes | 2 | 1, 1 | GT + PT |
| Switzerland | 50–69 | | 50 | Possible | 2 | All | GT, Pr |
| Greece | 40/50–64 | < 25 | 40 | Yes | 2 | 2, 2 | GT + PT |
| Germany | ≥ 50 | 2 | | Yes | 1 | 2, 2 | S (80%) + Pr |
| Hungary | 50–64 | | | | 1 | 2, 2 | |
| Japan | ≥ 30 | 30 | 15 | Possible | 1 | 1 1 | GT + S |
| Uruguay | ≥ 45 | 20 | | Possible | 2 | | PT |

From: del Moral Aldaz et al. (1994); Giordano et al. (1996); Ancelle-Park et al. (1997), Ancelle-Park & Nicolau (1999); Mammography Screening Evaluation Group (1998); Shapiro et al. (1998a); Ballard-Barbash et al. (1999);  Dean & Pamilo (1999); National Health Service Breast Screening Programme (2000); de Landtsheer et al. (2000); Klabunde et al. (2001a,b); Fracheboud et al. (2001a); de Wolf (2001); Wang et al. (2001); Autier et al. (2002)
GT, general taxes; PT, pay-roll taxes; S, self-pay; C, charity money; Pr, private insurance
[a] Proportion of national population of eligible women who have access to the programme
[b] Proportion screened
[c] As defined in Chapter 1
[d] Modified some years after implementation, or for women already in programme
[e] For women aged 40–50

later transformed into regional or national programmes financed by the country's health system. The Netherlands and the United Kingdom did not propose projects for the network as their nationwide programmes were ready to be implemented; however, they were represented in the network and served as experts for other countries. Specific guidelines were prepared by a specially appointed working group, some of them in each of the official languages of the European Union (Day et al., 1989; Kirkpatrick et al., 1993; de Wolf & Perry, 1996; National Health Service Breast Screening Programme, 1993, 1997, 1998). The guidelines were designed to help standardize procedures, increase quality assurance and improve reporting of results. A consultant visited all pilot centres. Screening performance and

## Breast cancer screening in Europe

- Most European countries have established nationally or regionally organized programmes, although many administer screening facilities regionally.

- Most emphasize screening women aged 50–69.

- Almost all include invitation to mammography every 2 years, and some include clinical breast examination of participants.

- The number of screening views used in practice is reduced from two to one after the initial screening.

- The proportion of women who have been screened in organized screening programmes varies. Most programmes have intermediate to high rates of use (50–89%).

- In all the organized European programmes, the main indicators of performance and effectiveness can be estimated, but with a wide variety of methods, periodicity and precision.

quality assurance were defined and standardized. With the exception of France and Luxembourg, none of the countries involved in the network had begun nationally organized programmes.

The type of delivery system is directly related to the country's health care system. In countries with health care systems supported mainly by the national government, screening is centrally organized and distinct from the delivery of general medical care. Opportunistic screening is relatively rare, and the screening tests are provided in distinct, fixed or mobile specialized units. Mammography is always offered and is sometimes complemented by clinical examination. The programme is administered at either national or local level. When the health care system is both public and private, screening is done in the context of general medical care, screening tests being provided either in specialized structures or in centres such as private radiological units. In the latter system, the role of the national government extends from no plan to strictly reg-

ulated programmes that follow guidelines, professional and structured accreditation, regulations, laws and continuous evaluation.

In organized programmes, whatever the type of organization, direct mail invitations are generally sent to women in previously defined age groups, offering them free screening. The requirement for an up-to-date list and recall system has been met more or less, except in Germany. Publicity campaigns through media advertising, pamphlets, newspapers, radio and television and referrals from general practitioners are frequently used with the mailings. In only two countries are media campaigns and direct referral the only recruitment tool. Physicians' referrals facilitate appropriate follow-up of a positive result.

Of the 19 European programmes described in Table 10, only four recommend beginning breast cancer screening at the age of 40, one (Spain, Ascune et al., 1994) at the age of 45 and 14 at the age of 50. Much greater variation among countries is seen with respect to the

upper age limit, which varies from 59 to 74; 10 programmes have set this limit at 69 years and three (the new French national programme, The Netherlands and Sweden) at 74 years.

The screening interval for women over 50 years of age is 2 years in almost all the programmes and once a year for women under the age of 50 and for those with a family history of breast cancer. In the United Kingdom, women aged 50–64 are offered screening every 3 years. All countries except Belgium and Spain require two views at the initial mammography (some countries recently modified their policy from one view to two to increase the sensitivity of the test). Furthermore, seven programmes require two views at both the initial and subsequent screening.

Expert radiologists recommended double reading of mammograms to improve the quality of the interpretation, and doing so increases sensibility and specificity (McCann et al., 1997; see Chapter 2). Many programmes have implemented this procedure for all screens, Iceland for 95% of cases, France (in its new programme) only for women with a negative result after the first reading and the United Kingdom in 80% of screens. Each programme in which double reading is used has an established policy for arbitration of discordant interpretations.

The results, whether positive or negative, are always sent to the woman, except in Luxembourg where a notice is sent only to the referring physician. In half the countries, the results are not sent to the physician.

In order that women obtain the maximum benefit from a breast cancer screening programme, an accurate recall system must be in place to avoid losing women to follow-up after an abnormal result. All programmes except the Danish one are responsible for ensuring the follow-up of women with a positive result. The follow-up includes full assessment for diagnosis, biopsy and treatment when necessary. In all programmes, there is reporting on the collection of data, computerized or not, and on the results of additional diagnostic procedures and cancers detected at screening.

### Financing

Screening mammography is offered free in some countries, and in others it is reimbursed either by the government or by the health insurance system. The organization is funded from various sources: the government (general tax), public or private insurance (payroll tax), research funds (Europe Against Cancer) and charity funds (de Wolf, 2001). Table 10 shows that there is a mix of approaches. Money from taxes covers the financing of the administration of centres and direct delivery of care (i.e. radiologist and mammography fees).

### Extent of use and access

As noted in Table 10, access and participation vary by country. The availability of organized screening varies widely, from 2% in Germany to 100% in Finland, Iceland, Sweden and the United Kingdom. The Netherlands reported 75–100% access, and Luxemburg, 98%. The proportion of women who receive a mammogram when it is recommended (participation) also varies widely, from very high rates of 89% in Finland to 28% in Belgium. Levels of overall use by country are not recorded systematically.

### Methods for assuring quality

Several factors in a screening programme are expected to contribute to reducing mortality from breast cancer, such as the participation rate of the targeted population, the quality of the radiological process, the follow-up of women with abnormal results, the quality of the diagnostic procedures and initial treatment. Several initiatives have been made to develop and promote quality assurance standards, and guidelines have been published, such as those

sponsored by the Europe Against Cancer Programme (de Wolf & Perry, 1996). Most European countries have implemented quality assurance by following the European guidelines (Perry et al., 2001) or national guidelines. Quality assurance programmes include external controls and technical, process and outcome components (Donabedian, 1980; Klabunde et al., 2001a). In Europe, breast screening programmes include extensive quality assurance and quality control components with regard to mammography but little control of the whole screening process.

External controls for quality assurance involve laws, mandatory or voluntary accreditation and surveillance and evaluation, including site visits and mandatory data collection (Table 11). Differences in external controls are linked to the type of programme, but the organization of quality assurance does not necessarily reflect the organization of the programme. Quality assurance of national breast screening programmes is more likely to be based on legislation or require mandatory accreditation of screening facilities (National Health Service Breast Screening Programme, 1998), but regionally organized programmes may include a national quality assurance programme, as in Norway and Sweden. In at least 14 countries, a special committee is appointed to control data on quality regularly, but the periodicity of their meetings varies from every week to once a year. Six countries have national laws for quality assurance, and they apply to all mammography units. Accreditation processes for cytology and pathology also exist in six countries. Periodic site visits to radiological units are organized in 13 programmes at various intervals, and external audits and guidelines exist for pathological units in six countries (National Health Service Breast Screening Programme, 1993, 1997).

Technical quality control of radiological equipment and procedures is the baseline of all the breast cancer screen-

ing programmes. Regular monitoring of mammography facilities and films, including processor sensitometry, screen–film contact, beam collimation and automatic exposure was reported for most programmes (Bassett et al., 1994a). Cassette cleaning, tube voltage accuracy and reproducibility and beam quality were measured regularly in all programmes. One or two countries do not routinely perform other tests, such as for developer temperature, phantom image quality, compression force, film viewing conditions and beam entrance exposure. Some tests are not performed everywhere (Hendrick et al., 2002). All programmes have a requirement for documentation of the policy and procedure for breast positioning, but five did not require documentation for women with breast implants. Qualifications and experience were mandatory for radiographers and radiologists in seven programmes, and training was required in 15.

Quality control of pathological laboratories is less common than quality control of radiological equipment and training. Only six European countries require accreditation for cytology and pathology laboratories, and regular site visits are made in only six programmes (Table 11).

The process components comprise (Donabedian, 1980; Klabunde et al., 2001a):

- monitoring of invitations to women (not performed in four programmes);
- monitoring of mammography procedures (double view, double reading, standardized reading and report) generally at periodic site visits;
- monitoring of notification of results to women and/or the referring physician (means of communication, time), mentioned in all the programmes; and
- assessment after abnormal results according to specified policies (not included in quality control activities in only three programmes).

## Table 11. Organization of quality assurance in breast cancer screening programmes

| Country | Organizational level | Quality assurance committee | External controls | | |
|---|---|---|---|---|---|
| | | | Radiological units: A/site visit | Guidelines[a] | Pathology laboratory: A/site visit |
| Australia | National | 4/year | Yes / Mandatory | National | Yes / Yes |
| Finland | National | No | No / Mandatory | National | No / No |
| France | National | Varies | Yes/ Mandatory | European | No / Yes |
| Iceland | National | No | Yes / Mandatory | National | No / No |
| Israel | National | 2/year | Yes / Mandatory | National | No / No |
| Luxembourg | National | Monthly | Yes / voluntary | European | No / No |
| Netherlands | National | 4–6/year | Yes / Mandatory | National | Yes / Yes |
| Norway | National | 2/year | No / Mandatory | National | No / No |
| Sweden | National | 2/year | Yes / No | National | Yes / No |
| United Kingdom | National | 2/year | No / Mandatory | European | No / Yes |
| Canada | Regional | Varies | Yes / No | National | No / No |
| Belgium | Facilities | No | No / Mandatory | European | No / No |
| Denmark | Regional | 6/year | No / No | European | Yes / No |
| Ireland | Both | 4–6/year | Yes / Yes (?) | | No / No |
| Italy | Regional | Annually | No / voluntary | European | No / No |
| Portugal | Regional | Weekly? | No / voluntary | European | Yes / No |
| Spain | Regional | Weekly? | No / Mandatory | European | No / Yes |
| Switzerland | Regional | | Yes/ Mandatory | European | |
| Greece | Regional | 4/year | No / Mandatory | European | Yes / Yes |
| Germany | Both | 2/year | Yes / Mandatory | European | No / Yes |
| Hungary | Regional | 4/Year | No / No | National | Yes / No |
| Japan | Regional | No | No | National | Yes / No |
| Uruguay | Facilities | Monthly | Yes / Mandatory | American College of Radiology | Yes / No |

From Chappelon and Jestin (1998); Mammography Screening Evaluation Group (1998); Ballard-Barbash et al. (1999); Dean and Pamilo (1999); de Koning (2000a); National Health Service Breast Screening Programme (2000); de Landtsheer et al. (2000); Fracheboud et al. (2001b); Klabunde et al. (2001a, b); Wang et al. (2001); Autier et al. (2002); Hendrick et al. (2002)

A, one or regular accreditations
[a] Guidelines for quality control

A time limit for diagnosis assessment is defined and monitored in nine programmes and varies from 1 week to 1 month. Few programmes define a minimum percentage of abnormal results that should lead to fine-needle aspiration, core biopsy or open biopsy.

Quality assurance in data collection is based on recommendations about the type of data needed and the management of the data while maintaining confidentiality (Klabunde et al., 2001b). Nearly all programmes have computerized systems for: identification of eligible women, screening mammography test results, follow-up of women with abnormal results, results of diagnostic procedures, cancers detected at screening and treatment outcomes. Linkage to a population-based cancer registry was reported for all but three programmes. In half the programmes, the staff collecting data receive training. Standardized definitions (national or international) and coding manuals are generally used.

### Performance indicators

Performance measures (Sancho-Garnier, 1993; de Koning et al., 1995b; Moss et al., 1995; van den Akker-van Marle et al., 1999; Blanks et al., 2000; de Koning, 2000a) reflect activities ranging from the process of care (participation rate, recall rate) to outcomes (cancer detection, interval cancer rate) (Table 12). Eleven programmes specify a maximum recall rate (based on both technical and additional imaging for diagnosis), varying from 2% (Netherlands) to 8% (United Kingdom) for the initial screening test and from 1% to 7% for subsequent examinations.

Screening performance indicators are used in all the programmes, whatever the type of organization. The most commonly estimated indicators in the initial and subsequent rounds (Table 12) are: the participation or uptake rate, the recall rate, the positive predictive value of imaging, the positive predictive value of biopsy, the benign:malignant ratio, the cancer detection rate, the percentage of screen-detected DCIS, the tumour size and the percentage of node involvement. The interval cancer rate and incidence can be estimated when a population-based registry is linked with the programme, and these allow an estimate of the sensitivity of the programme. Mortality data are available for all programmes.

Some programmes, like those in The Netherlands and the United Kingdom, allow identification of other indicators, taking into account the entire targeted population, like overall sensitivity and specificity, impact and costs. Those countries can estimate such indicators because they have a longer experience in screening and greater ease in collecting the necessary data because of the national health system and more flexible confidentiality laws.

The entries in Table 12 show that the programmes are variable, reflecting factors such as the epidemiology of the disease in the country, the characteristics of the programmes (target, procedures, data processing, quality) and the way in which the estimate was made (numerators and denominators used). Such indicators should be interpreted with caution in view of the differences in the programmes and operational definitions.

## Americas

This section summarizes the available data on the delivery of screening services in Canada, Latin America and the Caribbean and the USA. The breast cancer screening techniques used in the regions reflect the differences in health care delivery systems and cultural, political and economic realities. The type of organization varies from the comprehensive breast cancer screening programme of Canada, through the provider-based screening funded from work-based and federal insurance plans in the USA to the mixture of the two in Latin America and the Caribbean. There has been growing interest in mammography during the past decade, with heavy documented use in North America, where nearly 80% of women aged 50–69 have had at least one mammogram. Clinical breast examination is also used, but the use is not well documented. Summaries of how screening is organized, financed and reviewed for quality and the level of screening achieved in the three regions are summarized below.

### How screening is delivered
*Canada*
*Organization*
In Canada, breast screening is offered within a national programme but also outside the programme (opportunistic screening) (Minister of Public Works and Government Services Canada, 1999). Organized breast screening programmes are now operational in each province, which are responsible for health care in Canada. The programmes began gradually, on the basis of a recommendation of a national workshop in 1988 (Workshop Group, 1989). Women in defined age groups receive direct invitations by post for free mammography screening. All the programmes include women aged 50–69, and most accept women in their 70s but do not actively seek their participation. Throughout the history of the Canadian national programme, women aged 40–49 were actively recruited only in British Columbia, but that was abandoned in 2000. Although women aged 40–49 are not actively recruited in the programme, young women are not turned away if they seek screening, and they are then offered annual re-screening.

*Mammography*
Two-view (cranio-caudal and medio-lateral–oblique) mammography is offered every 2 years in all programmes. Five also offer clinical breast examinations, in two programmes by a nurse, in two by a technician and in one by either a nurse or a technician. The latest report on the programmes is available at www.hc-sc.gc.ca/hpb/lcdc/publicat/obcsp-podcs98/.

Opportunistic screening for breast cancer consists of examinations by private radiologists outside the provincial programmes. Women may be referred to a radiologist for a mammogram by their family physician or go by themselves.

*Clinical breast examination*
Family physicians are expected to offer clinical breast examination as part of annual physical examinations. They may refer women for mammography at that time, but they also refer women without a physical examination.

*Breast self-examination*
Breast self-examination is promoted by the Canadian Cancer Society and by other groups interested in women's health; however, it is often poorly performed, and special instruction is rarely given, except in special projects (Baines & To, 1990).

## Breast cancer screening in Canada

- Canada has a nationally organized programme that is financed and delivered by provincial organizations. Care is monitored within the programmes, but use and performance outside the programmes are not routinely monitored or reported.

- Two-view (cranio-caudal and mediolateral–oblique) mammography is offered every 2 years in all programmes; five also offer clinical breast examination.

- Mammograms are submitted to quality control in facilities involved in the provincial programmes on the basis of standards adopted by the Canadian Association of Radiologists. Performance is also monitored, but the results are not published.

- Ever having had a mammogram was reported by 79% of respondents to a national survey of women aged 50–69, 54% within the previous 2 years.

*Financing*

Mammography is offered free within the national programme according to its guidelines. Those who seek opportunistic screening are reimbursed for the mammogram through provincial health scheme funding, so that the woman need not pay at the time of the examination.

*Latin America and the Caribbean Organization*

Health services and systems for screening vary widely across the region, from universal coverage in Cuba to a highly fragmented system in Paraguay. The degree to which any country can offer breast cancer screening is contingent on the financing scheme and the local availability of expertise. Typically, most specialized physicians remain in the largest cities, limiting access or the possibility of organizing a screening programme. In decentralized systems, decisions about the content and type of services offered are left to the provider, who is often responsible for either a geographically defined population or subscribers.

Recommendations on how screening should be done also vary widely. In order to regulate multiple providers and decentralized services, governments issue specific guidelines, some of which have legal status, as in the case of Mexico and Colombia. However, many ministries of health have no mechanism for guaranteeing implementation of or monitoring compliance with recommendations for breast cancer screening (PAHO, 1998). Reviews in 1998 and 2000 showed that 11 of 23 countries reported having official guidelines (Robles & Galanis, 2002). Three countries, Argentina (Argentina Ministry of Health, 2001), Mexico (Secretariat of Health, 2000) and Costa Rica (Costa Rica Ministry of Health, 2000), updated their guidelines during 2000–01. Table 13 summarizes the guidelines in 11 countries.

*Mammography*

Mammography is offered by clinics at the secondary level of care in most countries, but there are many private mammography services, which charge the full cost of the test. In Argentina, 81% of women identified a gynaecologist as the person who ordered a mammography, which implies attending a specialized service (Mejia *et al.*, 1999). Mammography is recommended in all countries except Colombia. Two countries, Bolivia and Cuba, recommend mammography as early as 25 and 30 years of age, respectively, and three others, Ecuador, Mexico and Panama, start mammography in women aged 40. In Argentina, although the basic target group is women aged 50–70, the guidelines indicate that, if the resources are available, screening by mammography can be begun at the age of 40 and extend through 74. In addition, the guidelines of Argentina and Costa Rica indicate that screening of women who have a first-degree relative who had breast cancer can begin at 35 years of age in Argentina and 40 in Costa Rica, or 10 years earlier than the age at which cancer was diagnosed in the relative. In Mexico, if a woman has two or more risk factors, she may be screened from the age of 40; however, the risk factors are not named. Mammography is recommended every 2 or 3 years, except in Ecuador, Panama and Uruguay, where annual screening is advised. In several countries, private clinics and radiologists advertise mammography services for a fee, to which women do not need referral.

## Table 12. Performance indicators for breast cancer screening programmes

| Country and indicators | Period | Participation (%) | Recall rate (%) | PPV of surgical biopsy[a] | Invasive cancer | | Reference |
|---|---|---|---|---|---|---|---|
| | | | | | Detection rate per 1000 | Screen-detected DCIS (%) | |
| Finland | 1987–97 | | | | | | Dean & Pamilo (1999) |
| All screens (age 50–59) | | 88 | 3.3 | 33–66 | 3.7 | 11 | |
| Initial screens | | 88 | 4.5 | | 4.7 | | |
| Subsequent screens | | 89 | 2.3 | | 2.2 | | |
| Netherlands | 1993 | | | | | | de Koning et al. (1995a) |
| All screens | | 78 | | | | | Fracheboud et al. (1998) |
| Initial screens | | 79 | 1.3 | 50 | 6.5 | 14 | |
| Subsequent screens | | 77 | 0.7 | 54 | 3.5 | | |
| Sweden | | | | | | | Thurfjell & Lindgren (1994; |
| All screens | 1988–89 | | | | | | Uppsala 1988–89); |
| Initial screens (n = 2) | 1991–93 | 87–89 | 4.6–2.1 | 53–42 | 4.8 | 11 | Lenner & Jonsson (1997; Nordbotten, |
| Subsequent screens | | 78–84 | 5.7–1.8 | | 4.8 | | 1991–93) |
| United Kingdom | 1998–99 | | | | | | National Health |
| All screens, age ≥ 50 | | 76 | 5.4 | | 6.2 | 22 | Service Breast Screening Programme |
| Initial screens, age 50–64 | | 74 | 8.2 | | 5.2 | 19 | (2000) |
| Subsequent screens | | 87 | 3.9 | | 4.3 | | |
| France[b] | 1989–97 | | | | | | Ancelle-Park & |
| All screens | | 50 | | | | | Nicolau (1999) |
| Initial screens | | 37 | 7.7 | 52 | 5.5 | 14 | |
| Subsequent screens (n = 18) | | 40 | 4.4 | 64 | 4.2 | 14 | |
| Denmark[c] | 1991–95 | | | | | | Mammography |
| All screens | | | | | | | Screening Evaluation |
| Initial screens (n = 2) | | 71–88 | 6.8–2.7 | 60–74 | 12–9.8 | 12–16 | Group (1998) |
| Subsequent screens (n = 1) | | 69 | 4.6 | 70 | 6.4 | 8 | |
| Italy | 1994 | | | | | | Giordano et al. (1996) |
| All screens | | | | | | | |
| Initial screens (n = 15) | | 32–72 | 1.6–8.4 | | 3.8–11 | 5.1–17 | |
| Subsequent screens (n = 6) | | 59–88 | 1.8–6.7 | | 4.4–6.3 | 5.9–23 | |
| Norway | 1996–97 | | | | | | Wang et al. (2001) |
| All screens | | | | | | | |
| Initial screens | | 80 | 4.2 | 74 | 6.7 | 20 | |

## Table 12 (contd)

| Country and indicators | Period | Participation (%) | Recall rate (%) | PPV of surgical biopsy[a] | Invasive cancer | | Reference |
|---|---|---|---|---|---|---|---|
| | | | | | Detection rate per 1000 | Screen-detected DCIS (%) | |
| Spain (Navarra)[d] | 1990–94 | | | | | | van den Akker-van Marle *et al.* (1997) |
| All screens | | | | | | | |
| Initial screens | | 85 | | 44–64 | 5.9 | | |
| Subsequent screens | | 86 | | 70–78 | 2.9 | | |
| Germany (Aurich and Brunswick) | 1990–93 | | | | | | Robra *et al.* (1994) |
| All screens | | | 4.8 | 34 | 3.3 | | |
| Initial screens | | | 5.1 | 34 | 3.4 | 14 | |
| Belgium (Flemish region) | 1989–92 | | | | | | van Oyen & Verellen (1994) |
| Initial screens | | 28 | 4.1 | 52 | 2.9 | 30 | |
| Ireland | 1989 | | | | | | Codd *et al.* (1994) |
| Initial screens | | 62 | 4.2 | 50 | 7.2 | 12 | |
| Portugal[d] | 1986–90 | | | | | | Rocha Alves *et al.* (1994) |
| Initial screens | | 35 | 13–2.3 | 64 | 1.1–3.2 | 17–20 | |
| Greece (southern) | 1989 | | | | | | Garas *et al.* (1994) |
| Initial screens | | 51 | 5.5 | 47 | 3.9 | 3.5 | |

PPV, positive, predictive value; DCIS, ductal carcinoma *in situ*
[a] Referral or performed
[b] Results from 26 regional programmes for initial screening and 18 for subsequent screening
[c] Copenhagen 1991–93 and Fyns 1993–95
[d] Age 45–65

*Clinical breast examination*

In general, primary care providers are expected to conduct clinical breast examination and teach breast self-examination, if recommended. The extent to which this actually occurs is unclear and varies by country. In Mexico, guidelines were developed by consensus among all institutions that provide health care, of which the main ones are the Secretariat of Health and the Mexican Institute of Social Security; others include the Social Security and Services Institute for State Workers, several Army services and nongovernmental organizations. In principle, this means that all these institutions guarantee implementation of the guidelines and coverage of services at minimum cost to women. In Colombia, where there is a highly decentralized system, insurers must offer a basic package of preventive services, which include clinical breast examination. Brazil's 'Viva Mulher' programme includes cervical and breast cancer screening by municipal and State departments of health, coordinated by the National Cancer Institute. In Argentina, clinical breast examination is recommended with mammography and not separately. Uruguay has a screening programme based on clinical breast examination for women aged ≥ 30 (Ministerio de Salud, 2000) and also recommends mammography after the age of 50. Clinical breast examination is also the main method of screening for breast cancer in Chile (Ministerio de Salud, 1998) and is recommended for women aged 35–64 every 3 years,

## Table 13. Guidelines for breast screening in 11 Latin American countries

| Country | Breast self-examination | | Clinical breast examination | | | Mammography | | |
|---------|-------------|------|-------------|------|-----------|-------------|------|-----------|
| | Recommended | Age | Recommended | Age | Frequency | Recommended | Age | Frequency |
| Argentina | No | – | Yes | 50–70 | Yearly | Yes | 50–70 | 2 years |
| Bolivia | Yes | 15–75 | Yes | 25–75 | Yearly | Yes | 25–75 | 2 years |
| Chile | Yes | ≥ 35 | Yes | 35–64 | 3 years | Yes | 50–74 | 3 years |
| Colombia | No | – | Yes | – | NR | No | NR | – |
| Costa Rica | No | – | No | – | – | Yes | 50–70 | 2 years |
| Cuba | Yes | ≥ 30 | Yes | ≥ 30 | Yearly | Yes | 30–49 | 2 years |
| | | | | | | | 50–65 | 2–3 years |
| Ecuador | Yes | ≥ 12 | Yes | ≥ 12 | Yearly | Yes | 40–49 | 2 years |
| | | | | | | | ≥ 50 | yearly |
| Mexico | Yes | ≥ 12 | Yes | ≥ 25 | Yearly | Yes | ≥ 40 | 2 years |
| Panama | Yes | ≥ 20 | Yes | 20–59 | Yearly | Yes | ≥ 40 | Yearly |
| Uruguay | Yes | ≥ 30 | Yes | 30–39 | 3 years | Yes | 50–64 | Yearly |
| | | | | 40–65 | Yearly | | | |
| Venezuela | Yes | 12–64 | Yes | 35–74 | Yearly | Yes | NR | NR |

NR, not reported

in conjunction with a Pap smear; mammography is being introduced in a second phase. Screening by clinical beast examination is begun for girls of 12 years of age in Ecuador and for women aged 20 in Panama and 25 in Bolivia and Mexico.

*Breast self-examination*

Most countries, except Argentina, Colombia and Costa Rica, recommend breast self-examination. In addition, several externally funded family planning programmes have introduced teaching of breast self-examination as part of women's health packages. As shown in Table 13, there is no consistency about the age at which women are supposed to start practising breast self-examination.

The age range or frequency of screening is not related to the incidence of or mortality from the disease in the various countries or with the resources of the health care system.

In fact, countries with low mortality rates from breast cancer, such as Ecuador, recommend screening by breast-self examination and clinical breast examination at menarche. Most notably, the guidelines of many countries are clearly not based on evidence.

*Financing*

In general, countries that have developed guidelines for breast cancer screening offer the test at no cost, and it is incorporated in health care delivery systems by a range of financing mechanisms, including health insurance, social security and government revenues. Financing is not universal. In Trinidad and Tobago, a country with one of the highest rates of mortality from breast cancer in the region, high cost was the main reason cited by women for not having had mammography (Modeste *et al.*, 1999). Chile has a dual system of financing, with a minimum of 7% of income contributed by individuals.

Part of the system is run by the State and approximately 30% by private insurers, which charge more than the minimum rate, on the basis of individual risk. Public health clinics are offered incentives if they perform periodic health examinations that include screening for cancers of the cervix and breast.

In most countries, the main problems arise when diagnostic work-up and treatment are required. Several countries do not cover the full extent of services or have cooperative payment schemes. Policy-makers in developing countries regard breast cancer control as expensive, but a study in São Paulo, Brazil, suggested that the total national cost of case management of breast cancer is US$ 1646 per case (Arredondo *et al.*, 1995). The cost of breast cancer management consists of 30% for human resources, 7.8% for diagnostic services and 43% for treatment. Although no data on the cost of services for breast cancer control were available for other countries, a study in Jamaica showed that 50% of cancer patients had to forego treatment because of an inability to pay (Henry-Lee & Yearwood, 1999). In several Caribbean countries, screening services are available but treatment has to be sought elsewhere, even at Government expense. Three countries, Argentina, Chile and Mexico, have information systems that allow monitoring of follow-up and mechanisms to ensure that women with positive results at screening undergo diagnostic work-up and treatment. Although the Costa Rican guidelines do not address this component of the programme, the social security system offers full coverage for diagnosis and treatment, and the population-based cancer registry has national coverage. Cuba, Uruguay and Venezuela can also provide full follow-up. Assistance for non-medical costs comes from the nongovernmental sector in many countries.

*Collateral financing*
In several countries, cancer care is provided through a public–private partnership, with strong participation from the nongovernmental sector and volunteer organizations. In Ecuador, a country that spends only 5.3% of its gross national product on health, a law mandates that 0.1% of credit transactions be assigned to cancer control by the 'Society against Cancer'. Although the Government participates,

the Society is in essence a nongovernmental organization, with semi-autonomous chapters based in major cities. In Brazil, the Ministry of Health has delegated the cancer control programme to the National Cancer Institute. A non-profit foundation channels resources to the Institute, thus maintaining high standards of care. In its preventive programme, the Institute, in turn, works through State and municipal health services. Its breast cancer screening programme is expected to reach all the population at risk of Brazil. Costa Rica, although it has a social security system covering nearly 90% of the population and devotes 8.5% of its gross national product to health, funds its national cancer institute through a lottery. As stated above, guidelines were developed recently and a cancer control department created within the Social Security system. Implementation of the programme is in the initial stages. In all cases, most of the income generated is spent on curative services. This financing scheme, which other countries are emulating, allows for expansion of the available resources and provides an opportunity for introducing preventive services.

*USA*
*Organization*
Health care providers in the USA offer clinical breast examination, mammography and teaching of breast self-

examination to screen for breast cancer. As reflected in Table 14, there is disagreement on how those techniques should be used, although all groups recommend mammography at some interval among women aged 50–64. No single group in the USA establishes the national standard.

*Mammography*
Mammography is almost always done in a facility that offers an array of radiology services, although those services may occasionally be provided by a primary care practice, a mobile unit or a specialized centre. Facilities that seek reimbursement for the procedure from the Federal Government must meet specific requirements, including use of qualified radiologists and technicians, use of dedicated mammography equipment that produces high quality images and record keeping (Food & Drug Administration, 1997).

*Clinical breast examination*
Most clinical breast examination is provided by primary care providers during a complete physical examination or at the time of a woman's health examination which includes a Pap smear and pelvic examination. Breast self-examination instruction is exceptionally provided during the visit. There are no organized programmes of screening based on geographic

| Table 14. Guidelines for breast screening in the USA | | | | |
|---|---|---|---|---|
| National group | Age group | Clinical breast examination | Mammography | Breast self-examination |
| Preventive Services Task Force | 40–49 | No recommendation | Every 1–2 years | No recommendation |
| | 50–69 | Annually | Every 1–2 years | No recommendation |
| | ≥ 70 | No recommendation | No recommendation | No recommendation |
| American Cancer Society | 40–49 | Annually | Annually | Monthly |
| | 50–69 | Annually | Annually | Monthly |
| | ≥ 70 | Same as above; cessation based on morbidity | | |

## Breast cancer screening in Latin America

- Mammography is available on demand in Latin America. Nonetheless, the national policies are not always based on available scientific evidence.

- Organized breast cancer screening programmes have been attempted in Uruguay, with clinical breast examination and mammography.

- The mortality rates from breast cancer in Argentina and Uruguay are as high as those in industrialized countries, and the trend continues upwards.

- In Jamaica, 50% of cancer patients had to forego treatment as they were unable to pay.

region, although some programmes exist within organized health plans (Rimer et al., 1988; Taplin et al., 1997). Most women are first screened by clinical breast examination and then referred for mammography. Women must take the initiative to schedule a visit with their primary care provider, although some health plans send reminders to schedule that examination or a mammography, or women may refer themselves for a mammogram.

*Breast self-examination*
Some national groups recommend instruction in breast self-examination, but this is not universally endorsed. The extent of the practice in the USA is unclear but is thought to be low. In one study of women doctors, only 21% reported breast self-examination at least monthly (Frank et al., 2000).

*Financing*
How screening is financed in the USA depends on whether a woman has health care insurance, what type of insurance she has and the practice of the community in which she lives. While

the national standard for care is improving, geographic variation still exists. Lobbying in state legislatures secured reimbursement for mammography through commercial insurance in all 50 states by 2000 (Fowler, 2000; Rathore et al., 2000). Insurance plans provide reimbursement for care of individuals on the basis of what they use (fee for service) or to their health care providers on a fixed rate per person under their care (capitation). Before the lobbying of the late 1980s, preventive care was not necessarily reimbursed. In parallel with the effort to secure reimbursement from commercial insurance, increasing efforts were made to obtain reimbursement through Federal insurance programmes (Medicare/ Medicaid) (Blustein, 1995). The latter provides reimbursement for health care of individuals aged ≥ 65, disabled individuals and low-income families. People covered by commercial insurance, Medicare or Medicaid represent a median of 84% of the state populations (Chattopadhyay et al., 1999). Medicare began coverage for mammography every 2 years in 1991 and annually in 2001.

*Extent of use and access*
*Canada*
All women who meet the age requirements of the provincial programmes have access to mammography. By 1996, the proportion of women aged 50–69 who had participated in the seven organized programmes of Canada varied from 11 to 54% (Paquette et al., 2000). Between 1981 and 1994, the annual number of mammograms performed in Canada increased from fewer than 200 000 to more than 1.4 million (Gaudette et al., 1996). Data from the 1996–97 National Population Health survey were analysed to determine the extent to which women in the target group for the provincial programmes (aged 50–69) receive mammography from all sources. Of the respondents, 79% reported ever having had a mammogram, 54% within the previous 2 years (Maxwell et al., 2001). The latter proportion varied by province, ranging from 41% in Newfoundland to 69% in British Columbia. Predictors of never having had a mammogram included higher age, residence in a rural area, Asia as place of birth, no involvement in volunteer groups, no regular physician or recent medical consultation (including recent blood pressure check), current smoking, infrequent physical activity and no hormone replacement therapy. The proportion of women aged 40–49 who had never had a mammogram was 44%. Among those who had recently had a mammogram, 80% had done so for screening purposes. The corresponding proportions for women aged ≥ 70 were 36% and 83%, respectively.

Corresponding data for breast self-examination and clinical breast examinations by a health professional have not been published.

*Latin America and the Caribbean*
Most women are reimbursed for screening by clinical breast examination and mammography, but the availability of facilities and personnel varies widely. No published data for a probabilistic population-based sample were available with

regard to use of breast cancer screening services in Latin America, but some information can be derived from studies of specific populations. For example, women in Puerto Rico with higher educational status are more likely to have had a mammogram or clinical breast examination. In this group, no relationship was found between knowledge and screening practices, whereas beliefs did play an important role (Frazier *et al.*, 1996a; Oliver-Vazquez *et al.*, 1999). A study of preventive practices in five low-income settings in Latin America confirmed that beliefs, including fear of cancer, are an important determinant of preventive behaviour (Agurto, 2001). Women in this group considered that health services are important only during their reproductive years; thus, middle-aged women were likely to attend only if they felt ill. In addition, women were more likely to attend screening services when their peers had done so and had had a positive experience.

Two independent studies showed that breast cancer was diagnosed at stage I in only 9.8–10% of women. The first study was based on the records of the histopathology registry of Mexico (Rodriguez-Cuevas *et al.*, 2001) and the other on data from three major hospitals in Mexico City (Lopez-Carillo *et al.*, 2001). Although these are not population-based studies, their results compare unfavourably with those of similar studies in developed countries, emphasizing the low rate of early diagnosis in these settings. Women of higher socio-economic status may have access to screening services recommended by their physician, especially a gynaecologist, but access to diagnostic and treatment facilities, necessary to complete the screening process, may be limited.

## USA

In the USA, the extent of screening is affected by the proportion of women who have some reimbursement for primary care and/or mammography. As noted above, the mean percentage of adults in the USA who have some type of insurance is 84%; however there is geographic variation in the availability of insurance, such that 9% of the Wisconsin population and 24% of that in Texas is uninsured. Populations with lower socioeconomic status are more likely to have insufficient insurance, but there are specific programmes to serve low-income populations (Chattopadhyay *et al.*, 1999). Once income is accounted for, differences in use by race and other factors are harder to identify (Lawson *et al.*, 2000).

### Mammography

The proportion of women aged ≥ 40 who report having had at least one mammogram has grown steadily since the late 1980s, to 85% (Figure 28; Blackman *et al.*, 1999). Similarly, the proportion of women who had a mammogram within the previous 2 years grew to 71%. Both estimates were based on telephone surveys. A recent report based on household surveys, not dependent on having access to a telephone, showed a comparable but lower level of mammography use (67%) within the previous 2 years among women aged ≥ 40 (Breen *et al.*, 2001). There are no national measures of the proportion of women who have had a first and subsequent screens.

Despite the growing use of mammography within the USA, it is not evenly distributed. For example, a smaller proportion of Hispanic women than white women reported having had a mammogram, and they were less likely than blacks or whites to have had clinical breast examination (Frazier *et al.*, 1996a). Women in the oldest (≥ 70) and youngest (40–49) age categories had the lowest rates of any use (80% and 82%, respectively). Native Americans and Hispanics in the USA also had somewhat lower rates of any use

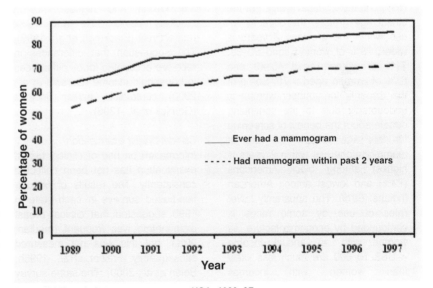

**Figure 28 Trends in mammogram use, USA, 1989–97**

Percentage of women aged ≥ 40 years in 38 states who reported ever having had a mammogram, having their most recent mammogram as part of a routine check-up and having had a mammogram within the past 2 years; Behavioral Risk Factor Surveillance System; adjusted to the 1989 age distribution for women

From Blackman *et al.* (1999)

## Breast cancer screening in the USA

- Screening is opportunistic, except for some programmes organized within health care plans.

- Screening by mammography is usually done after referral by a primary care physician who has performed clinical breast examination.

- Mammography is free of charge for the 84% of women with health care coverage.

- An increasing proportion of low-income women without health care insurance may have mammograms at federally-financed screening organized through state health departments.

- Treatment is available through private or government-based insurance to all women in whom breast cancer is diagnosed.

- Use of mammography is assessed in state-based telephone surveys.

- Cancer occurrence is monitored by state registries, but high-quality case ascertainment is most reliable in populations living within regions served by the nine organized cancer registries funded by the National Cancer Institute.

(79% and 82%, respectively). For the oldest age groups, the disparity for use within the previous 2 years is wider: 78% of women aged 50–59, 71% of women aged 40–49 and 67% of women aged > 70. Some of the disparity for younger women is undoubtedly due to the continuing debate about the benefit of screening for this age group. The rate of mammography use within 2 years is highest among black Americans (73%) and lowest among American Indians (60%). The apparently lower rates of use by some races is confounded by economic factors, as women with an annual income < US$ 10 000 are much less likely than women with incomes > US$ 50 000 to have ever had a mammogram (77% and 90%, respectively) (Qureshi et al., 2000). The disparity for use within 2 years increases with extremes of income, mammography use among women in

the lowest and highest income brackets being 58% and 79%, respectively (Blackman et al., 1999). The suggestion that differences in race are accounted for by differences in household income (Qureshi et al., 2000) contradicts earlier findings (Gornick et al., 1996).

*Clinical breast examination*
Information on use of clinical breast examination has not been collected consistently. The results of population-based surveys in each state in 1993 suggested that clinical breast examination was frequent (median, 90%), but this was not measured subsequently (Frazier et al., 1996b; Bolen et al., 2000). The same survey technique showed the frequency of clinical breast examination within 2 years to be lower in 1993 (73%) and only slightly higher by 1997 (77%) (Bolen et al., 2000). Use of clinical breast examination differs

by race, with a rate as low as 20% among American Samoans in 1993. However, race and economic factors may be confounded in these reports as the rates were higher (45%) among individuals earning > US$ 20 000 per year (Mishra et al., 2001).

***Methods for assuring quality***
*Canada*
*Mammography*
Mammography performed in facilities in the provincial programmes is controlled to ensure that it is of high quality, based on standards adopted by the Canadian Association of Radiologists, which are similar to those in the USA. However, quality control may be deficient for radiologists who are not part of provincial programmes. Details of the quality control programmes have not been published.

*Clinical breast examination*
Family physicians are not trained consistently in performing a clinical breast examination and may neglect to offer it. There are no standards for quality.

*Latin America and the Caribbean*
*Mammography*
Guidelines in Argentina and Mexico mention quality assurance for mammography in general terms but make no reference to a specific programme or to standards. In Mexico, provision is made for internal and external quality assurance for all screening methods, but no detailed description is given. A study of the use of mammography for diagnosis in Mexico suggested that the quality may be deficient (Poblano-Verastegui et al., 2000).

*Clinical breast examination*
No standards for quality are available. Training of health personnel varies across countries, and no detailed

description is presented in any of the guidelines.

## USA

### Mammography

The United States Congress passed the Mammography Quality Standards Act in 1991 to ensure high-quality mammography. The Act established parameters for the technical and clinical quality of the image. The technical assessment includes evaluation of imaging equipment with a standardized test object (phantom), evaluation of the processor to ensure that it is appropriately set for the film used and measurement of the dose of radiation to the breast (Hendrick et al., 1995). Clinical assessment involves review of the films produced by a facility and consideration of positioning, breast compression, contrast, exposure, noise, sharpness, artefacts and labelling (Bassett, 1995; Food & Drug Administration, 1997). The Mammo-graphy Quality Standards Act established a mammography certification programme that includes evaluation of facility personnel, procedures and technical image quality at annual site inspections and clinical quality review at least every 3 years through an accreditation body (Hendrick et al., 1995; Food & Drug Administration, 1997). Since implementation of the Act, there has been a demonstrable improvement in technical quality (Hendrick et al., 1998).

### Clinical breast examination

There are no standards for the quality of clinical breast examination and no regular reviews of performance. Physicians may receive instruction in clinical breast examination at medical school and during residency training, but it is not systematic and is rarely, if ever, reviewed (Barton et al., 1999).

### Performance indicators

Table 15 shows performance indicators for mammography in Canada and the USA. Similar data were not available for Latin America and the Caribbean.

### Canada

The information in Table 15 for Canada for 1997–98 is derived from a report on the national screening programme. The programme's database allows a comparison of the performance of initial and subsequent screens separately. As expected, the proportion of abnormal results or cancer decreased at subsequent screens. Of the cancers found through the programme, the proportion without nodal involvement was high for women aged 50–59 and 60–69 (78% and 79%, respectively). The proportion of tumours ≤ 10 mm was lower among women aged 50–59 than among those aged 60–69 (35% and 40%, respectively).

**Table 15. Performance indicators for breast cancer screening in Canada and the USA**

| Outcome | Canada | | USA | |
| --- | --- | --- | --- | --- |
| | Age 50–59 | Age 60–69 | Age 50–59 | Age 60–69 |
| Women attending when invited (%) | 12–55 | 12–55 | | |
| Abnormal recalls: | | | | |
| Initial screen (%) | 12 | 10 | 12 | 11 |
| Subsequent (%) | 6.4 | 6.0 | NA | NA |
| Cancer detection rate (per 1000) | | | | |
| Initial screen | 5.6 | 8.7 | 4.8 | 7.4 |
| Subsequent | 3.5 | 4.8 | NA | NA |
| PPV of abnormal screen | 5.0 | 8.8 | 3.6 | 6.2 |
| Benign:malignant open biopsy ratio | 2.0 | 1.2 | 2.5 | 1.4 |
| Ductal carcinoma in situ (%) | 22 | 17 | 23 | 19 |

From Organized Breast Cancer Screening Programs in Canada—1997 and 1998 report (available on www.hc-sc.gc.ca/hpb/lcdc/publicat/obcsp-podcs98/) and Kerlikowske et al. (2000)

*Latin America and the Caribbean*

Performance indicators for mammography are not available throughout Latin America and the Caribbean; however, they are available from a screening programme in Uruguay based on clinical breast examination (Robles & Galanis, 2002). The guidelines for the programme recommended clinical breast examination for women aged ≥ 30. Data from 14 health care delivery centres in which 10 266 women were examined during 1999–2000 showed that 3813 (37%) required further study, but 14% were lost to follow-up. The average age of the women studied was 52 years. It is not clear whether the screens were initial or subsequent ones or if women were actively invited for screening. The detection rate was 19 per 1000, for a total of 193 confirmed malignant neoplasms of the breast during this period. The detection rates varied substantially across centres, ranging from 4.6 to 41 per 1000. The follow-up of women with negative results at screening is not described. Overall, the positive predictive value was 5.1%. Half (51%) of the women in whom breast cancer was diagnosed had no node involvement, and 33% had invasive tumours measuring ≤ 10 mm. Mammography is offered parallel to this programme, but there was no indication of whether women participating in the clinical breast examination programme were also screened by mammography. The programme continues and may provide an opportunity to evaluate the use of clinical breast examination in a developing country with high rates of incidence of and mortality from breast cancer.

Performance indicators for mammography screening in Latin America may be difficult to obtain, as much of the screening is opportunistic. If the Chilean and Mexican guidelines were fully implemented and the corresponding information systems generated good data, evaluation would be feasible. The new programme in Costa Rica is also based on mammography; however the incidence and mortality rates in this country are still low, and the population of women at risk is less than 200 000.

*USA*

Performance indicators are available from one report on seven sites of the Breast Cancer Surveillance Consortium (Kerlikowske *et al.*, 2000). The Consortium is a collaborative effort to link information from mammography and tumour registries for women in geographically diverse sites (Ballard-Barbash *et al.*, 1997). The data in Table 15 represent those collected up to 1996 and are therefore somewhat earlier than the Canadian data. Although the data mainly reflect initial mammograms, the sample also included women who had had prior mammography. The proportion of abnormal results and the cancer detection rate are somewhat lower than from the initial screens in Canada, partly because of the inclusion of women who had had more than one mammogram.

## Oceania and Asia

For countries with no known breast cancer screening programme, a search was undertaken for a cancer society affiliated with UICC or a cancer registry affiliated with IARC, or both. If the country had one or both, a further search was carried out for evidence of a cancer control, and possibly a screening, policy. Two health networks organized under the auspices of WHO provided information about South-East Asia and the Western Pacific.

The publication *Cancer Survival in Developing Countries* (Sankaranarayanan *et al.,* 1998) contains brief comments about cancer control programmes, including mention of screening in countries of Asia and Oceania. Four regions of Asia have or have had trials of screening: of clinical breast examination in Shanghai, China, of clinical breast examination and mammography in Japan, of clinical breast examination in the Philippines and a trial in progress of clinical breast examination and breast self-examination in Mumbai, India (funded by the United States National Cancer Institute).

The WHO Cancer Database for the Western Pacific Region (WHO, 1999a; hereafter referred to as the 1997 WPRO survey) shows that 15 of 29 countries surveyed for cancer control activities in 1997 responded 'Yes' to the question "Has screening for breast cancer been routinely available to women?". The countries that replied 'Yes' were American Samoa, Australia, China (and Hong Kong), Japan, Malaysia, New Zealand, the Philippines, Republic of Korea and Viet Nam. Apart from this response, no other information was available for Guam, Mariana Islands, Niue, Palau and Tokelau.

### Countries with organized mammographic screening
*How screening is delivered*
*Australia*
  *Mammography*
  Organized mammography was begun in three states of Australia in mid-1991 and was available to most women by mid-1994, with the last units in place nationwide by the end of 1995. In addition to the organized programme, medical practitioners can refer women for mammography within the private health system.

  A review of international evidence led to the establishment of six pilot screening programmes in Australia in 1989 and the National Program for the Early Detection of Breast Cancer in 1991. The organized programme, called BreastScreen Australia since 1996, is funded jointly by the national Government and the States and Territories. The description of Breast-Screen Australia and its organization given below is based on information in two national reports (Australian Institute of Health and Welfare, 1998, 2000), five state reports (Breast-

## Organized breast cancer screening programmes in Oceania

- The BreastScreen Australia programme began gradually. It targets women aged 50–69, but all women ≥ 40 years who attend are screened. It has national accreditation requirements which were first published in 1991 and revised in 1994 and 1999–2000, and has a nationally agreed minimum data set for reporting.

- In BreastScreen Aotearoa, implemented nationally in New Zealand, only asymptomatic women 50–64 years of age are screened. The programme had interim national quality standards at commencement and receives agreed data items from providers as part of their contract.

Screen SA, 1999; (BreastScreen NSW, 2000; BreastScreen Queensland, 2000; BreastScreen Victoria, 2001; BreastScreen WA, 2001) and a review of the national accreditation requirements in BreastScreen Australia (National Quality Management Committee of BreastScreen Australia, 2001).

BreastScreen Australia targets asymptomatic women aged 50–69 years, who are screened with two-view, 2-yearly mammograms read by two independent readers, of whom one is a radiologist; women aged 40–49 and ≥ 70 may also attend. Individual services differ with regard to their policy on screening women with symptoms. Initial invitation letters are sent to women listed on the Australian electoral roll, and reminders for re-screening are sent to those who have attended. The programme's services are free. Before BreastScreen commenced, all mammograms were done in the private health care system and reimbursed by Medicare, the national health insurance scheme of the Health Insurance Commission. BreastScreen overcomes the challenge of distance in Australia with a combination of fixed-site, mobile, relocatable and satellite services.

Mammography is still available outside the BreastScreen services, mainly reimbursed by Medicare, although private radiology services also offer mammograms for which women pay the full cost. While the Medicare-reimbursed mammogram was intended for diagnostic purposes only, the large numbers suggest its use in screening.

### Clinical breast examination
Most women have clinical breast examination at their own request or as part of a health check at a visit to their primary health-care provider or at a health centre, at the time of a Pap test in the national cervical screening programme. Visits by individuals to a general practitioner are reimbursed under the national compulsory medical scheme, Medicare.

### Breast self-examination
A number of large public health information programmes in Australia were designed to encourage women to practise routine breast self-examination. Cancer societies, mammographic screening services, cancer support groups and various public and private organizations involved in disseminating health messages have developed statements about the benefits of breast self-examination,

although few offer instruction. Financing of such instruction depends on an organization's conviction about the benefits of breast self-examination and its commitment and financial resources. In 1996, 53% of women surveyed nationally reported that a general medical practitioner had recommended that they practise breast self-examination (Barratt et al., 1997a).

An expert advisory group of the National Breast Cancer Centre (2001) recommended in 2001 that women should know how their breasts look and feel normally and to have changes investigated promptly by their doctor.

### New Zealand
### Mammography
National screening began within Breastscreen Aotearoa with six lead providers in December 1998. Mammography is also readily available outside the programme from private medical practitioners. The Cancer Society of New Zealand and the Department of Health invited a working group to make recommendations about screening in 1987. The report concluded that New Zealand's shortage of appropriately specialized professionals was too great, and it recommended waiting for the outcome of pilot programmes before deciding on a routine screening programme (BreastScreen Aotearoa, 1998). Two pilot programmes began in 1991 and continued to December 1996, while the national programme began in December 1998. Information about BreastScreen Aotearoa is available on its website (www.cancer-soc.org.nz) or through contact with the National Screening Unit, Ministry of Health, Wellington.

The programme is funded by the Government through the Ministry of Health, which allocates funds, in competition with other resources, to the National Screening Unit, an independent business unit. BreastScreen contracts directly with six lead provider services (four public health and two private units) that cover the regions of 22 district health boards.

Asymptomatic women aged 50–64 are invited by letter, can attend voluntarily or may be referred by a general practitioner to the organized screening programme and are offered free, 2-yearly, two-view mammography within a network of fixed and mobile screening units and fixed assessment centres. Women with symptoms are advised to consult their usual medical practitioner. As the programme does not have access to a population register, there is no way of identifying and inviting all eligible women. Women outside the age range of the programme are eligible for Government-funded mammograms, provided they meet certain criteria or, if they do not, can pay for mammograms in the private health system. The lead providers send a reminder letter to women to attend for re-screening.

*Clinical breast examination*
The New Zealand Cancer Society encourages doctors to offer a breast check to women who are concerned about breast cancer, especially those 40 years of age and older, although it does not recommend regular clinical breast examination. The Breast Cancer Screening Policy Advisory Group acknowledged the role of clinical breast examination in clinical practice for women with symptoms or those recalled with abnormalities detected through mammographic screening.

*Breast self-examination*
Breast self-examination is not taught within BreastScreen Aotearoa, but the New Zealand Cancer Society, in recognition of the need to optimize women's chances of finding

symptomatic changes and reporting them promptly to their doctors, supports a concept of 'breast awareness', recommending that women, especially those over the age of 40, know what is normal for their breasts and to look and feel for changes regularly (www.cancer-soc.org.nz).

*Financing*
Organized mammographic screening in Australia and New Zealand is financed from general taxes. A fixed part of the cost of mammograms outside organized screening is paid from general taxes, while the individual pays the difference between the fixed rebate from the Government and the amount charged by the private provider of the service.

### Extent of use and access
*Australia*
BreastScreen services are available to all women in Australia aged 50–69, although women aged 40–49 and ≥ 70 years who approach BreastScreen services are also screened; the expected participation rate by age group is 40% of women aged 40–49, 70% at 50–69 and 15% at 70–79 years. BreastScreen monitors several indicators of its coverage of population groups: indigenous women, women from non-English-speaking backgrounds, women in metropolitan, rural or remote areas by socio-economic status. While the programme

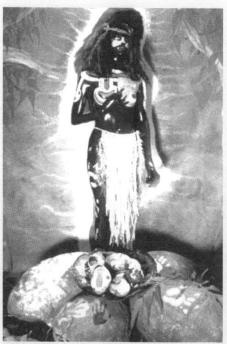

*A mannequin, named Merindah Bibi (meaning beautiful women, breast) as the centerpiece to the work is dressed in traditional costume. One breast is painted in an anatomical style and the other displays an Aboriginal design which represents breast paintings used in traditional dance. The backdrop is a silhouette of Merindah Bibi, the aura of this woman is shown by splashes of colour which represent her spiritual health and well-being. At her feet a turtle shell is filled with painted emu eggs, showing what health and well-being means to each individual woman.*

**BreastScreen Victoria project in partnership with the Victorian Aboriginal Health Service to raise awareness of breast screening and to inspire Koori women to think and feel positively about their bodies and their health.**

was designed primarily for asymptomatic women, some women present with a symptom and are screened. State-based programmes vary in their approach to these women, most advising or encouraging consultation with the woman's medical practitioner outside the programme.

Australia has universal health insurance coverage of its population by Medicare, which is funded by the Commonwealth Government and includes a levy on taxpayers in higher income brackets. Medicare reimburses its scheduled fee to women who have a medical practitioner's referral for mammography in the private sector; the women themselves must fund the difference in the provider's fee. Women who attend private radiology services for mammography without a referral do not qualify for fee reimbursement.

*Mammography*
By 1998, 54% of women aged 50–69 had participated in the national programme (Table 16). No national data are available on attendance for re-screening, but State-based programmes reported rates of 74% in Western Australia and 82% in Queensland for index screens in 1995 or 1996. The proportion of women attending for initial (range, 15–40%) and subsequent screens (range, 60–85%) varied among states, depending on the length of time since implementation and the geographic spread of services to be established. Uptake of screening by women with symptoms was reported to range from < 1% in Western Australia in 1995–96 to 4.7% in Victoria in 1997 and Queensland in 1998 and 8.4% in South Australia in 1995.

Most of the women who were screened (≥ 80%) were from an English-speaking background, the percentage screened varying across states but close to the population proportions in the 1996 census.

Participation was greater in areas outside metropolitan regions in all states. The percentage of women who were identified as Aboriginal and Torres Strait Islander was low but in line with the population proportions in the 1996 census in three states.

Use of mammography in the private sector peaked in 1992. More than 300 000 bilateral mammograms were reimbursed in Medicare each year from 1996 to 1999, of which 40% were for women aged 50–69.

*Clinical breast examination*
In the 1996 national breast health survey, 68% of women aged 30–69 reported having had a clinical breast examination by a health professional within the past 2 years, whereas only 35–50% had been examined in the past 3 years in earlier studies. In 1996, more younger than older women reported having had a clinical breast examination within the past 12 months (Barratt *et al.*, 1997a).

*Breast self-examination*
In the 1989–90 national health survey, 63% of women aged 18–64 reported performing breast self-examination 'regularly' (Barratt *et al.*, 1997b). By 1996, however, only one-third of women between 30 and 69 years of age reported performing monthly breast self-examination.

*New Zealand*
BreastScreen Aotearoa covers all areas in New Zealand and all symptomatic women 50–64 years of age. At the end of the first complete 2-year round of mammography in December 2000, the participation rate was 54% of women aged 50–64 years (Table 16). Participation was lower than the overall rate among Maori (35%) and Pacific Islander (34%) women and higher (56%) among all other women. The extent of use of clinical breast examination and breast self-examination is unknown.

*Methods for assuring quality*
*Australia*
*Mammography*
A national committee advises Breast-Screen Australia on specific policy, quality, data management, clinical aspects and administrative issues in programme management; five working groups report to the committee. In addition, a national quality management committee oversees accreditation issues in a comprehensive system to ensure that all BreastScreen services operate under a common set of standards. Each service is assessed every 3 years by an independent team of expert reviewers to ensure that service delivery complies with the national accreditation requirements, a set of minimum standards and requirements covering all aspects of service delivery.
In addition, the services must meet the equivalent of the national performance indicators, depending on the number of screens delivered, the cancer detection rate, the small-cancer detection rate, the number of interval cancers (invasive only) and detection of DCIS. To ensure that the standards remain relevant and current, the requirements were comprehensively updated in 2000–01 by the National Breast Cancer Centre, which collated evidence-based reviews undertaken by expert multidisciplinary teams appointed for the purpose.

Data are monitored independently of the accreditation process. Performance indicators were agreed at the national level, under the guidance of the National Advisory Committee, initially in relation to participation, cancer detection, small-cancer detection, programme sensitivity (interval cancers) and incidence and mortality. Services collect data in accordance with the BreastScreen Australia minimum data set, on the basis of nationally agreed definitions and classifications. Data

## Table 16. Performance indicators of breast cancer screening in Oceania: Age-standardized percentage and rates of participation per 10 000 women screened at 50–69 and ≥ 40 years

**Country and indicator**

**Australia, 1997–98[a]**

| | 50–69 years | ≥ 40 years |
|---|---|---|
| Participation (%) | 54 (54–54) | 36 (36–36) |
| Invasive cancer detection rate | | |
| First round 1998 (/1 000) | 5.9 (5.5–6.3) | 6.0 (0.7–6.4) |
| Subsequent round 1998 (/1 000) | 3.6 (3.4–3.8) | 3.4 (3.3–3.6) |
| Small invasive cancer (≤ 10 mm) detection rate | | |
| First round 1998 (/1 000) | 1.9 (1.6–2.1) | 1.8 (1.6–2.0) |
| Subsequent round 1998 (/1 000) | 1.5 (1.4–1.6) | 1.4 (1.3–1.5) |
| Interval cancer rate | | |
| (invasive cancers only) | | 0.65/1000[b] |

| Re-screening rates | Year of index screen | Rate in women 50–69 years (%) |
|---|---|---|
| Victoria | 1997 | 81 |
| New South Wales | 1996 | 75 |
| Queensland | 1996 | 82 |
| South Australia | 1995 | 79 |
| Western Australia | 1995/96 | 74 |

| Percentage DCIS of all cancers | Year | Women 50–69 years |
|---|---|---|
| Victoria | 1999 | 22 |
| New South Wales | 1998 | 23 |
| Queensland | 1997 | 22 |
| South Australia | 1997 | 25 |
| Western Australia | 1997–98 | 21 |

**New Zealand, 1998–2000[c]**

| | 50–64 years |
|---|---|
| Participation (%) | |
| All women | 54 |
| Maori | 35 |
| Pacific Islander | 34 |
| Other | 56 |
| | |
| Assessment (%) | 6.8 |
| False-positive rate (%) | 6 |
| Specificity (%) | 94 |
| Cancer detection rate | 7.0 / 1000 |

[a] BreastScreen SA (1999); Australian Institute of Health and Welfare (2000); BreastScreen NSW (2000); BreastScreen Queensland (2000); BreastScreen Victoria (2001); BreastScreen WA (2001)
[b] Crude rate in asymptomatic women screened in 1996 during 12 months' follow-up

are supplied by the six state and two territorial programmes to the Australian Institute of Health and Welfare for collation and analysis and reported jointly by BreastScreen, the Institute and the Commonwealth Department of Health and Aged Care.

*Clinical breast examination*
There are no standards of quality for clinical breast examination. Studies have shown an effect of training in clinical breast examination on the skill of clinicians (see Chapter 2), and some evidence was found that those performing clinical breast examination do not feel confident in their skills.

*Breast self-examination*
No standards for teaching breast self-examination were available. In 1996, 28% of women in Australia who had ever practised breast self-examination reported that their practice was correct (Barratt et al., 1997b).

*New Zealand*
*Mammography*
As part of the programme, the Government convened a group of national and international experts to develop interim national quality standards that all providers must meet. The standards, which were in place when the programme commenced, reflect six key areas: radiology, medical radiation therapy, medical physics, nursing, pathology and surgery. A current review will add standards relating to programme management, data management and health promotion and education.

The BreastScreen Aotearoa Independent Monitoring Group monitors and evaluates the programme under contract with the Ministry of Health, assessing performance against indicators specified by the Ministry. Lead providers are contractually bound to supply specified data regularly to the independent monitoring group. The first monitoring report appeared in February 2000, and quarterly reports had been produced up to September 2001 (BreastScreen Aotearoa Independent Monitoring Group, 2001).

The lack of a population register currently precludes complete enumeration of all eligible women and accurate calculation of registration and participation rates. BreastScreen Aotearoa may be able to use the electoral roll to identify eligible women in the future.

*Clinical breast examination*
The New Zealand Cancer Society acknowledges the importance of the quality of clinical breast examination, and its statement on the matter repeats the message of the 1997 National Institutes of Health Consensus Development Conference, that clinical breast examination requires proper quality control and monitoring before it can be regarded as a satisfactory screening tool.

*Breast self-examination*
The New Zealand Cancer Society has acknowledged the barriers to women practising breast self-examination regularly and competently and the fact that its practice can lead to unnecessary anxiety and medical investigations, particularly among younger women. Although no quality assurance strategies have been reported, women participating in focus group research in New Zealand admitted to a lack of confidence in doing breast self-examination and greater confidence in doing 'casual' checks. The message of familiarity with one's breasts was considered compatible with encouraging women to continue casual checks and increase their confidence. The researchers reported that women were comfortable with the breast awareness message, but the level of

practice is unknown(http://www.healthywomen.org.nz/bsa/default.asp).

*Performance indicators*
*Australia*
The national performance indicators in BreastScreen Australia are the rates of participation, cancer detection, small-cancer detection and programme sensitivity (interval cancers) in women 50–69 years of age (Table 16). The national participation rate was 54% (age-adjusted) in 1997–98, whereas the programme target is 70%. No reliable estimates are available of the proportion of mammograms conducted in women of these ages under Medicare that might be de-facto screening. The invasive cancer detection rate was 5.9 per 1000 women screened, and the rate of small cancers detected in the first screening round was 1.9 per 1000 (age-standardized rates). The minimum standards for cancer detection set in the 1991 national accreditation requirements included invasive cancers and DCIS, but the standards have since been revised to exclude DCIS. The minimum standard for sensitivity of the programme was less than 0.6 interval cancers per 1000 women screened. Nationally, a rate of 0.65 per 1000 was achieved in 1996 in all screening rounds in asymptomatic women of all ages in the 12 months after a negative result. Although BreastScreen Australia does not report the percentage of DCIS, these figures are calculated in five States for comparison with programmes in other countries (Table 16).

*New Zealand*
The agreed performance indicators are rates of participation, technical recalls, technical repeats, assessment, false-positives, open surgical biopsies and benign biopsy sample weighing < 20 g (BreastScreen Aotearoa Independent Monitoring Group 2001). The target participation rate is 70%, as in other programmes internationally. Accurate calcu-

lation of the participation rate requires a population-based register to identify eligible women. BreastScreen Aotearoa is also making progress in complete and timely data collection to enable monitoring of cancer rates by size, stage, nodal status and grade.

***Countries or regions with no organized mammographic screening***
Information from China (Shanghai), India (Mumbai), Japan, the Philippines and Singapore, indicated that some type of screening programme or a screening trial existed.

*China*
It is uncertain whether there is screening in China, although the 1997 WPRO survey indicated that breast cancer screening had been offered routinely since 1975 and that mammography was part of the procedure. Health education, well-developed and accessible health services and public awareness have been mentioned as necessary in the early diagnosis of breast cancers in China (Sankaranarayanan et al., 1998).

In a trial of breast self-examination in the absence of mammography was conducted in the Shanghai Textile Industry Bureau in 1989–9, it was concluded that the efficacy of breast self-examination is unproven (Thomas et al., 1997). Contact with the Women's Health Institute in Shanghai (Gao Xiao Ling, Deputy Director, personal communication) indicated that the Institute is responsible for 100 teams who supply breast and cervical screening to 400 000 women aged 25–60. Breast screening is carried out by clinical examination by teams of doctors and health workers. Women may come into contact with the team during a team visit to the workplace or when individual women attend a team clinic, e.g, in one of 19 maternal and child health centres in Shanghai. The visit is recorded on a card (extent of detail unknown) which is held by the woman, by the workplace or by the clinic.

Repeated visits at worksites are made to women seen at past visits and newly eligible women, and it would appear that women are eligible (criteria unknown) for repeat visits to clinics.

When a suspect sign or symptom is detected, the woman is referred to a hospital for mammography. A doctor from the team may accompany the woman to the hospital, although they are usually unaccompanied. Women can also attend the hospital directly (Gao Xiao Ling, personal communication).

## India

A Government-funded national cancer control programme associated with the Indian Cancer Society offers various activities across States, constituted mainly of health education programmes for early detection of cancers, including breast cancer, but there is no organized screening programme (Sankaranarayanan et al., 1998).

The Preventive Oncology Division of the Tata Memorial Centre offers regular cancer screening services (clinical examination and training in breast self-examination) to 3000–4000 women, who are screened annually at outpatient clinics, and to similar numbers who are screened at community-based cancer camps (www.tatamemorial centre.com).

A randomized intervention trial funded by the US National Cancer Institute is under way at the Tata Memorial Centre, Mumbai, to evaluate clinical breast examination and the teaching of breast self-examination in the control of breast cancer in that city; it is in its fourth year (I. Mittra, personal communication). The trial includes 150 000 women in suburban Mumbai in four rounds of screening at approximately 18-month intervals; cancer awareness messages are delivered to women in both arms of the trial in addition to the screening intervention, which also includes cervical screening.

## Japan

Clinical breast examination, which has been used for screening in Japan since about 1975, was incorporated into mass screening in 1987, with annual clinical examinations of women aged $\geq$ 30 years. The intervention was reported to cover approximately 8% of the population in 1995 (Abe et al., 1983; Ballard-Barbash et al., 1999). A screening trial in Miyagi Prefecture, Japan, in 1989–91 comprised one-view mammography every 2 years, at first to women aged $\geq$ 50 years and later to younger women. An improved cancer detection rate was found when compared with clinical examination alone (Ohuchi et al., 1993; Yokoe et al., 1998). The Ministry of Health and Welfare supported a study to analyse the cost-effectiveness and sensitivity of mammographic screening. After 1997, the group planned guidelines for a national mammographic screening programme, setting up training and assessing the quality and sensitivity of mammography (N. Ohuchi, personal communication).

Guidelines for quality assurance of mammography were drafted in 1999 (Klabunde et al., 2001b). In 2000, the national guidelines for breast cancer screening were changed to recommend one-view mammography every 2 years for women aged $\geq$ 50 (N. Ohuchi, personal communication). The programme targets 30% of the eligible population and has available two mammography facilities and three radiology units (Klabunde et al., 2001b). Population-based mammographic screening for women 40–49 years of age is still under consideration (Morimoto et al., 2000). The International Breast Cancer Screening Network, of which Japan is a member, has published summary information on the screening initiative in Japan (Ballard-Barbash et al., 1999; Klabunde et al., 2001b).

## Philippines

A randomized controlled trial of screening for breast cancer by clinical examination performed by trained nurses was established in 1995 in Greater Manila, with support from the United States Army Medical Research Development Command. A total of 202 health centres were randomized, with 219 000 women in the intervention and 190 000 in the control arm. The first round of examinations was completed by the end of 1997. Because of a very low rate of compliance with referral among women who had a positive result at clinical examination, the trial was discontinued after the first screening round, and follow-up of the target population was undertaken. Overall, 105 new cases of invasive breast cancer were found in the study population after an average of 3 years of follow-up. The proportion of cases diagnosed at stage I or IIA increased by 9% after the intervention (Parkin et al., 2001).

## Singapore

The Singapore Cancer Society offers free screening at its headquarters and has a mobile breast screening unit (www.cancer.org.sg). The Breast Cancer Foundation, a non-profit organization, offers instruction in breast self-examination and screening by clinical breast examination for women < 40 years and by mammography for women $\geq$ 40 years (www.bcf.org.sg). Up to the mid-1990s, screening was offered to women attending Government clinics for ante- and postnatal visits, and they were given instruction in examining their breasts. From 1987, Well Woman Clinics offered a clinical breast examination and instruction in breast self-examination, and after 1989 women aged $\geq$ 40 were encouraged to attend for mammography, although by the mid-1990s no more than 25% of women 50–64 years of age were estimated to have ever had a mammogram, perhaps because of the high fee (Seow et al., 1997). The

National Breast Cancer Screening Project conducted in 1994–96 enrolled 28 231 women aged 50–64 for a single free mammogram at one of two large mammographic screening centres, with 97 294 women as controls (Ng et al., 1998). The project concluded with recommendations for quality assurance programmes to ensure consistent reporting and for the establishment of minimum standards (Tan et al., 2000)

The Singapore Ministry of Health is introducing a mammographic screening programme for asymptomatic women in 2002, offering annual screening to women aged 40–49 and screening every 2 years to women aged 50–64. The programme will be linked to a population register to invite eligible women aged 50–64 and will maintain a screening register. Women with symptoms will not be screened in the programme but advised to see a doctor for investigation. After having a screening mammogram with negative results, women will be reminded to continue monthly breast self-examination. The programme aims to screen 50 000 women in the early years, to increase its coverage every year, and to screen 70% of the population by 2008 (T. Yoong, Singapore Ministry of Health, personal communication).

### Countries or regions for which there is more limited information

#### American Samoa
Although the 1997 WPRO survey indicated that screening had been conducted since 1996, with 52% coverage of the target population, there is no mention of mammographic screening. In contrast, a recent paper noted very little screening (Mishra et al., 2001).

#### Bangladesh
Information on breast cancer detection in Bangladesh was abstracted from a conference presentation of Dr R. Sultana at the World Conference on Breast Cancer in Ontario, Canada, in 2000

(www.bangla2000.com). The key facts mentioned were the lack of free health services, health insurance or a systematic health monitoring system in Bangladesh; furthermore, the numbers of women who develop or die from breast cancer each year are unknown. The Cancer Institute and Research Hospital in Dhaka is the sole Government-funded facility for cancer patients. The hospital, in collaboration with the Bangladesh Cancer Society and some private clinics in Dhaka, offers mammography and other breast cancer services.

#### Hong Kong (China)
Hong Kong lacks an organized screening programme. Four local health centres offer screening by clinical breast examination and mammography to mostly asymptomatic women aged between 40 and 65–70 years who are self-referred and pay for the services themselves (Abdullah & Leung, 2001; T. Lee, Hong Kong Anti-cancer Society, personal communication). The centres all have registers and report attendance of 4000–6000 a year per centre, indicating that many women in Hong Kong do not use the screening services (Chan et al., 1998; Lau et al., 1998; Abdullah & Leung, 2001; Hong Kong Sanatorium, personal communication). A fifth clinic, conducted by the Department of Health, is restricted to women 45–64 years of age; it charges an annual fee for its health promotion and disease prevention programmes and a separate fee for mammography.

#### Taiwan (China)
Breast self-examination, clinical breast examination and mammography all appear to be used in Taiwan (Chie et al., 2000). Hospitals with websites mention general clinical screening for cancer in adults and three specialized breast clinics. The Department of Health's breast cancer control programme aims to increase the number of women who

carry out breast self-examination and to conduct examinations, presumably clinical examinations, of up to 1 million women over 35 years of age for breast cancer (www.gio.gov.tw).

#### Republic of Korea
The 1997 WPRO survey reported that screening had been available since 1996 and that mammography formed part of the procedure. Information on the Korean Breast Cancer Society website confirmed this observation and suggested increased detection of breast cancer by mammography. Mammographic screening has been available since 1994 at Yonsei University Medical Centre.

#### Thailand
The two population-based cancer registries, in Chiang Mai and Khon Kaen, reported no organized breast cancer screening programmes and indicated that breast cancer screening was a low priority because of a low, but increasing, incidence. Khon Kaen and Chiang Mai University Hospitals offer health education and a mammography service on demand (Sankaranarayanan et al., 1998).

#### Viet Nam
Training programmes in breast cancer screening supported by WHO have been mentioned on the WHO Western Pacific Region website in Ha Noi and Hue and three pilot projects in Ha Noi and Ho Chi Minh City. Two publications from the Ha Noi and Ho Chi Minh City cancer registries mention a high breast cancer incidence but do not refer to early detection programmes (Anh et al., 1993; Nguyen et al., 1998).

The only source of information for a number of other countries on routine breast cancer was the 1997 WPRO survey. The countries are:

*Guam*
Screening since 1985, coverage unknown, mammography offered.

*Malaysia*
Screening since 1985, 60% coverage of the target population, no mammography

*Mariana Islands*
Screening offered, no mention of year of commencement, mammography

*Niue*
Screening since 1983, coverage unknown, no mammography

*Palau*
Screening since 1980, coverage unknown, no mammography.

*Tokelau*
Screening since 1996, coverage unknown, no mammography

*Fiji*
The WHO website mentioned support from WHO to develop breast and other cancer screening programmes.

## Behavioural factors and the longer-term success of screening

Behavioural factors are fundamental to the longer-term success of a screening programme. They include communication about breast cancer and the screening process, psychological consequences of participating in screening and issues affecting participation in screening. Most research about behavioural factors and screening has focused on predictors of participation and evaluation of strategies designed to encourage higher rates of participation.

## Information and understanding
Cancer screening programmes target individuals without symptoms, with the aim of preventing deaths from the dis-

ease. However, participation in screening may have considerable negative sides for the individual in terms of increased anxiety, additional tests and treatment if cancer is detected. Furthermore, ethical and legal considerations in respect of informed consent require that women fully understand the process of screening. Participants should therefore be fully informed about the potential benefits and harms of a screening programme in order that they can decide whether or not they wish to take part.

### Understanding the benefits and harms of screening
Women's decisions about whether to take part in screening and their understanding of the experience are affected both by their views about their own risk for developing breast cancer and by their understanding of the risks and benefits of screening.

*Women's understanding of the risk for breast cancer*
Women have been shown to overestimate their own risk for developing breast cancer. In one study, women overestimated their risk for dying from breast cancer within 10 years by 20-fold (Black *et al.*, 1995). In an Australian population-based study, Barratt *et al.* (1997b) found that 65% of women overestimated the risk for developing breast cancer, and 15% believing that more than 50% of women will develop breast cancer at some time in their lives. Women also overestimated their own risk for developing breast cancer, and younger women believed themselves to be at greater risk than did older women. Information about screening is interpreted against a community belief that the rates of breast cancer and individual risk for the disease are high.

*Women's understanding of the accuracy of screening*
Women tend to overestimate the accuracy of screening. Black *et al.*

(1995) for example, found that women overestimated the reduction in relative risk due to mammographic screening by sixfold and the reduction in absolute risk by more than 100-fold. Thirty-two per cent of women in an Australian study substantially overestimated the accuracy of screening mammography, believing that over 95% of cancers are detected (Barratt *et al.*, 1999). All the women in this sample believed that screening mammography should pick up all cancers, and three-quarters believed that the sensitivity of mammographic screening should be over 90%. Forty-five per cent of women thought that compensation should be awarded if a breast cancer was missed because it was not found in the test (Barratt *et al.*, 1999). These beliefs are based on a misunderstanding of the accuracy of mammography rather than unrealistic perceptions about what is needed for a worthwhile test; women said they would still find the test worthwhile if it found only 50% of cancers. Schwartz *et al.* (2000) also reported that women were tolerant of false-positive results.

Overestimation of the accuracy of screening mammography may have significant consequences. If a woman has a negative result in a screening mammogram and then develops breast cancer, she may feel a sense of betrayal and may believe that she is entitled to financial compensation. If she believes that the screening mammogram is highly reliable, she may delay seeking advice about a symptom that develops between screens. If she hears that cancers have been missed in other women by the screening programme, she may be discouraged from attending, in a belief that the particular programme is ineffective. A strong belief in the accuracy of screening may cause her to place considerable reliance on a positive result; even if it is found to be a false-positive finding, she may maintain concern that 'the test could not have been completely wrong'.

*Understanding and informed consent*

The legal requirements for consent to screening vary between jurisdictions. In Australia, for example, State legislation requires signed consent for participation in screening and for each assessment test. In Italy, no written consent is required for screening or for additional mammography of lesions detected at screening, although written consent is required for biopsy.

In most jurisdictions, however, the concept of 'informed consent' is fundamental (Austoker, 1999). Informed consent means that the woman understands what is involved in the screening process and that clear, comprehensible information is given about the key issues of relevance for the woman, particularly in relation to potential benefits and harms.

*Providing better information about the benefits and harms of mammographic screening*

The challenge is to create more accurate understanding of screening and screening mammography among women in the community. There is growing pressure on screening programmes to provide fuller information about the sensitivity, specificity and potential harms and benefits of screening (e.g. Dixon-Woods *et al.*, 2001).

Relatively little is known about how best to communicate these sometimes complex issues in a way that is clear, accurate and relevant to women. Screening programmes rarely provide detailed information about the accuracy of screening mammography; in an Australian study of 58 pamphlets containing information about mammographic screening, only one-fourth gave information about sensitivity and none gave data about specificity (Slaytor & Ward, 1998).

Community understanding might be improved by describing the result of screening mammography as the 'magnitude of the risk' for having cancer rather

than a simple dichotomy of 'having cancer or not' (Goyder *et al.*, 2000). For example, a negative result in a screening test might be described as indicating a 'low risk' for breast cancer rather than 'no abnormality'. Goyder *et al.* (2000) analysed some of the questions that may be important to women in understanding screening for breast cancer and deciding whether or not to participate, as shown in the box below. Some research has been done of individuals' understanding of risk, both absolute and relative, and the preference for numerical or verbal information. Individuals clearly differ in the type and style of information they prefer and in their interpretation of verbal, numerical and graphical information (Sutherland *et al.*, 1991; Butow *et al.*, 1996; O'Connor *et al.*, 1998).

Another approach is to consider tailored printed communications which provide individualized information based on the risk and other characteristics of the individual. Rimer and Glassman (1999) reviewed five studies of communications designed to encourage participation in screening mammography and reported inconsistent results. However, this approach has been effective in providing information in relation to other health problems; it may be that the provision of more accurate information about mammographic screening will not necessarily increase participation rates but might provide women with an opportunity to assess better whether they wish to take part. At present, little is known about how best to assist women in understanding the harms and benefits of breast cancer screening.

***Other issues in communication and information***

Other communication issues of relevance to screening include:

---

### Questions women may ask in considering whether to participate in mammographic screening

- What is my chance of dying from breast cancer if I decide not to be screened?

- What is my chance of dying from breast cancer if I decide to participate in screening?

- What is the chance that my mammogram will be normal?

- If my mammogram is not normal, what is the chance that I have breast cancer?

- What further tests might I be advised to have if my mammogram is not normal?

- If my mammogram is normal, what is my chance of having breast cancer anyway (that is, cancer undetected by the mammogram)?

- What is the chance that I may be harmed by screening, by receiving unnecessary treatment or exposure to radiation?

Adapted from Goyder *et al.* (2000)

- *Information about tests:* There is good evidence that satisfaction with care and compliance with recommendations are increased if individuals are provided with adequate information before undergoing medical tests and procedures (e.g. Johnston & Voegele, 1993). Screening programmes should provide detailed information about the benefits and harms of the assessment and of diagnostic tests and about the experience of undergoing the test itself.

- *Understanding the consequences of a diagnosis:* The ways in which women are told they have breast cancer can affect their understanding of their illness and their long-term adjustment (e.g. Roberts et al., 1994). Screening results in higher rates of detection of non-invasive conditions such as DCIS, and this makes communication about the diagnosis particularly complex. Information about the likelihood of developing subsequent invasive disease must be conveyed, although little is known about the prognosis for some types of DCIS. Women with a diagnosis of ductal carcinoma are confused about their diagnosis and its consequences (Bluman et al., 2001).

## Psychological consequences of participation in screening

One of the potential harms of mammographic screening is increased anxiety for women. High levels of anxiety may also reduce the likelihood of regular participation in screening. Increased anxiety may be generated at several points in the screening pathway.

### Anxiety associated with mammography screening

A number of studies have explored anxiety and distress associated with mammographic screening; in general,

the studies had methodological problems, including small sample sizes, lack of comparability between attenders and control groups and lack of validated measures (Rimer & Bluman, 1997).

A review (Rimer & Bluman, 1997) addressed four studies in which anxiety associated with screening was measured and concluded that most studies showed increased anxiety among women attending for screening. One study (Fine et al., 1993) showed that 60% of women were anxious about having a mammogram and 20% were very anxious; another study (Walker et al., 1994) showed that 20% of women attending for screening had clinically significant anxiety levels. Some studies have suggested that women with lower levels of education, African Americans and women with a family history may be more vulnerable to anxiety (Rimer & Bluman, 1997). Women's anxiety appears to be more closely related to fear of an abnormal result than to the mammogram procedure itself (Mainiero et al., 2001).

Several studies have examined the impact of pain from mammography. Many women (73%; 66%) reported that mammography was painful (Hafslund, 2000; Keemers-Gels et al., 2000); however, most found the pain mild, and very few reported that the pain might deter them from participating in screening in the future.

### Anxiety associated with false-positive results

A number of studies have explored the psychological impact of a false-positive result, and most reported a short-term, moderate increase in anxiety and distress. There is no evidence that a false-positive result decreases subsequent participation in mammographic screening. The psychological effects of false-positive results are discussed in Chapter 5.

### Anxiety associated with a diagnosis of breast cancer

While most women with breast cancer experience some symptoms of anxiety, 12–30% have been found to experience clinically significant anxiety (Maraste et al., 1992; Pinder et al., 1993), and there are major psychological, physical and practical consequences of a diagnosis of breast cancer. While these problems are managed primarily by treatment teams, screening programme personnel often inform women of a diagnosis of breast cancer.

## Encouraging participation in screening

The long-term success of a screening programme depends on participation by a substantial proportion of eligible women. Considerable research has been conducted on the factors associated with participation in screening and strategies for increasing participation rates in relation to each of the programmes for breast cancer, as described below. The studies of predictors of participation rarely addressed the contribution of these factors to non-participation. Studies of the effectiveness of various intervention strategies may therefore contribute more to our understanding of participation in screening.

### Mammographic screening
*Predictors of participation*

High participation rates in mammographic screening make a major contribution to the cost–effectiveness of the entire screening programme. In order to identify factors associated with an increased likelihood of participating in mammographic screening, a literature search was undertaken with the search terms 'mammographic screening x participation, attendance and predictors'; a recent review of studies of participation in screening (Potter et al., 1996) was used as another source. The results are shown in Table 17.

**Table 17. Predictors of attending for mammographic screening**

*Prospective studies*

| Reference | Study type | Country | Study population | Key findings: Increased attendance associated with: |
|---|---|---|---|---|
| Sutton et al. (1994) | Prospective survey before invitation to attend breast screening for the first time; objective measure of attendance | United Kingdom | 3291 women aged 50–64 | Demographic: owning accommodation (compared with renting); married or single; black. No significant association with other indicators of socioeconomic status; education; age; distance from screening centre
Cognitive: Perceived importance of regular screening; intention to go for breast screening; beliefs about personal consequences of screening, effectiveness of screening and chance of getting breast cancer; attitudes of significant others; moderate anxiety (rather than low or excessive anxiety) |
| Turnbull et al. (1995) | Prospective interview of women invited to attend for screening; objective measure of attendance | Australia | 285 women aged 45–70 | Cognitive: no significant association with knowledge, attitudes, prior experience, perceived susceptibility, information about screening |
| Cockburn et al. (1997) | Cohort study with prospective interview before arrival of mobile van; objective measure of participation | Australia | 180 rural women | Demographic: higher education
Cognitive: perceiving a personal risk; intention to attend
Health care: no previous mammogram
Access: knowing location of service |
| Aro et al. (1999) | Prospective interview 1 month before invitation to attend first round of screening; objective measure of attendance | Finland | Attenders: 946
Non-attenders: 641 | Demographic: working, middle income, average education
Cognitive: overoptimism about sensitivity of mammography; perception of own risk as moderate
Health care: regular visit to gynaecologist; attend for Pap smears and practise breast self-examination |
| Aro et al. (2001) | Prospective interview; objective measure of attendance | Finland | 436 | Cognitive: lower levels of depression and anxiety; more social support
Health care: less compliance with health recommendations |

**Table 17 (contd)**

*Comparisons of attenders and non-attenders with objective measure of participation*

| Reference | Study type | Country | Study population | Key findings: Increased attendance associated with: |
|---|---|---|---|---|
| Donato et al. (1991) | Survey of sample of attenders and non-attenders at screening; objective measure of attendance | Italy | 429 non-attenders; 477 attenders | Demographic: lower educational level, married and widowed (compared with single, separated, divorced); Cognitive: family history of breast cancer |
| Ciatto et al. (1992) | Sample of attenders and non-attenders at screening; objective measure of attendance | Italy | 393 women: 227 attenders; 166 non-attenders | Demographic: aged 40–49 (compared with younger and older), marital status. No significant association with socioeconomic status or education; Cognitive: belief that screening is useful; Health care: attendance at gynaecologist; advice from doctor |
| Kee et al. (1992) | Sample of attenders and non-attenders at screening; objective measure of attendance | Ireland | 300 attenders; 300 non-attenders | Demographic: younger age; Access: attendance by private car (rather than public transport); accepted appointment during office hours |
| Margolis et al. (1993) | Women invited to attend scheduled mammography at a teaching hospital; objective measure of attendance | USA | 907 women | Demographic: aged $\geq 60$; race; insured women |
| McNoe et al. (1996) | Samples of attenders and non-attenders; objective measure of attendance | New Zealand | 191 attenders; 174 non-attenders | Demographic: not significantly associated with age, education, income, socioeconomic status |
| Lagerlund et al. (2000a) | Samples of attenders and non-attenders; objective measure of attendance | Sweden | 434 non-attenders; 515 attenders | Cognitive: lower emotional barriers; anxiety about breast cancer; perceived benefits of screening; more knowledge; Health care: physician recommendation |
| Lagerlund et al. (2000b) | Samples of attenders and non-attenders; objective measure of attendance | Sweden | 434 non-attenders; 515 attenders | Demographic: married, employed; Health care: greater use of health care services, other preventive behaviour and screening tests |
| Lostao & Joiner (2001) | Survey of attenders and non-attenders; objective measure of screening | Spain | 708 women 45–65 years; 512 participants and 196 non-participants | Demographic: aged 45–50 and 56–60; Cognitive: knowing someone with breast cancer; belief that breast cancer can be treated; anxiety about cancer; Health care: being in better health |
| Banks et al. (2002a) | All women invited to screening in two general practices; objective measure of attendance | United Kingdom | 1064 women aged 50–64 | Demographic: more affluent areas; Health care: having a prescription for hormone replacement therapy |

**Table 17 (contd)**

| Reference | Study type | Country | Study population | Key findings: Increased attendance associated with: |
|---|---|---|---|---|
| *Cross-sectional self-reported* | | | | |
| Bernstein *et al.* (1991) | Cross sectional survey; self-reported measure of attendance | USA | 4728 women ≥ 40 | Health care: being a member of a health management organization |
| Glanz *et al.* (1992) | Cross-sectional telephone survey at selected, diverse work sites | USA | 798 women ≥ 40 at 39 work sites | Cognitive: better knowledge; belief that cancer is curable, mammography is effective and mammograms necessary in the absence of symptoms; knowing someone with breast cancer<br>Health care: doctor's recommendation |
| Grady *et al.* (1992) | Population-based cross-sectional survey, randomly selected from census; self-reported | USA | 630 women aged 45–75 | Health care: physician encouragement to a greater degree than health status, health care use, attitudes or demographic characteristics. Older women no more likely to report physician encouragement |
| Zapka *et al.* (1992) | Cross-sectional survey of women aged 52–75; self-reported participation | USA | 1987: 838<br>1990: 601 | Cognitive: family history<br>Health care: having a regular physician |
| deBruin *et al.* (1993) | Cross-sectional survey; self-reported | Netherlands | 2702 | Health care: having recently had a Pap test |
| Calle *et al.* (1993) | Cross-sectional survey; self-reported | USA | 12 252 women | Demographic: higher income, non-Hispanic or other non-white background, higher education attendance, age < 65, living in urban area |
| Mandelblatt *et al.* (1993a) | Cross-sectional survey of attendees at public hospital clinic | USA | 271 women (average age, 75 years, 99% black) | Cognitive: intention to have a mammogram. No significant association with knowledge or attitudes<br>Health care: more than three chronic illnesses |
| Fox & Roetzheim (1994); Fox *et al.* (1994) | Medicare sample of older women plus cross-sectional population survey; self-reported | USA | Older sample: 724 women ≥ 65 years (5% Hispanic)<br>Population sample: 972 women ≥ 50 years | Ethnicity: Hispanic women reported greater concern than white or African American women. No significant differences in attendance rates.<br>Health care: physician endorsement of mammography |
| Urban *et al.* (1994) | Cross-sectional survey; 50–75-year-old women in four counties in Washington; self-reported | USA | Whole country, analysis by residential area | Demographic: higher income<br>Cognitive: family history of breast cancer<br>Health care: regular visits to gynaecologist or physician |
| van Gessel-Dauekaussen & de Konig (1995) | Cross-sectional survey | Netherlands | 1638 | Demographics: no association with education, income or marital status |
| Rosenman *et al.* (1995) | Cross-sectional survey of women in four farming communities; self-report | USA | 680 women | Demographic: higher education, income and insurance; same rates of screening as in urban women |

**Table 17 (contd)**

*Cross-sectional self-reported (contd)*

| Reference | Study type | Country | Study population | Key findings: Increased attendance associated with: |
|---|---|---|---|---|
| Frazier et al. (1996a) | Cross-sectional survey; self-reported | USA | 22 657 | Demographic: higher education<br>Health care: routine examination in past year |
| Thomas et al. (1996) | Cross-sectional interview; self-reported measure of participation | USA | 1011 women aged ≥ 65 | Cognitive: belief that screening 'eases the mind' |
| Barratt et al. (1997b) | Cross-sectional survey; self-reported measure of attendance | Australia | 3014 | Demographic: aged 50–69. No association with age or rural residence |
| McPhee et al. (1997) | Cross-sectional survey in Vietnamese-American communities; self-reported | USA | 258 women aged ≥ 40 | Demographic: years in USA; education<br>Health care: good health |
| Ali-Abarghoui et al. (1998) | Cross-sectional survey; self-reported measure of participation | USA | 915 | Demographic: higher education, health insurance |
| Fox et al. (1998) | Cross-sectional survey of church attenders | USA | 1517 | Health care: physician recommendation; having medical insurance<br>Ethnicity: African American white (rather than Hispanic). Compared with community sample, churchgoers more likely to be screened |
| Hoffman-Goetz et al. (1998) | Cross-sectional population surveys, 1987 and 1992; separate analyses by racial or ethnic group by income; self-reported | USA | 1987:22 043<br>1992:12 035 | Demographic: higher education and income in all racial groups (white, African American, Hispanic) |
| Paskett et al. (1998) | Cross-sectional survey of African–American women; self-reported | USA | 555 women aged ≥ 40 | Cognitive: better knowledge of mammography; belief that mammography is useful<br>Health care: regular visits to physicians; regular check-ups; having a medical condition |
| Friedman et al. (1999) | Cross-sectional survey in clinic population; self-reported | USA | 121 ethnically diverse low-income women recruited from hospital psychiatry clinic | Cognitive: knowledge of breast cancer<br>Health care: physician recommendation |
| Borràs et al. (1999) | Cross-sectional survey; self-reported | Spain | 5865 women aged ≥ 20 years | Demographic: age 40–49; higher education, membership of voluntary private health insurance, educational level in women over 40 |

**Table 17 (contd)**

| Reference | Study type | Country | Study population | Key findings: Increased attendance associated with: |
|---|---|---|---|---|
| *Cross-sectional self-reported (contd)* | | | | |
| Mandelblatt *et al.* (1999) | Cross-sectional population survey; quota sample stratified by age, using random-digit dialling to find 50 women per ethnic group; self-reported | USA | 1420 women from four Hispanic and three black groups | Demographic: born in USA or lived there for some time<br>Cognitive: positive attitudes to cancer<br>Health care: having usual source of care; having private health insurance |
| Michielutte *et al.* (1999) | Women attending seven primary care clinics; self-reported | USA | 719 women aged ≥ 60 | Cognitive: symptoms; perceived susceptibility; belief that mammography is useful<br>Health care: physician recommendation<br>Access: knowing where to get a mammogram |
| Maxwell *et al.* (2001) | Cross-sectional survey; self-reported | Canada | 8602 women aged 50–69 | Demographic: younger age, residence in urban area, born in Canada<br>Health care: regular doctor, recent doctor visit, not smoking |
| Rutledge *et al.* (2001) | Cross-sectional survey of members of women clubs; self-reported | USA | 538 women (average age, 60) | Demographic: older age<br>Health care: recommendation from doctor or nurse<br>Cognitive: knowledge of screening |
| Valdez *et al.* (2001) | Cross-sectional survey of self-identified Latinas; self-reported | USA | 583 women aged > 40 | Health care: having a regular doctor |
| *Other designs* | | | | |
| Conry *et al.* (1993) | Patients of family physicians; chart review | USA | 839 patients | Health care: first visit to that doctor; had a mammogram in the past; had a breast-related complaint; attending for an annual examination; considered by doctor as more likely to participate |
| Horton Taylor *et al.* (1996) | Response rates to special invitation by 65–74-year-olds compared with routinely invited women aged 50–64; pilot study on effectiveness of screening | United Kingdom | 65–74: 4836<br>50–64: 7446 | Demographics: aged 50–64 compared with older women |

Studies of women who had attended for screening and those who had not were included, as were studies in which actual attendance for screening and self-reported attendance were used. Nevertheless, more reliance should be placed on studies of actual attendance as the outcome measure, as there is likely to be some response bias in self-reported attendance. Studies in which 'intention to attend' was used as a surrogate measure were excluded. As community views about mammographic screening and its availability have changed considerably over the past decade, only studies published after 1990 were included.

Several studies (e.g. Sutton *et al.*, 1994; Cockburn *et al.*, 1997) were prospective surveys of women invited to screening, and the characteristics of those women who subsequently attended were compared with those who did not; these provide the most reliable data about predictors of screening. In several studies, non-attenders were interviewed to identify their reasons for not participating; some information from these studies has been included, where relevant, although individuals may not be able to explain reliably why they did not attend, and there may be response bias. Studies with very small sample sizes were also excluded, although it should be noted that there has been considerable qualitative research (e.g. Lagerlund *et al.*, 2001), on which the interventions described in the following chapter were based.

The review indicated at the outset that the characteristics of the health service delivery system (whether screening was offered opportunistically, whether it was free, whether it was population-based) would be related to the characteristics of the women who attended. However, in practice, there was remarkable similarity among countries and screening programmes in the characteristics of women who attended for screening.

## Demographic predictors of attendance
### Age
Most studies have shown that younger women, even within the range 50–70 years, are more likely to attend for screening than older women (Ciatto *et al.*, 1992; Horton Taylor *et al.*, 1996; Maxwell *et al.*, 2001).

### Socioeconomic status
Lower educational and income status were associated with lower rates of participation in many studies (e.g. Calle *et al.*, 1993; Urban *et al.*, 1994; Cockburn *et al.*, 1997; Ali-Abarghoui *et al.*, 1998; Hoffman-Goetz *et al.*, 1998; Borràs *et al.*, 1999). For example, Calle *et al.* (1993) found that 80% of women living below the poverty level had never had a mammogram, and Hoffman-Goetz *et al.* (1998) found that socioeconomic status was an independent predictor of attendance within racial or ethnic groups in the USA.

The apparent influence of socio-economic status on participation may, however, be due to the strategies used for recruitment and the characteristics of health service delivery. For example, in Italy, less well educated women were more likely to attend a public screening programme (Donato *et al.*, 1991), and socioeconomic status was not associated with attendance (Ciatto *et al.*, 1992). The authors postulated that more affluent women were screened in the private sector. In a large prospective study in the United Kingdom (Sutton *et al.*, 1994), women in rented accommodation were less likely than those in owned homes to attend for screening; no other indicator of socioeconomic status was important.

### Rural residence
The findings about whether living in rural areas affects attendance are inconsistent; some studies have shown that rural women are as likely to attend for screening as urban women (e.g. Rosenman *et al.*, 1995; Barratt *et al.*, 1997b), while others have shown lower attendance rates by rural women (Calle *et al.*, 1993; Maxwell *et al.*, 2001). The inconsistency of these findings may be due to confounding between rural residence and access to screening. In areas where mobile screening is available, rural residence appeared to be less important (e.g. Barratt *et al.*, 1997b), and distance from a screening centre has been shown to affect attendance (e.g. Sutton *et al.*, 1994).

### Marital status
Married and single women were more likely than divorced, separated or widowed women to attend for screening (e.g. Donato *et al.*, 1991; Ciatto *et al.*, 1992; Sutton *et al.*, 1994).

### Ethnic background
Most research suggests that ethnic background itself is not an important independent predictor of attendance at mammographic screening (e.g. Fox & Roetzheim, 1994; Fox *et al.*, 1994; Sutton *et al.*, 1994), and that factors like socioeconomic status and physicians' recommendation are important (Hoffman-Goetz *et al.*, 1998; Friedman *et al.*, 1999).

## Knowledge and attitudes as predictors of attendance
Studies of the effect of knowledge and attitudes on participation in screening are difficult to compare when different questions and measurement tools are used. Nonetheless, four factors can be distinguished:

### Knowledge of screening
Women who know about mammographic screening are more likely to attend (e.g. Glanz *et al.*, 1992; Friedman *et al.*, 1999; Lostao *et al.*, 2001; Valdez *et al.*, 2001).

## Predictors of participation in mammographic screening

The factors most consistently associated with participation in mammographic screening appear to be:

- an invitation or reminder to participate in an organized programme;

- a strong recommendation from a doctor;

- good understanding of the benefits of mammographic screening and a belief that breast cancer can be treated;

- a perception of personal risk and moderate anxiety about breast cancer; and having recently had a Pap test or other health intervention.

*Belief that screening is effective*
Women are more likely to attend for screening if they believe that mammographic screening is effective in finding small cancers that can be cured (Donato *et al.*, 1991; Ciatto *et al.*, 1992; Glanz *et al.*, 1992; Sutton *et al.*, 1994; Paskett *et al.*, 1998; Lagerlund *et al.*, 2000a; Lostao & Joiner, 2001; Lostao *et al.*, 2001).

*Fear that breast cancer will be detected*
Strong fear that breast cancer will be detected is associated with a decreased likelihood of attending for screening (Donato *et al.*, 1991; Ciatto *et al.*, 1992; Munn, 1993). Women who report being very concerned about breast cancer may not attend for screening (Ciatto *et al.*, 1992), whereas moderate anxiety (rather than little or excessive anxiety) about breast cancer is most likely to predict attendance at screening (Sutton *et al.*, 1994). In interviews of non-attenders, the reasons given for not participating in screening included 'apathy' or lack of concern (Donato *et al.*, 1991; Munn, 1993), fear of a positive result (Donato *et al.*, 1991; Munn, 1993; Sutton *et al.*, 1994), 'rather not know' (Kee *et al.*, 1992) and fear of

pain or embarrassment (Kee *et al.*, 1992).

*Perceived personal risk*
Perceived personal risk is also a key predictor of attending for screening. Women who believe they are more likely to develop breast cancer are more likely to attend (Donato *et al.*, 1991; Cockburn *et al.*, 1997), as are women who report breast cancer among family members (Donato *et al.*, 1991; Glanz *et al.*, 1992; Vernon *et al.*, 1992) or friends (Glanz *et al.*, 1992).

*Health care factors as predictors of participation*
A recommendation by a doctor to attend for screening appears to be very influential and has been shown to be associated with attendance in many studies (e.g. Glockner *et al.*, 1992; Zapka *et al.*, 1992; Fox & Roetzheim, 1994; Crane *et al.*, 1998; Paskett *et al.*, 1998; Friedman *et al.*, 1999; Lagerlund *et al.*, 2000a). For example, Fox *et al.* (1994) reported that women who said that their physician had recommended a mammogram were 4.5 times more likely to participate. Grady *et al.* (1992) found that encouragement by a physician was more important than any other variable explored.

Many studies have shown that women who participate in other screening programmes, such as those for cervical cancer, or who practise breast self-examination are more likely to attend for mammographic screening (e.g. Vernon *et al.*, 1992). This apparent association might reflect a belief in the value of early detection and screening. It might also be linked with access to health services: women who have a usual source of care are more likely to have a mammogram (Urban *et al.*, 1994; Mandelblatt *et al.*, 1999; Maxwell *et al.*, 2001; Valdez *et al.*, 2001). This hypothesis is supported by the finding that doctors are more likely to order a mammogram for women who have had a previous mammogram or clinical breast examination (Glanz *et al.*, 1992; Conry *et al.*, 1993); the medical record may prompt a doctor to order a mammogram. The value of prompting a doctor to recommend mammographic screening is also reflected in the increased likelihood that women will have a screen after a check-up visit (Conry *et al.*, 1993).

*Access as a predictor of participation*
The role of structural factors, such as access, cost and health insurance, has been less thoroughly investigated, and inconsistent findings have been reported. All the studies listed in Table 17 were of predictors of attendance within a particular health system. Regular letters of invitation and reminders to attend, which are part of an organized approach to screening, were found to increase access and attendance (e.g. Irwig *et al.*, 1990; Sutton *et al.*, 1994; Somkin *et al.*, 1997).

Distance from the screening site was found to be important in some studies (Haiart *et al.*, 1990) but not others (Sutton *et al.*, 1994). The inconsistency may be due differences in distance, the availability of public transport and attitudes towards travel for health care. Access to private transport was found to be important in one study (Kee et al., 1992). Interviews of non-attenders indicated that poor access was often cited as a reason for not participating in screening (e.g. Glockner et al., 1992; Hopkins & Hensley, 1993; Munn, 1993).

The role of cost is more difficult to assess, and the findings about the extent to which socioeconomic status predicts attendance are mixed (Donato et al., 1991; Calle et al., 1993; Sutton et al., 1994). Income level is likely to be confounded by health service delivery characteristics, in particular whether screening is free and the availability and cost of private screening and insurance. Nonetheless, cost is often cited as a reason for not attending (Hopkins & Hensley, 1993; Munn, 1993). Cost might be important only below a certain income level. For example, Hopkins and Hensley (1993) found that women with annual incomes below US$ 15 000 were more likely to cite high cost as important, and Calle et al. (1993) found that women living below the poverty line were less likely to participate.

*Participation in re-screening*
Although most programmes have shown high re-screening rates (e.g. Fracheboud et al., 1998; BreastScreen Victoria, 2001), little is known about the factors that encourage regular mammographic screening. While these factors are probably different from those that cause women to attend for a first screen, first screens were not differentiated from subsequent screens in most studies.

Several studies have been conducted of re-attendance. In the United Kingdom, Orton et al. (1991) explored the reasons for non-attendance among the 11% of women who did not return for re-screening. These women were more likely to report the test as having been embarrassing or distressing and significantly less likely to have found the clinic staff helpful or to report that they considered their attendance worth-

while or reassuring. Women who had received a false-positive result were not less likely to attend for subsequent screening. Baines et al. (1990) found that women who did not return for re-screening were less likely than regular participants to report that they had received prompt, courteous, competent examination.

Cockburn et al. (1997) followed a group of women from first to second screening rounds. They found that 'reluctant attenders' at the first screening were least likely to come back. The predictors of returning for a second screening were initially being invited through a community campaign rather than by letter and having had a previous mammogram before the screen. O'Byrne et al. (2000), in a study of women in Australia invited for second-round mammographic screening, found that women were less likely to attend the second time if they were from a non-English-speaking background, indigenous or reported breast symptoms at the first screen.

*Strategies to encourage participation in mammographic screening*
As participation in mammographic screening is less than optimal in most countries, many approaches have been tested to encourage attendance. However, as yet, no recommendations can be made about the most effective strategies for public health screening programmes, for several reasons. Few studies have been conducted on the cost of the various recruitment strategies, although, in a population progamme, the cost–effectiveness of the approach is of critical importance. A statistically significant increase in participation found in a randomized trial to be due to a particular intervention may be of little consequence to a population programme if the cost is high.

Furthermore, little information is available about the effects of community-based strategies or programmes for

specific populations. During the initial phase of a new screening programme, community-based strategies are often implemented to raise awareness. As the screening programme becomes established, specific strategies may be needed for specific groups whose attendance is low. Although such strategies are of considerable interest to the providers of public health programmes, they are difficult to assess in randomized trials and are therefore not included in systematic reviews.

Comparison of studies is difficult because of the differences in interventions, populations and methods. Differences in health service delivery systems may also confound the effectiveness of an intervention; for example, a strategy may be differentially effective depending on whether the system is population-based or whether mammograms are provided free of charge.

The types of intervention that have been investigated include strategies targeting individual women, community-based strategies, health care provider programmes and strategies for specific groups.

*Strategies targeting individual women*
Many studies have been conducted of strategies to encourage individual women to participate in mammographic screening. These were summarized in a Cochrane Collaboration review (Bonfill et al., 2001), which highlighted the limitations of many studies of the effect of such strategies: of the 151 studies located, only 16 met the criteria for inclusion in the review. The review showed that five active strategies were effective in encouraging women to participate in population-based mammographic screening relative to controls with no intervention: a letter of invitation (odds ratio [OR] 1.66; 95% CI, 1.43–1.92), mailed educational material (OR, 2.81; 95% CI, 1.96–4.02); letter of invitation plus phone call (OR, 2.53; 95% CI, 2.02–3.18);

phone call (OR, 1.94; 95% CI, 1.70–2.23) and training plus direct reminders (OR, 2.46; 95% CI, 1.72–3.50). Neither home visits nor letters of invitation to multiple examinations with educational material increased participation.

Four studies included in the review explored the effect of receiving a letter of invitation (Irwig et al., 1990; Turnbull et al., 1991; Sutton et al., 1994; Somkin et al., 1997). All the studies reported higher rates of participation among women who received the letter. On average, the invitation letter increased attendance by about 30%, with greater increases when an appointment time or medical chart reminder were included with the letter.

Three studies explored the effect of an invitation letter plus a phone call (Lantz et al., 1995; Janz et al., 1997; Bodiya et al., 1999). All the studies found that adding a telephone call to the invitation letter increased participation; in one study (Lantz et al., 1995), the rate of attendance was four times greater among women who received a phone call. However, the costs of a telephone invitation are clearly greater than those of an invitation alone; it was estimated in one study that the phone call increased costs by about US$ 9 per mammogram (Bodiya et al., 1999).

In several studies in the review, multi-component strategies were compared with a single strategy. The multi-component approaches were found to be more effective, but the relative cost–effectiveness of the different approaches could be evaluated in few of the studies. For example, Davis et al. (1997) compared a birthday-card reminder, a personalized letter and a multi-component phone call including reminder, counselling and scheduling of appointments. The third strategy was the most effective in increasing participation rates; however, although no data on cost were provided, it would also have been the most expensive. The importance of considering cost–effectiveness was

illustrated in a comparison of three strategies: reminder postcard, reminder telephone call and motivational phone call (Fishman et al., 2000). The marginal cost–effectiveness was US$ 22 per woman screened for the postcard and US$ 92 for the reminder call.

Several studies in the review showed that inclusion of an appointment increases participation, an appointment functioning as a behavioural prompt to attending for screening. For example, Irwig et al. (1990) reported participation rates of 38% for a group who received an appointment with the screening letter and 24% for those without an appointment. Another study showed a 132-fold increase in attendance when an appointment was included (Hurley et al., 1994).

Overall, most recruitment strategies targeting individual women were more effective than no intervention in encouraging participation in mammographic screening. Although combinations of effective strategies resulted in greater participation, more data are needed about relative cost–effectiveness.

### Programmes with health care providers
#### Effect of a recommendation from a health care provider

Several studies have shown that a recommendation from a doctor is strongly associated with participation in mammographic screening (Grady et al., 1992; Fox & Roetzheim, 1994), as have most randomized trials. In Australia, two studies (Cockburn et al., 1990; Clover et al., 1992) showed high rates of attendance after a verbal recommendation by a doctor to attend for screening. Fox et al. (1994) and Kohatsu et al. (1994) showed that the enthusiasm with which a doctor recommends screening is a key predictor of attendance; women who perceived their physicians as having some enthusiasm for mammography were 4.5 times more likely to be screened.

Several studies have shown that a personal letter from a woman's doctor increases participation; for example, Turner et al. (1994) found that inclusion of a letter from the woman's general practitioner with the standard second invitation letter doubled the number of women attending for screening. Mayer et al. (1994) found that a reminder on the doctor's letterhead resulted in a greater participation rate than one on a standard letterhead. In Italy, Giorgi et al. (2000) found that in some but not all towns the involvement of a general practitioner increased participation. Sharp et al. (1996) reported that a personal letter from a general practitioner was at least as effective as a home visit from a nurse and certainly more cost–effective. However, two studies showed that a personal letter from a woman's doctor did not increase participation over that with a standard letter from the programme (Taplin et al., 1994; O'Connor et al., 1998). A personal telephone call from a doctor increased participation (e.g. Hoare et al., 1994; Bodiya et al., 1999).

Despite their potential effectiveness, doctor-based strategies might be costly and therefore of limited use in public health programmes. Other health care workers may be equally effective in encouraging participation and perhaps more cost–effective. For example, Mohler (1995) found that a call from a medical assistant was more cost–effective (US$ 3 per mammogram) than either a doctor's letter alone (US$ 14 per mammogram) or a call from the doctor (US$ 52 per mammogram). The cost of doctor-based strategies might be reduced by minimal interventions. Two studies showed that brief interventions can be as effective as more extensive, costly interventions. Clover et al. (1992) found that 82% of women attended for screening after a simple recommendation from their doctor and 91%

attended after a more intensive educational programme. Likewise, Taplin et al. (2000) found that a brief reminder call from a counsellor was as effective as a motivational call of nearly three times the length.

*Strategies to encourage doctors to recommend mammographic screening*

Although a recommendation from a doctor is highly effective in encouraging screening, many women have reported that their doctor had not recommended participation. For example, only 35% of Australian women of the target age for screening reported that their doctor had recommended it (Barratt et al., 1997b), and only 50% of women in the USA reported that their physician had encouraged them to attend (Paskett et al., 1998).

A meta-analysis of the effect of strategies to encourage health professionals to recommend screening (Mandelblatt & Yabroff, 1999) was conducted of studies from the USA of randomized or non-randomized design with concurrent controls; 35 studies that met the inclusion criteria were located. Behavioural, cognitive and sociological interventions with health professionals increased participation rates to a similar extent (13.2%; 95% CI, 7.8–18.4; 18.6%; 95% CI, 12.8–24.4; 13.1%; 95% CI, 6.8–19.3). Strategies targeting doctors and women were usually no more effective than those targeting doctors alone. In this review, the sociological interventions were heterogeneous, including interventions by nurses; the behavioural strategies included reminders or office prompts. Several studies showed that prompts to doctors based on medical records or computer files increased participation in mammographic screening among their patients. For example, Burack et al. (1994) found that including a reminder form for mammography in the medical record

prompted physician referral and increased participation in screening. Ornstein et al. (1991) tested computer-generated reminders to patients, to their doctors or to both patients and their doctors. The greatest increases were seen when both received a reminder, with a doubling in participation in mammographic screening. The cognitive interventions included provision of educational materials or audit and feedback; for example, Dietrich et al. (1992) found that educational sessions plus office system planning resulted in increased rates of mammographic screening, as did the educational sessions alone.

Cost–effectiveness must also be considered in strategies for encouraging health care providers to recommend screening. Over time, it may be cost–effective to target those doctors who regularly do not refer women to screening; it may be possible to identify these doctors from the low attendance rates of their patients (Lane & Messina, 1999).

*Community strategies*

Community strategies may be particularly important for announcing the establishment of a screening programme, creating a context for other recruitment strategies and recruiting women from specific groups. The few studies of the effect of community strategies were not randomized trials, but some included a control community. Unfortunately, in few of these studies were the costs of these potentially expensive, resource-intensive strategies assessed.

The media were the most commonly cited source of information about mammographic screening (Metsch et al., 1998), and media coverage can affect attendance (Clover et al., 1996; Yanovitzky & Blitz, 2000). However, the media alone are less effective than community development, health professional or telephone strategies (Clover et al., 1996;

Barr et al., 2001). Barr et al. (2001) found that routine media publicity was as effective as a mail strategy.

Community participation and development programmes increase participation in screening more than media strategies or the provision of free screening in a mobile van (Clover et al., 1996; Flynn et al., 1997). Nevertheless, community development and participation programmes are expensive, resource-intensive and likely to result in long- rather than short-term gains. The role of such strategies for specific groups warrants further investigation, as community development programmes might have other health benefits beyond the issue of interest.

Strategies to modify access and cost can also be implemented at community level. The provision of vouchers for free screening increases participation rates (Stoner et al., 1998); however, cost probably interacts with a range of other variables, such as income level and insurance. The effect of cost might be modified by other variables; for example, Rimer et al. (1992) compared the effect of providing free screening with that of providing free screening and improving access and education. Women in the communities receiving the more extensive intervention were much more likely to participate in screening. The authors concluded that the provision of free mammography alone is not sufficient to generate attendance.

*Strategies for specific ethnic groups*

The few studies of strategies to encourage attendance among women from specific ethnic groups were not based on a trial method. Community-based programmes appeared to be effective among African American women (Paskett et al., 1999), and use of health workers of the same ethnic group increased attendance in some communities (e.g. Bird et al., 1998) but not in others (Hoare et al., 1994). A media programme targeting Vietnamese American women increased their knowledge about mammography but did not affect their attendance (Jenkins *et al.*, 1999).

Several studies have shown that programmes run by health care providers are particularly effective. For example, Atri *et al.* (1997) in the United Kingdom randomized doctors' receptionists to receive training in encouraging participation in screening by patients from minority ethnic groups. The overall rate of participation by these women was very low (4%), and the training resulted in a modest but statistically significant increase. The intervention was more effective in certain ethnic groups: the participation of Indian women increased by 14% as compared with an increase of 5% in the total intervention sample. A study in Wales showed that special programmes in a general practice increased the attendance of women in specific ethnic communities (Bell *et al.*, 1999). Nurse practitioners were found to be effective in encouraging attendance by poor, elderly black women (Mandelblatt *et al.*, 1993b). However, a primary care programme for women with low income and of minority groups did not increase screening rates (Manfredi *et al.*, 1998).

As participation rates increase in the community as a whole, cost–effective strategies to reach such groups will become more important.

### Clinical breast examination

Various approaches have been taken to investigating clinical breast examination, with differences among studies in the population and the age of the women, the frequency of clinical breast examination and measures of practice (e.g. self-report, chart review). There is little information for countries outside Europe, North America and Australasia about the practice of clinical breast examination.

Studies in western countries suggested higher rates of practice of clinical breast examination than of breast self-examination. The annual rates of clinical

breast examination ranged from 42% in Michigan, USA (Ruffin *et al.*, 2000), to 54% in Australia (Barratt *et al.*, 1997b) and 87% (20–40 year-olds) and 70% (over 40 years) in the USA (Vincent *et al.*, 1995). Two-thirds of female physicians in the USA reported undergoing annual clinical breast examination (Frank *et al.*, 2000).

Several studies have been conducted with health professionals to explore predictors of offering clinical breast examination. Male but not female doctors reported that women's embarrassment prevented them from offering clinical breast examination (Desnick *et al.*, 1999), and there is some evidence that screening is commoner among the patients of female doctors (Burns *et al.*, 1996).

There also appear to be woman-specific factors that increase the likelihood of receiving clinical breast examination, but it is not clear whether these factors increase the likelihood that women will request examination or that doctors will offer it. Women receiving clinical breast examination were more likely to perceive that the examination was of value and to have greater health motivation (Fung, 1998; Mandelblatt *et al.*, 1999; Rutledge *et al.*, 2001; Tanjasiri & Sablan-Santos, 2001); they were more likely to have seen a specialist for routine examination in the previous year, to have a usual source of care and to have had more than a high-school education (Frazier *et al.*, 1996a; Mandelblatt *et al.*, 1999; Tanjasiri & Sablan-Santos, 2001). An Australian study (Barratt *et al.*, 1997b) found that a clinical breast examination in the previous 2 years was commoner among women aged over 50 than in younger women, and a study of Hispanic-American women found clinical breast examination to be associated with knowledge of breast self-examination, being a non-smoker and having recently had a Pap smear and mammogram (Zambrana *et al.*, 1999).

Strategies targeting doctors increase the frequency with which clinical breast examination is offered. For example, in randomized trials, the numbers of women receiving clinical breast examination was increased after introduction of a computer prompt system (Williams *et al.*, 1998) and an office reminder system (Manfredi *et al.*, 1998).

### Breast self-examination

Programmes to encourage breast self-examination were first established in Europe, Australasia and North America in the 1950s, and major sustained public information programmes were implemented up to the late 1990s to encourage women to practise monthly breast self-examination (see also Chapter 2). By the mid-1990s, however, surveys in most western countries indicated that only about one-third of women regularly practised this examination: for example, 31% in Virginia, USA (Giles *et al.*, 2001), 37% in Australia (Barratt *et al.*, 1997b), 27% in Seattle, USA (Strickland *et al.*, 1997), 28% in Ireland (Murray & McMillan, 1993), 15% of Chinese-American women (Lu, 1995) and 27% of Chamorro women in the USA (Tanjasiri & Sablan-Santos, 2001). The rates of monthly breast self-examination were low even among female physicians, who might be expected to practise preventive health measures more commonly; for example, 30% of Norwegian (Rosvold *et al.*, 2001) and 21% of American (Frank *et al.*, 2000) female physicians reported practising monthly breast self-examination.

Many studies have been conducted of the characteristics of women who practise breast self-examination, and a range of indicators was found. Comparison between studies is difficult, however, because of the different populations and assessment of different measures; various questions have been used to assess practice, and it is not possible to evaluate the extent to which women's reports of breast self-examination are accurate. Taking these factors into account, women appear to be more likely to practise breast self-examination if they are very anxious about breast cancer (e.g. Abdel-Fattah *et al.*, 2000) or have a significant family history of the disease (e.g. Brain *et al.*, 1999). In general, women who were better educated and had more knowledge were more likely to practise breast self-examination (e.g. Murray & McMillan, 1993; Friedman *et al.*, 1999). Women who were more confident about how to undertake breast self-examination were also more likely to practise it (e.g. Murray & McMillan, 1993; Friedman *et al.*, 1999;

Rutledge *et al.*, 2001), as were women whose doctor had recommended the practice (e.g. Friedman *et al.*, 1999). Women under 50 (Murray & McMillan, 1993), married women and those working outside of the home were more likely to practise breast self-examination (Murray & McMillan, 1993). In Hong Kong, breast self-examination was associated with being more health-conscious (Abdullah & Leung, 2001).

The small number of studies of the practice of breast self-examination in non-western countries, outside of organized cancer control activities, found low rates: 1.3% of women reported

practising breast self-examination in Malaysia (Chan, 1999), 10% in Egypt (Abdel-Fattah *et al.*, 2000) and 16% in Hong Kong (Fung, 1998).

Studies in developed countries found that few women practised breast self-examination competently (Coe *et al.*, 1994; Bragg Leight *et al.*, 2000). Training improved the frequency of practice, confidence and objective proficiency as rated by others (Clarke & Savage, 1999; Bragg Leight *et al.*, 2000).

# Chapter 4
# Efficacy of screening

## Methodological and analytical issues in assessing efficacy

### Issues in evaluating the efficacy of screening

Efficacy was defined by Last (1995) as "the extent to which a specific intervention, procedure, regimen or service produces a beneficial result under ideal circumstances." This contrasts with the related term 'effectiveness', defined by Last (1995) as "a measure of the extent to which a specific intervention, procedure, regimen or service, when deployed in the field in routine circumstances, does what it is intended to do for a specific population." In practice, studies to evaluate breast screening have rarely assessed efficacy or effectiveness as defined, but rather a mixture of the two, depending on the design used and the circumstances of the study. To avoid being exclusive, the term 'efficacy' is used in this chapter according to this common usage, but an attempt is made to characterize each study in accordance with Last's (1995) usage.

The process of screening is illustrated in the box on the right.

A number of issues should be noted in evaluating screening. Almost invariably, individuals identified with disease as a result of screening will live longer than those in whom disease is diagnosed in the normal way. The first issue is 'lead time', considered in Chapter 1. The second issue, which accounts for improved survival of cases detected at screening, is 'length-biased sampling' (see Chapter 1). This bias is most obvious at the first or prevalence screen, but length bias also affects the type of cases detected at

re-screening, the more rapidly progressing cancers being diagnosed in the intervals between screens. Hence, in evaluating the total effect of screening, both the interval cases and the screen-detected cases must be identified and taken into consideration. The third issue is 'overdiagnosis' bias. Some lesions identified and counted as disease would not have presented clinically in those individuals during their lifetimes in the absence of screening. This is, in practice, an extreme example of length bias. The fourth bias which can artefactually improve survival

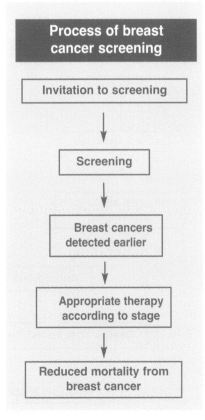

### Process of breast cancer screening

Invitation to screening

↓

Screening

↓

Breast cancers detected earlier

↓

Appropriate therapy according to stage

↓

Reduced mortality from breast cancer

is selection bias. Women who accept invitations for screening are volunteers and are almost invariably more health-conscious than those who decline to enter. This means that they are likely, even in the absence of screening, to have a better outcome of their disease than the general population.

If mortality attributable to the disease (i.e. deaths related to the person–years of observation, or cumulative mortality) is used as the end-point, rather than survival, lead time, length-biased sampling and overdiagnosis biases are eliminated. To eliminate selection bias, the design of choice for evaluation of changes in mortality is the randomized controlled trial (see below). If, for some reason, individual or cluster randomization is not possible, a less desirable method is the quasi-experimental study, in which screening is offered in some areas, and unscreened areas as similar as possible are used for comparison. However, this design is not a cheap and easy substitute but demands the same methodological rigour as required for randomized trials. Further, as substantially larger populations may have to be studied than in randomized trials, it may prove to be more expensive than the preferred design. In addition, difficulties in analysis may ensue if the baseline mortality rates in the comparison areas differ (UK Trial of Early Detection of Breast Cancer Group, 1988).

In general, it is difficult to evaluate the effectiveness of screening by historical comparisons of mortality rates, because biases associated with changes in the accuracy of staging and in therapy can confound the effect of screening (see Chapter 5).

## Use of randomized controlled trials in evaluation of screening

The randomized controlled trial with mortality as the outcome is the only type of study designed specifically to eliminate the effects of the biases discussed above (Prorok et al., 1984). Thus, lead time and selection bias are not issues. The latter is eliminated by the equal distribution of subjects with respect to risk factors for death from breast cancer by the randomization process. The former is eliminated as screening was started for all women at the same time, and all cases that occur during follow-up are included in the evaluation.

A randomized screening trial can be of efficacy or of effectiveness. Trials of efficacy are based on randomization of the screening test and are designed to answer the biologically relevant question of whether mortality is reduced among those who are screened. Trials of effectiveness are based on randomization of invitations to attend for screening and more nearly replicate the circumstances that pertain in practice in a population. The designs of the trials used by the Working Group to evaluate the efficacy of breast cancer screening are summarized in Chapter 1. Trials of effectiveness are discussed in Chapter 5.

The women in such a trial who participate in screening are volunteers. Among the women who are invited to attend for screening, some will refuse, depending on their perception of the value of the tests offered. All trials, therefore, should be analysed according to the intention to screen, i.e. both those who accept the invitation and those who refuse it should be included in the assessment of outcome. A number of issues must be considered in the design and analysis of screening programmes.

### Adequacy of randomization

Randomization is designed to ensure that no observable characteristic influences the selection of the groups selected for comparison. However, even in large trials, especially if cluster randomization is used, comparability cannot be assumed.

### Comparability between groups

The difference in the rate of mortality from breast cancer in groups randomized to screening or no screening cannot be measured directly if the intervention is effective. It can be inferred by comparing the risk factors for death from breast cancer (potential confounders) in the two groups; however, most of the variation will be unpredictable and due to differences between the groups in unknown predictors of death from breast cancer (unknown confounders). The comparability of the known potential confounders in the two groups can be assessed and indeed adjusted for, but the comparability of unknown confounders cannot. Randomization is used to ensure the comparability of unknown confounders between groups. Comparison of mortality rates from all causes other than breast cancer, after adjustment for known confounders if indicated, can give assurance that the two groups are comparable.

It is important to separate two concerns:

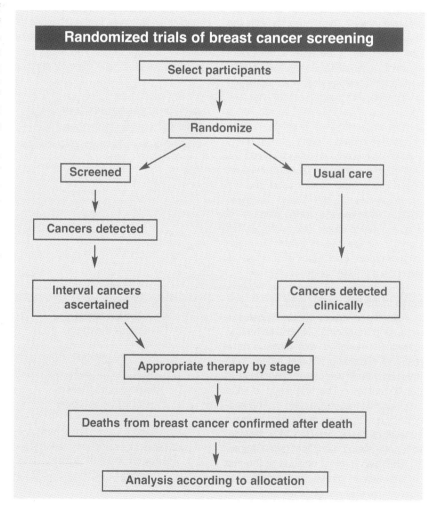

**Randomized trials of breast cancer screening**

Select participants

↓

Randomize

↙ ↘

Screened      Usual care

↓                ↓

Cancers detected

↓                ↓

Interval cancers ascertained      Cancers detected clinically

↘                ↙

Appropriate therapy by stage

↓

Deaths from breast cancer confirmed after death

↓

Analysis according to allocation

## Potential confounders

Even if trials have adequate randomization, there may still be an imbalance in some potential confounders, owing to chance. This is more likely in small trials or even in large trials randomized by cluster. Potential confounders are important if the imbalances are large enough to distort the estimates of the effect of screening. The extent of confounding is determined by how strongly the potential confounder predicts outcome (mortality) and the magnitude of the imbalance in the distribution of the potential confounder between the screened and unscreened groups. An imbalance of potential confounders between screened and unscreened groups can be predicted to result in under- or overestimation of the difference in mortality, and that bias can be adjusted for if the potential confounder has been measured. In practice, age is likely to be the most important such confounder.

## Measuring an underlying problem with the process of randomization

In this case, the concern is that there is maldistribution of unknown confounders, which is due not solely to chance. As the direction of any potential bias is unknown, it cannot be corrected for. The adequacy of the process of randomization can be judged by checking whether a range of variables measured in the trial are distributed equally between the groups or by examining mortality rates from causes other than breast cancer in the two groups. However, if there is evidence of imbalance of randomization, adjusting for these observed imbalances may not necessarily adjust for the true underlying problem. The criterion for determining the presence of imbalances is statistical significance, irrespective of the magnitude of the difference: about 1 in 20 comparisons can be expected to be significant by chance.

## Types of randomization

In breast cancer screening trials, women have been randomized by individual and by cluster. The advantage of individual randomization is that, when large numbers of women are randomized, balance with regard to the risk factors is more likely to be achieved. Recruitment of subjects is often simpler in cluster randomized than in individually randomized trials, but, if the number of units randomized is small, there will be greater potential imbalance (Berry, 1998). In addition, generalized linear models have to be used, with extra variation to account for the cluster randomization (Moore & Tsiatis, 1990; Nixon et al., 2000). In the breast screening trial in Edinburgh (see Chapter 1), for example, a difference in social class was found between the randomized groups, which affected the risk for death from cardiovascular disease (Alexander et al., 1989). Reports of randomized screening trials should confirm that balance was achieved through randomization. A potential advantage of cluster randomization is that, under some circumstances, contamination of the control group with screening can be reduced.

## Post-randomization exclusions

The subjects eligible for a screening trial should ideally not have had a previous diagnosis of the disease of interest (e.g. breast cancer) at the time of randomization. This criterion can be achieved directly in an individually randomized trial with volunteers at the time of enrolment, but may be difficult with cluster randomization based on population registers unless linkage can be made with a population-based cancer registry serving the whole area. Other exclusions should be kept to a minimum and restricted to women who were initially ineligible. If the number of cases of breast cancer excluded is not similar to that in the comparison group, the randomization porcess did not result in groups at equal risk for breast cancer.

## Compliance and contamination

Lack of compliance with the intervention will reduce the estimated efficacy of screening and should therefore be documented.

Contamination, i.e. screening of control women, will also reduce the estimated efficacy. This is more difficult to measure than lack of compliance and may require surveys or annual questionnaires. Contamination may be difficult to define, however, as mammography is also used for diagnosis, and data to distinguish between screening and diagnostic mammograms may not be available.

Methods to adjust for poor compliance and contamination in screening trials have been proposed (Cuzick et al., 1997). Similar methods were applied by Glasziou (1992), who found that the reduction in relative risk was larger than that based on observed numbers.

## Therapy

The efficacy of screening depends not only on early detection of cancer but also on effective treatment. It is a requirement of a good randomized trial design that therapy should be equivalent in the two arms of the trial for equivalent stage of disease. Stage-specific treatment should therefore be described in trial reports.

## Frequency of screening

The frequency of re-screening (annual, every 2 years) should be documented. The longer the interval between screens, the larger the proportion of cancers that will present clinically in the intervals and the lower the overall sensitivity of the screening approach will be.

## Design of interventions to be compared

Differences in the duration of the intervention in the trials of mammography considered in this chapter and in whether the control group was also screened affects the subsequent analysis of mortality.

The design of the Health Insurance Plan study in New York, USA, and of the Canadian trials prescribed four annual screens, followed by no further screening in either group. In this situation, rates of death from breast cancer should theoretically be based on all cases of breast cancer that are diagnosed between randomization and the time at which the curves of cumulative incidence in the two arms converge (Connor & Prorok, 1994).

In the trials in Malmö, Sweden, and Edinburgh, Scotland, no limit was placed on the duration of screening for women who received invitations to screening, and no decision was taken to screen women in the control arm. In such a situation, the cumulative incidence will be greater among women invited for screening throughout the trial, as lead time will have a continuous effect. The cumulative rates of death from breast cancer in the two arms should be compared for all periods after randomization, with no limitation on which cases of breast cancer are to be included.

In the other trials in Sweden, the control group was also invited to screening 4–9 years after the women in the screening arm had received their invitations. In this situation, the comparisons of mortality rates should reflect the fact that the two arms differed for only a short time.

### Cancer detection

As indicated in Chapter 1, it is anticipated that screening will result in diagnosis of breast cancer cases at an earlier stage. This is a necessary but not a sufficient indication of possible efficacy. Cancer detection rates should be reported by tumour size, nodal status (stage) and, if possible, grade. It is expected that, with effective screening, the absolute (cumulative) rate of advanced breast cancer will be lower in the screened group than in the control group. This difference has been proposed as a proxy for mortality; however, as suggested by Prorok et al. (1984),

metastatic disease presenting during follow-up is a preferable measure.

Cumulative mortality from breast cancer after randomization is the primary outcome measure of interest in randomized trials. Annual rates of death from breast cancer after initial screening are also of interest, as the time at which differences in rates emerge between the two arms is important in evaluating the effects of newly introduced population-based programmes.

### End-point of screening trials

The outcome of all the trials of breast cancer screening was death due to breast cancer as the underlying cause. Cause of death can be determined either by an independent committee or from official statistics. Review of the cause of death by independent reviewers was pioneered in the Health Insurance Plan trial (Shapiro et al., 1988). Reviews of causes of death are generally conducted in order to determine these causes in an unbiased way. The cause of death of women with breast cancer should be ascertained in the absence of knowledge about which arm of the study they were in. If official statistics are used, it may be necessary to assess their accuracy, as was done, e.g., in Sweden. Garne et al. (1996) found a discordance in 4.6% of cases, mainly due to coding errors, in a sample with a high autopsy rate. Furthermore, causes of death in official statistics were compared with those determined by an independent committee who were unaware of which arm of the study cases were found in. A high degree of concordance was found (Nyström et al., 1995; see below). It should be recognized that the accuracy of death certificates can change over time, with factors such as autopsy rates, place of death and the criteria used by the doctors issuing the certificates (Lindstrom et al., 1997).

*Breast cancer as the underlying cause of death* is attributed to patients with disseminated or locally advanced

breast cancer. Biological evidence should be available indicating cancer as the most important reason for the death, which can include suicide, lung emboli, acute heart disease and sepsis for patients with advanced breast disease and deaths due to treatment. *Breast cancer present at death* covers all deaths among patients with recurrence or whose tumour was not removed radically, irrespective of whether the breast cancer was of biological importance in the death. This category also includes breast cancer cases detected accidentally at autopsy.

All causes of death among women with breast cancer is not a valid measure. Although in younger women with limited follow-up, mortality is due mainly to the breast cancer, in older women and with longer follow-up, an increasing number of intercurrent deaths unrelated to breast cancer will occur. Early diagnosis of breast cancer in the invited group due to lead time implies that the women with breast cancer were at greater risk for intercurrent death during a longer period. Some authors (Wright, 1986; Olsen & Gotzsche, 2001; Black et al., 2002) have proposed that deaths from all causes are the preferable end-point. Use of this end-point avoids the problems of ascertaining cause of death precisely and the concern that some deaths not apparently due to the cancer of interest were a consequence of treatment for the cancer or of the screening process as a whole. However, measuring this end-point would require very large trials, because even a disease as common as breast cancer constitutes only a small component of deaths from all causes, and the difference in all-cause mortality would be very small. For example, even the combined data from the screening trials would be too few by an order of magnitude to achieve reasonable power.

Lenner (1990) proposed use of an 'excess mortality rate', which is based on the rate of death from all causes among the women with breast cancer minus the similar rate of death among the women without breast cancer in the screened population. The excess death rate in the invited group can then be compared with that in the women not offered screening. The method avoids the necessity of determining cause of death, and, in screening trials, is considered to be unbiased with regard to lead time and overdiagnosis. The measure should capture any deaths caused by treatment for breast cancer and unrecognized as such, but not deaths caused directly or indirectly by the screening procedure and associated diagnostic interventions for women without breast cancer. Nyström et al. (1993) used both this approach and the conventional approach in the Swedish overview analysis (see below) and obtained very similar results. The method has so far not been used in other breast cancer screening trials.

## Use of cohort (observational) and case–control studies in evaluating screening

Cohort study designs have been suggested for estimating the effect of screening. In these studies, mortality from the cancer of interest in a group of individually identified and followed-up screened women (the cohort) is compared with that of a control population, often derived from the general population. Cohort studies of individuals who choose to be screened or not to be screened suffer from potential selection bias, however. In addition, differential ascertainment of deaths due to breast cancer in screened and unscreened women can bias estimates of efficacy.

Thus, observational studies based on individual screening history, no matter how well designed and conducted, should not be regarded as providing evidence of an effect of screening. In order to establish a causal association between screening and a reduction in mortality, the evaluation must take into consideration not only the type of study

but also the magnitude of the association, the consistency of the results in independent studies, the biological plausibility of the result, possible response relationships and the absence of alternative explanations.

It has been suggested that case–control studies could be used to evaluate screening, provided that the programme was introduced sufficiently long before the study so that an effect can be expected to have occurred (Weiss, 1983; Sasco et al., 1986). The ideal design is one that mimics randomized controlled trials as far as possible, especially in terms of the cases (ideally, in this instance, deaths due to breast cancer or advanced disease as a surrogate for deaths). The screening histories of the cases are compared with those of comparable controls drawn from the population from which the cases arose. Individuals with disease, if sampled during the control selection process, would be eligible as controls if the date of diagnosis was not earlier than that of the case, as diagnosis of disease truncates the screening history.

Commonly, the exposure of interest is ever having had a screening mammogram. The odds ratio is then an estimate of the effect of screening on the risk for advanced or fatal breast cancer. The odds ratio is intended to measure the efficacy of screening, i.e. a comparison of the odds for fatal disease in women who did and who did not complete a screening examination. In contrast, a randomized trial is typically designed to compare the mortality experience of two groups of women who differ with regard to whether they received an invitation to screening.

The case–control approach is appealing in terms of its simplicity and cost; however, even if such a study is perfectly designed and conducted, the inherent bias is important potential baseline differences in the screened and unscreened groups with respect to factors that are associated with the risk for fatal breast cancer. There is empirical

evidence that the survival rate of women who decline screening is worse than that of women who accept screening (see e.g. Tabár et al., 1999). This may be due to differences in the distribution of lifestyle factors associated with tumour progression in the two groups, but is more likely the consequence of differences in tumour stage at presentation.

In the studies in Malmö and the Health Insurance Plan study, in which case–control studies were performed within the trials, although women who refused invitations for screening had a breast cancer incidence similar to that of controls, their mortality from breast cancer was greater than that of controls (Janzon & Andersson, 1990; Friedman & Dubin, 1991; Güllberg et al., 1991). Estimates of the effect of screening in such case–control studies will therefore be higher than would be expected in the total population. The bias is best explored by comparing the results of high-quality trials and case–control studies conducted within them. In the Malmö study, the odds ratio in the case–control study was 0.42 (Janzon & Andersson, 1990; Demissie et al., 1998), whereas the relative risk in the trial was 0.96, or 0.92 (Glasziou, 1992) when the results were adjusted for non-compliance and contamination to estimate efficacy. In the Health Insurance Plan study, the odds ratio in the case–control study was 1.07, whereas the relative risk in the trial was 0.80 (Friedman & Dubin, 1991). The difference was shown to be due to a lower rate of mortality from breast cancer among women who refused screening than among those allocated not to be screened.

## Efficacy of screening by conventional mammography

### Randomized trials

The basic characteristics of the randomized trials of the efficacy of mammography screening are shown in Table 18, and the overall results of these trials are summarized in Table 19. The designs of the trials are described in Chapter 1.

### Health Insurance Plan of Greater New York

Shapiro (1994) reported that, after exclusion of breast cancers ascertained after randomization but diagnosed before the date of randomization, there were 30 239 women in the study group and 30 756 in the control group. Gotzsche and Olsen (2000) considered that the randomization in this trial was adequate but were concerned about the use of radiotherapy and about the review of causes of death, and suggested that the exclusions after randomization may have led to lack of comparability. Miller (2001) pointed out that the trial was performed at a time when breast cancers in North America were much larger than became usual in the subsequent two decades. Lumpectomy was not performed in this era, although radiotherapy was used frequently, for locally advanced disease. If radiotherapy was the unrecognized cause of death and was labelled as cardiovascular disease, such labelling would have been applied without bias as to assignment to screening. The decisions made on the deaths reviewed were entirely masked. A difference in the numbers of women with breast cancer excluded from the two arms of the trial arose because previously diagnosed breast cancers were identified in women in the screened group when they attended for screening, but this was not possible for the controls. The 18-year follow-up, however, allowed identification of deaths from breast cancer in the two groups; determination of the date of diagnosis was then possible from hospital records. Women who had died from breast cancers diagnosed before randomization were then excluded (Miller, 2001).

[The relative risks for death from breast cancer 18 years after recruitment were estimated by the Working Group

from the data of Shapiro et al. (1988) to be 0.77 (0.52–1.13) for women aged 40–49 at recruitment, 0.79 (0.58–1.08) for women aged 50–64 at recruitment and 0.78 (0.61–1.00) overall. The Working Group concluded that the Health Insurance Plan study was valid, but could not be included in its evaluation of mammography alone, as the screening included clinical breast examination.]

### The Edinburgh trial

Alexander et al. (1989) reported that the cluster randomization in the Edinburgh trial resulted in differences by socioeconomic category and also in rates of mortality from all causes between the two comparison groups. A report based on 14 years of follow-up and 577 518 woman–years in the initial cohort showed a rate ratio for breast cancer mortality of 0.87 (95% CI, 0.70–1.06). After adjustment for socioeconomic status, the rate ratio was 0.79 (95% CI, 0.60–1.02) (Alexander et al., 1999). The results for women aged 45–49 in all three cohorts, with 266 281 women–years of follow-up, showed a rate ratio of 0.83 (95% CI, 0.54–1.27) before adjustment for socioeconomic status and 0.75 (95% CI, 0.48–1.18) after adjustment.

[The results for all cohorts combined reported in Table 19 were estimated by the Working Group. Although adjustment for socioeconomic group lowered the relative risks slightly, possible confounding from other variables cannot be excluded. Therefore the Working Group did not include this trial in its evaluation.]

### The Canadian National Breast Screening trials

Concern has been expressed about possible subversion of the randomization in these trials, given the procedure described in Chapter 1, especially of women aged 40–49 (Tarone, 1995). However, the authors have pointed out that an abnormal result on clinical breast

examination was not an incentive for spurious allocation to mammography because the protocol required that all abnormal results be referred to the study surgeon for assessment. The surgeon ordered diagnostic mammography when appropriate. If abnormal results of clinical breast examinations had generated spurious mammography allocations, there should have been more referrals of women in the mammography group for review (Miller et al., 2000, 2002). This was not the case. Of the women aged 40–49 at the first screening, 3569 screened women and 3674 in the control group were referred after clinical breast examination for review (Miller et al., 1992a). For the women aged 50–59, the figures were 2164 and 2207, respectively (Miller et al., 1992b). A systematic external review of the randomization records showed no evidence of subversion (Bailar & MacMahon, 1997).

Women were recruited between 1980 and 1985. A separate trial was conducted for women aged 40–49 in order to evaluate the efficacy of screening in this group. The mammography used in these trials has been criticized (Moskowitz, 1992; Kopans, 1993; Kopans & Feig, 1993), but these criticisms have been addressed (Miller et al., 1990; Baines, 1994). The rates of cancer detection with mammography (alone or together with clinical breast examination) at the first screening of women aged 40–49 and 50–59 at entry were 2.54 and 5.48 per 1000, respectively (Miller et al., 1992a,b). Both rates exceed those reported in the Two-county study in Sweden (see below), which were 2.09 and 4.67 per 1000, respectively. The prevalence:incidence ratios were similar in the two studies (Fletcher et al., 1993; Baines, 1994). After 11–16 years of follow-up, the breast cancer mortality rate ratio was 1.06 (95% CI, 0.80–1.40) in the 40–49-year-old women (Miller et al., 2002) and 1.02 (0.78–1.33) in the 50–59-year-old women (Miller et al., 2000).

**Table 18. Basic characteristics of randomized controlled trials on mammography screening among women aged 40–74**

| Trial | Randomization | No. of women | Accrual period — Invited group | Accrual period — Control group | Age at entry | Intervention | No. of mammography views | Screening interval (months) | No. of rounds | Attendance rate (%)[e] | Determination of end-point[b] |
|---|---|---|---|---|---|---|---|---|---|---|---|
| Health Insurance Plan | Individual | 60 995 | Dec 1963–June 1996 | | 40–64 | M+CBE | 2 | 12 | 4 | 67 | Independent death review |
| Malmö I | Individual | 42 283 | Oct 1976–Sep 1978 | Oct 1990–Mar 1993 | 45–70 | M | 2[c] | 18–24 | 6–8 | 74 | Independent death review, official statistics |
| Malmö II | Individual | 17 793 | Sep 1978–Nov 1990 | Sep 1991–Apr 1994 | 43–49 | M | 2[c] | 18–24 | 1–7 | 75–80 | Official statistics |
| Two-county Kopparberg | Cluster Municipality, tax district, 7 triplets | 56 448 | Jul 1977–Feb 1980 | Sep 1982–Dec 1986 | 40–74 | M | 1 | 24, 33[d] | 2–4 | 89 | Death review |
| Östergötland | Cluster Municipality, parish, 12 pairs | 76 617 | May 1978–Mar 1981 | Apr 1986–Feb 1988 | 40–74 | M | 1 | 24, 33[d] | 2–4 | 89 | Death review, official statistics |
| Edinburgh | Cluster General practices, 87 | 44 268[e] | 1978–81[e] 1982–83 1984–85 | | 45–64 | M+CBE | 2 | 24 | 2–4 | 61 | Death certificates |
| Canada 1 (40–49) | Individual | 50 430 | Jan 1980–Mar 1985 | | 40–49 | M+CBE+P[f] | 2 | 12 | 4–5 | 100 | Independent death review |
| Canada 2 (50–59) | Individual | 39 405 | Jan 1980–Mar 1985 | | 50–59 | M+CBE+P[f] | 2 | 12 | 4–5 | 100 | Independent death review |
| Stockholm | Cluster Day of birth | 60 117 | Mar 1981–May 1983 | Oct 1985–May 1986 | 40–64 | M | 1 | 28 | 2 | 81 | Official statistics |
| Göteborg | Individual cluster Day of birth | 51 611 | Dec 1982–Apr 1984 | Nov 1987–June 1991 | 39–59 | M | 2[c] | 18 | 4–5 | 84 | Official statistics |
| Finland | Cluster Year of birth | 158 755 | 1987–89 | After 1990 | 50–64 | M | 2 | 24 | | 90 | Official statistics |

M, mammography; CBE, clinical breast examination; P, teaching of practice of breast self-examination; NA, not available
a First round
b In trials included in the first overview of the Swedish trials, both independent death review and official statistics were used to determine cause of death.
c From round 3, one or two views according to parenchymal pattern
d Averages for age groups 39–49 and 50–75, respectively
e Refers to the first cohort; 4867 and 5499 women aged 45–49 years were randomized during the first and second accrual periods, respectively.
f Controls had only one CBE at entry and P in Canada 1, and CBE and P in Canada 2.

**Table 19. Overall results of randomized trials of efficacy of screening for breast cancer by mammography with and without clinical breast examination, women of all ages (40–74 years)**

| Trial | Enrollment (years/age) | Intervention (invitations to screening) | Population x 1000 (screened/control) | Mean duration of follow-up (years) | Breast cancer mortality per 100 000 person-years (number) (screened/control) | | RR (95% CI) |
|---|---|---|---|---|---|---|---|
| Health Insurance Plan, USA | 1963–66/40–64 | 4 in 4 years | 30.1/30.7 | 18 | 23 (126)/29 (163) | | 0.78 (0.61–1.00) |
| Malmo I, Sweden | 1976–78/45–70 | 4 in 8 years | 21.1/21.2 | 19.2 | 45 (161)/55 (198) | | 0.81 (0.66–1.00) |
| Malmo II, Sweden | 1978–90/43–49 | 4 in 8 years | 9.6/8.2 | 9.1 | 26 (29)/38 (33) | | 0.65 (0.39–1.08) |
| Kopparberg, Swedish Two-county | 1976–78/40–74 | 3 in 6 years | 28.2/18.3 | 20 | 27 (152)/33 (121) | | 0.59 (0.47–0.75) |
| Östergötland, Swedish Two-county | 1978–81/40–74 | 4 in 8 years | 38.9/37.7 | 17.4 | 30 (177)/33 (190) | | 0.89 (0.72–1.09) |
| Edinburgh, UK | 1978–81/45–64 | 4 in 8 years | 28.6/26.0 | 12.6 | 49 (176)/57 (187) | | 0.78 (0.62–0.97) |
| Canadian National I | 1980–85/40–49 | 5 in 5 years | 25.2/25.2 | 13 | 32 (105)/33 (108) | | 1.06 (0.80–1.40) |
| Canadian National II | 1980–85/50–59 | 5 in 5 years | 19.7/19.7 | 13 | 42 (107)/41 (105) | | 1.02 (0.78–1.33) |
| Stockholm, Sweden | 1981–83/40–64 | 2 in 4 years | 39.1/21.0 | 14.9 | 15 (82)/17 (50) | | 0.90 (0.63–1.28) |
| Göteborg, Sweden | 1982–84/40–59 | 3 in 5 years | 21.0/29.2 | 13.3 | 23 (62)/30 (113) | | 0.78 (0.57–1.07) |
| Finland | 1987–89/50–64 | 2 in 4 years | 89.9/68.9 | 4.4 | 16 (64)/21 (63) | | 0.76 (0.53–1.09) |

0.0    1.0    2.0

RR, relative risk, CI, confidence interval

[The Working Group concluded that these trials were valid, but could not be included in its evaluation of mammography alone, as screening in both trials included clinical breast examination, and the design for that with 50–59-year-old women was different from those of all other trials.]

**Finnish national programme**

Hakama et al. (1997) compared deaths from breast cancer reported to the Finnish Cancer Registry and diagnosed over the period 1987–92 among women in birth cohorts invited for screening in the national programme before 1990 with those among women who were invited after 1990. The breast cancer mortality rate ratio was 0.76 (95% CI, 0.53–1.09). The effect was greatest among women aged less than 56 years at entry (rate ratio, 0.56; 95% CI, 0.33–0.95). When follow-up for newly diagnosed breast cancers was extended to 1995, the difference between the cohorts largely disappeared (mortality rate ratio, 0.93; 95% CI not available), presumably because of the effect of screening in the control cohorts (Hakama et al., 1999).

[Although this was not a classical randomized trial, the results provide evidence of similar quality].

### Swedish trials

#### The Malmö mammography screening trials
Imbalances were noted in two birth-year cohorts in these trials: because of an administrative error, the whole 1934 birth cohort was invited to screening, and the 1929 birth cohort participated in another research project in which they were offered mammography. Thus, only 663 women were invited instead of the intended 777 (Olsen & Gotzsche, 2001). With a follow-up of 19.2 years in the first trial (age, 45–70 years at randomization), the relative risk for death from breast cancer was 0.81 (95% CI, 0.66–1.00). The corresponding figures in the second trial (age, 43–49 years at randomization) after 9.1 years of follow-up were 0.65 (95% CI, 0.39–1.08). The results for the two trials were similar with and without inclusion of the 1929 and the 1934 birth cohorts (Nyström et al., 2002).

#### The Two-county trial (Kopparberg and Östergötland)
The first results from the trial were published in 1985 (Tabár et al., 1985) and were updated comprehensively in 1992 (Tabár et al., 1992). The follow-up has been continuous, the latest being through 1998, which showed a significant, 32% reduction in breast cancer mortality in the two counties combined (relative risk, 0.68; 95% CI, 0.59–0.80). After 20 years of follow-up, the relative risk for death from breast cancer in Kopparberg was reported to be 0.76 (95% CI, 0.42–1.40) for women aged 40–49 years, 0.46 (95% CI, 0.30–0.71) for women aged 50–59, 0.58 (95% CI, 0.39–0.87) for women aged 60–69 and 0.76 (95% CI, 0.44–1.33) for women

aged 70–74 at randomization (Tabár et al., 2000b). In the follow-up through 1996 (Nyström et al., 2002), only data for Östergötland were available. After 17.4 years of follow-up, the relative risk for death from breast cancer was 0.89 (95% CI, 0.72–1.09) for women aged 40–74.

Nixon et al. (2000) analysed the data for the two counties in four ways with various statistical assumptions, and found that the point estimates and the 95% confidence intervals in fixed-effect models for women aged 40–74 (relative risk, 0.72; 95% CI, 0.61–0.83) agreed closely with those derived from three random-effects models (0.70, 0.60–0.82; 0.70, 0.57–0.84; 0.70, 0.59–0.83), because the heterogeneity between clusters was small.

Olsen and Gotzsche (2001) described various potential problems with the Two-county trial. However, Nyström et al. (2002) reported that the breast cancer incidence and mortality rates in the screened and control arms in Östergötland County before the trial (1968–77) were similar. They suggested that there is no reason to believe that the cluster randomization in this component of the trial was biased, as any bias would have manifested in breast cancer incidence and mortality. Duffy and Tabár (2000) rebutted similar criticisms published in an earlier review by Gotzsche and Olsen (2000) of the trial in Kopparberg.

#### The Stockholm trial
After a median follow-up time of 14.9 years, the relative risk for death from breast cancer was 0.90 (95% CI, 0.63–1.28). Although the possibility of double counting of controls in earlier analyses has been raised, this was not done in the most recent analysis (Nyström et al., 2002).

#### The Göteborg trial
With a median follow-up of 13.3 years, the overall relative risk was 0.78 (0.57–1.07). [The results of the trial for

women aged 50–59 were described only in the overviews of Nyström et al. (1993, 2002).]

#### Methodological issues with respect to the Swedish trials
There have been three overviews of the Swedish trials (Nyström et al., 1993; Larsson et al., 1997; Nyström et al., 2002), and the methodological issues have been addressed in several publications (Nyström et al., 1995, 1996).

*Randomization:* As discussed above, individual randomization simplifies statistical analyses. This method was used in the Malmö trials and in the second part of the Göteborg trial (women born 1935–44), but not in the other trials (see Chapter 1).

*Inclusion and exclusion criteria:* In all the Swedish trials, women randomized to the intervention group were invited to screening with mammography alone. Women in whom breast cancer had been diagnosed before invitation to screening were excluded from the statistical analysis. As the overviews focused on the age group 40–74 years at entry, a small number of women under 40 and over 74 at randomization were excluded.

*Outcome measures:* The main outcome measure in all the trials was death from breast cancer. Both the Two-county study and the first Malmö trial had detailed protocols for determining the cause of death as breast cancer. The protocol of the Two-county study prescribed identification of women with breast cancer present at death, and the researchers themselves determined the cause of death. In the Malmö trial, two sources were used to determine the underlying cause of death: an independent committee and the Cause of Death Register at Statistics Sweden.

An independent end-point committee was appointed by the overview group, which consisted of a pathologist, a radiologist, an oncologist (chairman) and a surgeon, who were unaware of whether a case had been found at screening or otherwise. Breast cancer as the under-lying cause of death and breast cancer present at death were the outcome measures (see above). A total of 27 582 deaths occurred during the follow-up, between the date of randomization through December 1989 (Nyström *et al.*, 1995). Of these, 1299 were reported as due to breast cancer to the Cancer Registry, and 14 were reported to the Cause of Death Register with breast cancer as the underlying or contributory cause of death only (Table 20). All available information was collected on all 1313 deaths from breast cancer, including medical records, death certificates, autopsy protocols and histopathology reports. The mode of detection was not revealed, and only year of birth and year of death were available to the reviewer (Nyström, 2000). Medical records and/or autopsy protocols were available for 99% of cases, death certificates for 99%, histopathology reports for 90%, medical records for 86% and autopsy protocols for 39%. Autopsy was performed in 551 cases, according to the available information, but reports could be traced in only 511 cases (92%). The autopsy rate was 74% in the Malmö trial,

45% in Kopparberg, 31% in the Göteborg trial, 25% in Östergötland and 22% in the Stockholm trial. Fifteen cases were excluded because, although they were reported as being breast cancer, the end-point committee concluded that their cancer had arisen at another site. Out of 843 deaths in which the underlying cause was classified by the end-point committee as having been breast cancer, 829 (98%) were also classified as breast cancer present at death (Nyström *et al.*, 1995).

The relative risks for death from breast cancer in the invited group in comparison with the control group, with the various end-points measured by the end-point committee and Statistics Sweden, are summarized in Table 21. As there was substantial concordance between the relative risks, both by trial and by age group (Table 22), Statistics Sweden was used as the source of cause of death for the follow-ups through 1993 and 1996.

Although it has been suggested the total mortality should be the main outcome examined (Black *et al.*, 2002; see above), the Swedish studies did not have sufficient statistical power for this to be used as the primary outcome. In the follow-up through 1996, the relative risk for deaths from all causes was 0.98

## Table 20. Numbers of deaths from breast cancer in the Swedish trials

| Source of information | Number |
|---|---|
| Reported to Cancer Registry and Cause of Death Registry | 1299 |
| Reported to Cause of Death Registry only | 14 |
| Total | 1313 |
| *Excluded by end-point committee:* | |
| Not breast cancer | 15 |
| Lack of information | 2 |
| **Study population** | **1296** |

From Nyström *et al.* (1995)

(0.96–1.00) (Nyström *et al.*, 2002; Table 23).

*Model for statistical analysis:* In all the trials except for part of that in Malmö (women born between 1908 and 1922) and part of the Two-county trial (women aged 70–74 years at randomization), the controls were later also invited to screening. Deaths among women whose breast cancer was diagnosed after the controls had completed screening

## Table 21. Effect of source of information on cause of death and of end-point measure on the relative risk (RR) for death from breast cancer among women aged 40–74 years at entry; follow-up until 31 December 1989

| Source | Cause of death | No. of breast cancer deaths | | RR | 95% CI |
|---|---|---|---|---|---|
| | | Invited | Control | | |
| End-point committee | Breast cancer underlying cause | 418 | 425 | 0.77 | 0.67–0.88 |
| | Breast cancer present at death | 440 | 442 | 0.79 | 0.69–0.90 |
| Statistics Sweden | Breast cancer underlying cause | 419 | 409 | 0.80 | 0.70–0.92 |
| | Breast cancer underlying plus contributory cause | 480 | 472 | 0.79 | 0.70–0.90 |

From Nyström *et al.* (1995)
CI, confidence interval

**Table 22. Effect of source of information on cause of death and of end-point measure on relative risk estimate by trial and age at entry; follow-up until 31 December 1989**

| Trial | Age at entry | End-point committee | | Statistics Sweden | |
|---|---|---|---|---|---|
| | | Underlying cause | Present at death | Underlying cause | Underlying plus contributory cause |
| Malmö I | 45–70 | 0.81 | 0.85 | 0.83 | 0.82 |
| Kopparberg | 40–74 | 0.68 | 0.73 | 0.67 | 0.68 |
| Östergötland | 40–74 | 0.82 | 0.78 | 0.89 | 0.87 |
| Stockholm | 40–65 | 0.80 | 0.81 | 0.84 | 0.82 |
| Göteborg | 40–59 | 0.86 | 0.84 | 0.93 | 0.87 |
| Overview | 40–49 | 0.90 | 0.92 | 0.95 | 0.9 |
| | 50–59 | 0.72 | 0.71 | 0.76 | 0.74 |
| | 60–69 | 0.69 | 0.75 | 0.69 | 0.75 |
| | 70–74 | 0.98 | 0.92 | 1.05 | 0.86 |
| | *40–74* | *0.77* | *0.79* | *0.80* | *0.79* |

From Nyström *et al.* (1995)

**Table 23. Mortality from all causes among women invited to screening and controls in the Swedish trials; follow-up model; follow-up until 31 December 1996**

| Trial | Age at randomization | No. of woman–years x 1000 | | Total no. of deaths | | Relative risk | 95% CI |
|---|---|---|---|---|---|---|---|
| | | Invited | Control | Invited | Control | | |
| Malmö I | 45–70 | 360 | 362 | 5 672 | 5 796 | 0.99 | 0.97–1.01 |
| Malmö II | 43–49 | 113 | 86 | 402 | 300 | 1.03 | 0.89–1.20 |
| Östergötland | 40–74 | 589 | 572 | 10 357 | 10 036 | 0.98 | 0.95–1.01 |
| Stockholm | 40–65 | 534 | 296 | 4 537 | 2 572 | 0.99 | 0.95–1.03 |
| Göteborg | 40–59 | 268 | 373 | 1 430 | 2 241 | 0.94 | 0.88–1.00 |
| Overview | 40–49 | 697 | 620 | 2 622 | 2 325 | 1.00 | 0.95–1.06 |
| | 50–59 | 709 | 677 | 6 398 | 6 464 | 0.95 | 0.92–0.98 |
| | 60–69 | 397 | 332 | 9 637 | 8 542 | 0.94 | 0.91–0.97 |
| | 70–74 | 62 | 59 | 3 741 | 3 614 | 0.99 | 0.91–1.07 |
| | *40–74* | *1865* | *1689* | *22 398* | *20 945* | *0.98* | *0.96–1.00* |
| | *40–74* | | | | | *0.98 [a]* | *0.96–1.00* |

From Nyström *et al.* (2002); CI, confidence interval
[a] Age-adjusted estimate

cannot contribute useful information about the effects of screening (Nyström *et al.*, 1993). Therefore, in addition to the traditional approach of following all breast cancer cases diagnosed between the date of randomization and the date of follow-up, this 'follow-up' model was complemented by an 'evaluation' model, which, by ignoring deaths in breast cancer cases diagnosed after the first round of screening of the control group was completed, minimized the dilution of screening effects originating from cancers detected after completion of the first screening of the controls.

*Follow-up through 1996*
For this follow-up, the Kopparberg part of the Two-county trial was not available for analysis, but the continuation of the Malmö trial was (Nyström *et al.*, 2002). Statistics Sweden was used as the source for cause of death. Initially, a pooled analysis was performed; thereafter, the analysis was stratified by age group, trial and age group and trial. As the stratified analysis gave the same results as the pooled analysis, only the results of the pooled data analysis are presented below, and as the results of

the follow-up and evaluation models were similar, the results from the evaluation model are presented.

With a median trial time of 6.5 years (range, 3.0–18.1) and a median follow-up time of 15.8 years (5.8–20.2) (Table 24), there was a significant, 20% reduction in breast cancer mortality (RR, 0.80; 95% CI, 0.71–0.90) (Table 25). Table 25 also presents the results for all ages combined for each of the trials considered and the results for all trials combined by age.

With regard to total mortality, there were 22 398 deaths in 1 864 770 woman–years in the invited group and 20 945 in 1 688 440 woman–years in the control group, resulting in a relative risk of 0.98 (95% CI, 0.96–1.00) (Table 23).

[The Working Group considered that the latest published data from each of the Swedish trials were valid and should be included in its evaluation.]

### On-going trials
#### United Kingdom
In 1991, a national, multicentre randomized controlled trial was set up by the United Kingdom Coordinating Committee on Cancer Research (Moss, 1999). The aim was to recruit 195 000 women aged 40–41 years, with 65 000 forming a study group and the remaining 130 000 a control group. Women in the study group are invited for annual screening by mammography and become eligible for the National Health Service Breast Screening Programme after the age of 50.

#### Singapore
During a 2-year period starting on 1 October 1994, 67 656 women in Singapore aged 50–64 were randomized to two-view mammography and 97 294 to the control group. Only 28 231 (42%) participated in the first screening round, suggesting that issues related to acceptability require further study (Ng et al., 1998). No evaluation of the effect on breast cancer mortality has been reported.

#### Slovenia
In 1989, 12 400 women aged 50–64 living in three regions of Slovenia were randomized to clinical breast examination, instruction in breast self-examination and a single medio-lateral view mammogram or to a control group with no intervention. The women in the intervention arm were then offered clinical examination and mammography at a screening interval of 24–36 months. The first follow-up of breast cancer mortality is planned to cover the period 1989–2000 (Rudolf, 1994).

### The Working Group's overview of all trials
Table 19 summarizes the most recently published results from the trials described above for women aged 40–74. Altogether, the trials included over 350 000 women in the intervention groups and 306 000 in the control groups, who were followed for an average of 14.1 years, giving a total of 9.2 million woman–years of follow-up. There were 1241 deaths from breast cancer in the intervention groups and 1331 in the control groups.

Among the women included in the randomized trials of mammography alone versus no screening, 107 700 were aged 40–49 at recruitment and 336 300 were aged 50–69 (Tables 26 and 27). The total number of deaths from breast cancer in the intervention and

**Table 24. Trial time for women invited to screening by age at randomization and trial, i.e. from date of randomization until the control group had undergone the first round of screening, or follow-up time until 31 December 1996**

| Trial | Age group | Trial time (years) | | Follow-up time (years) | |
|---|---|---|---|---|---|
| | | Median | Range | Median | Range |
| Malmö I | 45–70 | 18.8 | 13.9–20.2 | 19.2 | 18.3–20.2 |
| Malmö II | 43–49 | 5.8 | 3.1–18.1 | 9.1 | 5.8–18.3 |
| Östergötland | 40–74 | 7.7 | 6.5–10.9 | 17.4 | 15.8–18.6 |
| Stockholm | 40–65 | 4.4 | 3.2–4.8 | 14.9 | 13.6–15.8 |
| Göteborg | 40–59 | 6.7 | 4.8–7.5 | 13.3 | 12.7–14.0 |
| Overview | 40–49 | 6.6 | 3.0–18.1 | 14.8 | 5.8–19.8 |
| | 50–59 | 4.9 | 3.2–8.7 | 15.6 | 13.3–20.2 |
| | 60–69 | 7.0 | 3.2–10.9 | 17.4 | 13.6–19.8 |
| | 70–74 | 9.2 | 6.6–10.9 | 17.4 | 15.8–18.6 |
| | 40–74 | 6.5 | 3.0–18.1 | 15.8 | 5.8–20.2 |

From Nyström et al. (2002)

**Table 25. Numbers of 1000 woman–years and numbers of cases of breast cancer as the underlying cause of death according to Statistics Sweden among women invited to screening and controls by age at randomization; evaluation model; follow-up until 31 December 1996**

| Trial | No. of woman-years | | No. of deaths | | Relative risk | 95% CI |
|---|---|---|---|---|---|---|
| | Intervention | Control | Intervention | Control | | |
| Malmö I | 360 | 362 | 161 | 198 | 0.81 [a] | 0.66–1.00 |
| Malmö II | 113 | 86 | 29 | 33 | 0.65 [a] | 0.39–1.08 |
| Östergötland | 589 | 572 | 177 | 190 | 0.89 [a] | 0.72–1.09 |
| Stockholm | 535 | 296 | 82 | 50 | 0.90 [a] | 0.63–1.28 |
| Göteborg | 268 | 373 | 62 | 113 | 0.78 | 0.57–1.07 |
| Overview (age at randomization) | | | | | | |
| 40–49 | 697 | 620 | 140 | 155 | 0.80 | 0.63–1.01 |
| 50–59 | 709 | 677 | 206 | 235 | 0.84 | 0.70–1.01 |
| 60–69 | 397 | 332 | 133 | 168 | 0.67 | 0.53–0.84 |
| 70–74 | 62 | 59 | 32 | 26 | 1.18 | 0.71–1.97 |
| 40–74 | 1865 | 1688 | 511 | 584 | 0.80 [a] | 0.71–0.90 |

From Nyström et al. (2002); CI, confidence interval
[a] Age-adjusted estimate

control groups in these trials were 166 and 173, respectively, among women aged 40–49 and 496 and 549, respectively, among women aged 50–69. The combined estimates of relative risk for death from breast cancer in these trials were 0.81 (0.65–1.01) and 0.75 (0.67–0.85), respectively.

In the trials in which one-view mammography was used (Kopperberg, Östergötland and Stockholm), the relative risk for death from breast cancer in the group given mammography versus the unscreened group was 0.77 (95% CI, 0.62–0.92). In the trials with pre-dominantly two-view mammography (Göteborg, Malmö I and II and Finland), the corresponding figure was 0.78 (95% CI, 0.62–0.94). The exclusion or inclusion of any particular trial in the evaluation did not materially alter the overall estimates in Table 26 or 27. Further, addition of the Health Insurance Plan study, in which mammography plus clinical breast examination was compared with no screening,

did not significantly change the overall estimate of effect for women aged 50–69 (OR, 0.80; 95% CI, 0.73–0.87). However, addition of the Health Insurance Plan study and the study in Canada of women aged 40–49 to the trials of mammography alone among women age 40–49 resulted in an odds ratio of 0.88 (95% CI, 0.74–1.04).

The results of the trials in which the outcomes for women invited for mammography alone were compared with those for women given no screening can be used to estimate the absolute reduction in the number of deaths from breast cancer among women some time after screening. The results shown in Tables 26 and 27 indicate that the reduction in mortality from breast cancer over a 10-year period after first invitation for screening would be 0.5 per 1000 women aged 40–49 and 0.9 per 1000 women aged 50–59. Figure 29 gives the relevant results from the Swedish overview.

The estimate of reduction in breast cancer mortality from an 'intention to treat' analysis can be translated into an estimate of the reduction for women who are actually screened by taking account of lack of compliance in the invited arm and dilution in the control arm (Cuzick et al., 1997). The reduction in breast cancer mortality among women aged 50–69 presenting for screening was estimated to be about 39% on the basis of the early results of the Swedish trials (Day, 1991).

[Similar calculations based on the most recently published data from the Swedish trials give an estimate of 35% for women aged 50–69 at entry to the trial, who presented for screening.]

### Age-specific effects of screening

Only the Canadian trial in women aged 40–49 was designed to estimate the effect of screening during a limited age interval. The hypothesis that there might be a differential effect of screening by age was raised in the early analyses of

## Table 26. Efficacy of screening for breast cancer by mammography alone in women aged 40–49

| Trial | Enrollment (years/age) | Intervention (invitation to screening) | Population x 1000 (screened/control) | Breast cancer mortality per 100 000 person-years (number) (screened/control) | | RR (95% CI) |
|---|---|---|---|---|---|---|
| Malmo I, Sweden | 1976–78/45–49 | 4 in 8 years | 4.0/4.1 | 34 (24)/45 (33) | | 0.74 (0.44–1.25) |
| Malmo II, Sweden | 1978–90/43–49 | 4 in 8 years | 9.6/8.2 | 26 (29)/38 (33) | | 0.65 (0.39–1.08) |
| Kopparberg, Swedish Two-county | 1976–78/40–49 | 3 in 6 years | 9.5/5.1 | 14 (26)/18 (18) | | 0.76 (0.42–1.40) |
| Östergötland, Swedish Two-county | 1978–81/40–49 | 4 in 8 years | 10.3/10.5 | 18 (31)/17 (30) | | 1.05 (0.64–1.71) |
| Stockholm, Sweden | 1981–83/40–49 | 2 in 4 years | 14.3/8.0 | 17 (34)/11 (13) | | 1.52 (0.80–2.88) |
| Göteborg, Sweden | 1982–84/40–49 | 3 in 5 years | 10.9/13.2 | 16 (22)/28 (46) | | 0.58 (0.35–0.96) |
| **All trials** | | | 58.6/49.1 | 19 (166)/24 (173) | | **0.81 (0.65–1.01)** |

Tests for heterogeneity between trials $\chi^2_5$ = 7.34; $p$ > 0.1; not significant

the Health Insurance Plan trial (Shapiro et al., 1971). Subsequently, as summarized earlier in this chapter, all the trials were analysed by age. Several biological phenomena are relevant to screening of women aged 40–49 that might explain the lower efficacy of screening, including greater breast density, resulting in lower sensitivity of mammography (see Chapter 2), and the lower detection rates on screening, with lower prevalence and incidence ratios and higher proportionate rates of interval cancers (Fletcher et al., 1993).

Although the only trial to include women aged 70–74 did not find a significant effect of mammographic screening (Tabár et al., 1992), the participation rate of this group was poor, and

only two screens were offered. However, there is no biological reason to expect less effectiveness in this age group than among women aged 60–69, apart from the slower growth rate of tumours in older persons.

[The Working Group decided not to present a pooled estimate for all age groups, because of the differences in potential efficacy for women under and over the age of 50.]

### Frequency of mammographic screening

In most of the randomized controlled trials, a 1–2-year screening interval was used. In the Swedish Two-county trial, a 24-month interval was used for women aged 40–49 and a 33-month interval for

women aged ≥ 50. Although no formal comparison has been made, Tables 26 and 27 suggest no major difference in efficacy by screening interval.

The effect of annual versus 3-yearly mammography screening in increasing the likelihood of an improved outcome was tested in one trial (Breast Screening Frequency Trial Group, 2002). The measured outcomes included tumour size, nodal status and histological grade of invasive tumours. These data were fitted into two models to predict breast cancer mortality. Although the tumours diagnosed in the women in the study arm were significantly smaller than those in the control arm, there was no difference in terms of nodal status and histology grade. The relative risks for predicted

**Table 27. Efficacy of screening for breast cancer by mammography alone in women aged 50–69**

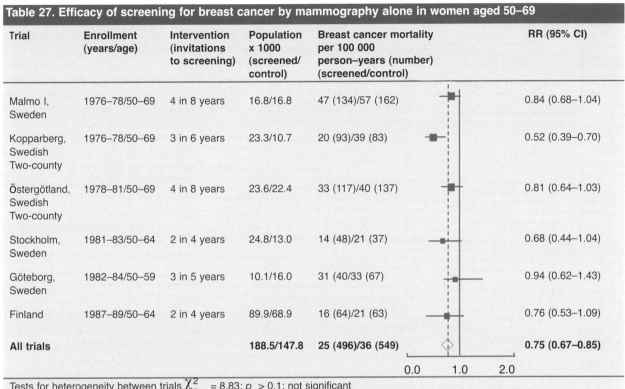

| Trial | Enrollment (years/age) | Intervention (invitations to screening) | Population x 1000 (screened/ control) | Breast cancer mortality per 100 000 person–years (number) (screened/control) | RR (95% CI) |
|---|---|---|---|---|---|
| Malmö I, Sweden | 1976–78/50–69 | 4 in 8 years | 16.8/16.8 | 47 (134)/57 (162) | 0.84 (0.68–1.04) |
| Kopparberg, Swedish Two-county | 1976–78/50–69 | 3 in 6 years | 23.3/10.7 | 20 (93)/39 (83) | 0.52 (0.39–0.70) |
| Östergötland, Swedish Two-county | 1978–81/50–69 | 4 in 8 years | 23.6/22.4 | 33 (117)/40 (137) | 0.81 (0.64–1.03) |
| Stockholm, Sweden | 1981–83/50–64 | 2 in 4 years | 24.8/13.0 | 14 (48)/21 (37) | 0.68 (0.44–1.04) |
| Göteborg, Sweden | 1982–84/50–59 | 3 in 5 years | 10.1/16.0 | 31 (40/33 (67) | 0.94 (0.62–1.43) |
| Finland | 1987–89/50–64 | 2 in 4 years | 89.9/68.9 | 16 (64)/21 (63) | 0.76 (0.53–1.09) |
| **All trials** | | | **188.5/147.8** | **25 (496)/36 (549)** | **0.75 (0.67–0.85)** |

Tests for heterogeneity between trials $\chi^2_5$ = 8.83; $p$ > 0.1; not significant

deaths from breast cancer for annual versus 3-yearly screening were 0.95 (95% CI, 0.83–1.07) and 0.89 (95% CI, 0.77–1.03) in the two models.

## Cohort and nested case–control studies

In 1973, the American Cancer Society initiated the Breast Cancer Detection Demonstration Project, a collaborative effort with the National Cancer Institute, to demonstrate the feasibility of large-scale screening for breast cancer (Beahrs et al., 1979; Baker, 1982). A total of 280 000 volunteer women aged 35–74 were recruited at 27 locations and screened annually for 5 years with two-view mammography, clinical breast examination and, up to 1977, thermography. The project was not designed for evaluation of the effectiveness of mammography screening; however,

Morrison et al. (1988) followed-up 55 053 white women for 9 years and, by calculating the 'expected' mortality from breast cancer for women without diagnosed breast cancer at the start of observation, they estimated ratios (observed: expected deaths from breast cancer) of 0.89, 0.76 and 0.74 for women aged 35–49, 50–59 and 60–74 years, respectively, at entry. [No confidence intervals or p values were reported.]

In 1974, de Waard et al. (1984a) set up a population-based study of periodic screening of women aged 50–64 years in Utrecht, The Netherlands. Of 20 555 invited women, 14 796 (72%) attended the first of four rounds (ended in 1987 when the national programme was launched). The intervals between successive screening rounds were 12, 18, 24 and 48 months. The effect of the programme on mortality from breast can-

cer was evaluated in nested case–control studies (Table 28), which showed a significant reduction in mortality for women who had ever been screened when compared with those who had never been screened (OR, 0.30; 95% CI, 0.13–0.70) (Collette et al., 1984). The odds ratios for women aged 50–54, 55–59, 60–64 and 65–69 at diagnosis were 1.13, 0.31, 0 and 0.10, respectively. These estimates were based on small numbers, and no confidence intervals were given.

In 1975, a population-based screening programme was set up in the city of Nijmegen (150 000 inhabitants), The Netherlands (Peeters et al., 1989a). The first screening round, in 1975–76, involved 23 000 women born in 1910–39, who were thus 35–64 years old. In the subsequent screening rounds, the same birth cohort was invited, as well

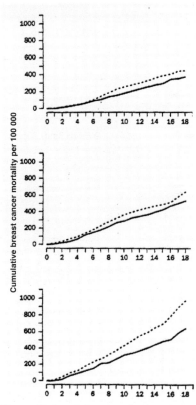

**Figure 29** Cumulative mortality from breast cancer per 100 000 among women aged 40–49, 50–59 and 60–69 years at time of invitation to screening and among controls in the Swedish overview; evaluation model; follow-up until December 1996

From Nyström et al. (2002)

as 7700 women born before 1910. The odds ratio for death from breast cancer estimated in a case–control analysis were 1.2 (95% CI, 0.31–4.8) for women aged 35–49, 0.26 (95% CI, 0.10–0.67) for those aged 50–64 and 0.81 (95% CI, 0.23–2.8) for women aged ≥ 65 (Verbeek et al., 1985).

Between 1970 and 1980, 33 000 women aged 40–70 years living in 24 municipalities in Florence, Italy, were invited to mammographic screening with cranio-caudal and mediolateral–oblique views every 2.5 years. In 1989, the study area was extended to include the city of

Florence. Palli et al. (1986, 1989) used a nested case–control approach to estimate the impact on breast cancer mortality (Table 28). The odds ratios for women aged 40–49 and ≥ 50 at diagnosis were estimated to be 0.63 (0.24–1.6) and 0.51 (0.29–0.89), respectively. [The estimates of risk by age at diagnosis instead of age at initiation of screening are confounded by lead time.]

The nested case–control approach was also used by Thompson, R.S. et al. (1994) to evaluate the effect of a screening programme in Washington State, USA, in 1982–88. The cohort consisted of 94 656 women aged ≥ 40 years. During the study, there were 1144 incident cases of breast cancer, including 126 deaths. A randomly selected subsample representing 2.4% of the cohort constituted the control group. With a mean follow-up of 3.5 years after screening, the relative risk for mortality from breast cancer in screened as compared with unscreened women was 0.80 (0.34–1.8) for women aged ≥ 40 and 0.61 (0.23–1.6) for women aged ≥ 50.

Two of the randomized controlled trials, the Health Insurance Plan trial (Friedman & Dubin, 1991) and one Malmö trial (Janzon & Andersson, 1990; Güllberg et al., 1991), were also evaluated in nested case–control studies (Table 28). For a discussion of the methodological issues related to these nested case–control studies, see above.

A meta-analysis of the Utrecht, Nijmegen, Florence, United Kingdom and Malmö case–control studies resulted in an odds ratio of 0.44 (95% CI, 0.38–0.50) for screened versus unscreened women, with a slightly lower odds ratio for women in programmes in which mammography was combined with clinical breast examination (OR, 0.37; 95% CI, 0.30–0.45) as compared with mammography alone (OR, 0.49; 95% CI, 0.42–0.58) (Demissie et al., 1998).

[The estimates in Table 28 should be treated with caution as they may be biased (see above).]

## Quasi-experimental study

In the Trial of Early Detection of Breast Cancer in the United Kingdom, set up in 1979, women aged 45–64 years were invited to screening at one of two centres, in Edinburgh and Guildford, every year for 7 years, by mammography and clinical breast examination every 2 years and by clinical breast examination only in the intervening years (UK Trial of Early Detection of Breast Cancer Group, 1988). Women in the same age range in the comparison centres were identified but were offered no additional services. The rate of mortality from breast cancer was 27% lower (rate ratio, 0.73; 95% CI, 0.63–0.84) in the two screening centres combined than in the control centres. The rate ratios for women aged 45–49, 50–54, 55–59 and 60–64 were 0.70 (0.57–0.86), 0.79 (0.62–1.0), 0.71 (0.51–0.90) and 0.72 (0.56–0.92), respectively (UK Trial of Early Detection of Breast Cancer Group, 1999).

## Efficacy of screening by clinical breast examination

Estimating the efficacy of clinical breast examination alone in reducing breast cancer mortality is hindered by the paucity of relevant data. No randomized trial of clinical breast examination compared with no screening has been completed. Indirect evidence of efficacy is based on comparisons by size, nodal status and stage of disease of tumours detected by clinical breast examination with others means of detection; comparison of the survival of women with cancers detected by clinical breast examination in contrast to mammography; and the results of a randomized trial in which breast cancer mortality was compared in women given breast examinations alone with that in women who received combined screening by mammography and clinical breast examination (Miller et al., 2000, 2002).

## Table 28. Results of selected case–control studies of mammography with and without clinical breast examination

| Reference | Study or location | Year of start | No. of start views | Clinical breast examination | Screening interval (months) | Age at entry | Attendance rate in rounds (years) 1 and 2 | Follow-up (years) | No. of women Cases | No. of women Controls | Odds ratio | 95% CI |
|---|---|---|---|---|---|---|---|---|---|---|---|---|
| Friedman & Dubin (1991) | Health Insurance Plan, USA | 1963 | 2 | Yes | 12 | 40–64 | 67, 53 | 16 | 95 | 380 | 0.54 | 0.24–1.23 |
| Palli et al. (1986, 1989) | Florence, Italy | 1970 | 2 | No | 30 | 40–70 | 60, NR | 7 / 10 | 57 / 103 | 285 / 515 | 0.53 / 0.53 | 0.29–0.95 / 0.33–0.85 |
| Collette et al. (1984, 1992) | Utrecht, Netherlands | 1974 | 2 | Yes | 12–48 | 50–64 | 72, 60 | 7 / 12 | 46 / 116 | 138 / 348 | 0.30 / 0.52 | 0.13–0.71 / 0.32–0.83 |
| Verbeek et al. (1984, 1985); van Dijck et al. (1994) | Nijmegen, Netherlands | 1975 | 1 | No | 24 | 35–64 / 65–74 | 85, 65 | 7 / 8 / 12 | 46 / 62 / 33 | 230 / 310 / 165 | 0.48 / 0.51 / 0.58 | 0.23–1.00 / 0.20–0.99 / 0.24–1.41 |
| Janzon & Andersson (1990); Güllberg et al. (1991) | Malmö, Sweden | 1976 | 2 | No | 1824 | 45–69 | 74, 70 | 12 | 60 | 300 | 0.42 | 0.22–0.78 |
| Moss et al. (1992) | Guildford, United Kingdom | 1979 | 1 | Yes | 24 | 45–64 | 72, NR | 7 | 51 | 255 | 0.51 | 0.27–0.98 |

CI, confidence interval; NR, not reported

The studies have found consistently that the percentage of tumours diagnosed at an early stage is higher with detection by clinical breast examination than those found by the women themselves but lower than with detection by mammography (Table 29). The largest of these studies was a nationwide study on mass screening for breast cancer involving clinical breast examination with or without instruction in self-examination, sponsored by the Ministry of Health and Welfare of Japan in 11 regions. Ota et al. (1989) compared the clinical stage and the survival rate of 728 patients with breast cancer detected during mass screening (726 by clinical breast examination) with those of 1450 patients in outpatient clinics, after matching on treatment facility, age and year of treatment. The proportion of cases detected at stage Tis, 0 or I was 41% with detection during mass screening and 29% of those diagnosed in outpatient clinics.

Nodal status at the time of detection in the Health Insurance Plan study (Shapiro et al., 1988), in the Breast Cancer Detection Demonstration Project (Beahrs et al., 1979) and in the Canadian National Breast Screening trial of women aged 50–59 (Miller et al., 1992b) is shown in Table 30. In the Health Insurance Plan study and in the Breast Cancer Detection Demonstration Project (in which both mammography and clinical breast examination were provided), clinical breast examination alone and mammography alone resulted in detection of similar proportions of node-negative tumours. However, the large proportions of cancers for which the mode of detection was unknown in the latter study makes the result questionable. Furthermore, the observations in these two studies probably reflect the lower quality of mammography in the 1960s and 1970s than in more recent years. In the Canadian National Breast Screening trial, annual clinical breast examination alone was associated with a lower pro-

## Table 29. Stage at diagnosis according to detection method

| Reference (country) | Definition of early disease | Mammography only | | Clinical breast examination only | | Not detected at screening | |
|---|---|---|---|---|---|---|---|
| | | Total no. of cases | % early stage | Total no. of cases | % early stage | Total no. of cases | % early stage |
| Smith et al. (1980) (USA) | In situ plus local | | | 54 | 64 | 57 | 58 |
| Seidman et al. (1987) (USA) | Intraductal plus in situ plus invasive < 1 cm | 1375 | 35 | 257 | 16 | 692 | 16 |
| Shapiro et al. (1988a) (USA) | Intraductal plus in situ plus local | 44 | 39 | 59 | 14 | 295[a] | 8.1 |
| Ota et al. (1989) (Japan) | TNM stage Tis or 0 or I | | | 728 | 41 | 1450 | 29 |
| Senie et al. (1994) (USA) | Axillary node negative | 30 | 90 | 101 | 73 | 598 | 56 |
| Ohuchi et al. (1995) (Japan) | In situ plus invasive < 1 cm | 35[b] | 26 | 44 | 9.1 | | |
| McPherson et al. (1997)[c] (USA) | Localized | 293 | 76 | 114 | 56 | 364 | 53 |
| Koibuchi et al. (1998) (Japan) | TNM stage Tis or 0 or I | | | 178 | 44 | 587 | 30.7 |
| Miller et al. (2002)[c] (Canada) | Invasive < 9 mm | 69 | 33 | 58 | 12 | NA | NA |
| Miller et al. (2000) (Canada)[d] | Invasive < 9 mm | 126 | 29 | 148 | 4.0 | NA | NA |

[a] Controls in randomized trial
[b] Includes cases diagnosed by mammography plus clinical breast examination
[c] Limited to women 40–49 years of age at enrollment
[d] Limited to women 50–59 years of age at enrollment

portion of node-negative tumours than was combined screening.

The survival rate was more favourable in cases detected by mammography than by clinical breast examination (Table 31). This is consistent with the data on stage of diagnosis shown in Table 29 and suggests that there is a longer lead time with detection by mammography than by clinical breast examination. The differences in the survival of women whose tumours were detected by clinical breast examination and by other means are small and not consistent among studies. The differ-

ence in 10-year survival reported by Ota et al. (1989) was not statistically significant, but the difference at 5 years was (92% for clinical breast examination; 86% for other modalities; $p < 0.01$).

The results of the Canadian National Breast Screening study (Miller et al., 1992a,b, 2000, 2002) are shown in Table 32. The survival rate after 7 years was only slightly better for women whose tumours were detected by mammography than for those whose tumours were detected by clinical breast examination. The absence of a difference in mortality from breast cancer after 13 years

suggests either that clinical breast examination was as effective as mammography plus clinical breast examination in reducing deaths from breast cancer or that neither affected breast cancer mortality in these trials.

In Japan, screening for breast cancer has been conducted mainly by breast examination by physicians. In a comparison of the change in age-adjusted death rate between 1986–90 and 1991–95, the average coverage rates for breast cancer screening per year for women aged 30–69 years were calculated for 3255 municipalities. Those with average

## Table 30. Nodal status at diagnosis according to method of detection (%)

| Nodal status | Detected during first 5 years in Health Insurance Plan Study | | | Canadian National Breast Screening Trial | | | Breast Cancer Detection Demonstration Project (first screening) | | |
|---|---|---|---|---|---|---|---|---|---|
| | Mammo-graphy | CBE alone | Both | Mammo-graphy | CBE alone | Both | Mammo-graphy | CBE alone | Both |
| Negative | 77 | 76 | 48 | 65 | 58 | 70 | 67 | 55 | |
| Positive | 16 | 19 | 41 | 26 | 36 | 10 | 17 | 26 | |
| Unknown | 7 | 5 | 11 | 9 | 5 | 20 | 17 | 19 | |

From Beahrs *et al.* (1979); Shapiro *et al.* (1988); Miller *et al.* (1992b)
CBE, clinical breast examination

## Table 31. Survival from breast cancer according to method of detection

| Reference (country) | Years of follow-up | Mammography only | | Clinical breast examination only | | Not detected by screening | |
|---|---|---|---|---|---|---|---|
| | | Total no. of cases | Survival (%) | Total no. of cases | Survival (%) | Total no. of cases | Survival (%) |
| Shapiro *et al.* (1982) (USA) | 12 | 44 | 68 | 59 | 56 | 294[a] | 43 |
| Seidman *et al.* (1987) (USA) | 10 | 1375 | 85 | 257 | 76 | 692 | 78 |
| Ota *et al.* (1989) (Japan) | 10 | | | 720 | 80 | 1440 | 78 |
| Senie *et al.* (1994) (USA) | 10 | 30 | 83 | 101 | 73 | 598 | 64 |
| McPherson *et al.* (1997)[b] (USA) | 8 | 293 | 88 | 114 | 71 | 364 | 75 |
| Koibuchi *et al.* (1998) (Japan) | 10 | | | 178 | 88 | 587 | 82 |
| Stacey-Clear *et al.* (1992) (USA) | 5 | 117 | 95 | 928 | 74 | NA | NA |

NA, not applicable
[a] Controls in randomized trial
[b] Limited to women 40–49 years of age at enrollment

coverage rates of 20–40% and more were each compared with two municipalities selected as 'controls' and matched on population, national health insurance rate and the age-adjusted death rate from cancer of the female breast in 1986–90. The percentage reduction in death rate in the high coverage-rate municipalities was statistically significantly greater than those in the control groups (Kuroishi *et al.*, 2000; Table 33).

Kanemura *et al.* (1999) conducted a case–control study of clinical breast examination in two Japanese prefectures (Miyagi and Gunma). Women who had died of breast cancer between January 1993 and December 1995 were identified from residential registers and medical records. Controls matched for year of birth (within 2 years), sex and address (administrative district) were

## Table 32. Outcomes in the Canadian National Breast Screening trials by method of detection of breast cancer

| | Women aged 40–49 | | Women aged 50–59 | |
| --- | --- | --- | --- | --- |
| | Mammography (n = 25 214) | Usual care (one clinical breast examination) (n = 25 216) | Mammography (n = 19 711) | Clinical breast examination only (n = 19 694) |
| *7-year survival after diagnosis (%)* | | | | |
| Mammography alone | 95 | NA | 92 | NA |
| Clinical breast examination alone | 89 | 91 | 89 | 87 |
| Both | 86 | NA | 86 | NA |
| *No. of deaths from breast cancer at 13-year follow-up* | 105 | 108 | 107 | 105 |

From Miller *et al.* (1992a,b, 2000, 2002)
NA, not applicable

## Table 33. Age-adjusted rates of death from cancer of the breast in areas of Japan with an average coverage rate ≥ 20% and control areas

| Coverage, by age | No. of municipalities | Coverage rate by screening (%) | 1986–90 | | 1991–95 | | Change in ADR (%) |
| --- | --- | --- | --- | --- | --- | --- | --- |
| | | | No. of deaths | ADR | No. of deaths | ADR | |
| All ages | | | | | | | |
| High coverage | 247 | 27 | 695 | 4.56 | 7.09 | 4.39 | −3.7* |
| Control | 494 | 8.5 | 5 144 | 5.09 | 6 346 | 5.62 | 10.6 |
| 30–69 years | | | | | | | |
| High coverage | 247 | 27 | 557 | 7.56 | 512 | 6.91 | −8.7** |
| Control | 494 | 8.5 | 4 133 | 8.18 | 4 884 | 8.84 | 8.2 |

From Kuroishi *et al.* (2000)
ADR, age-adjusted death rate per 100 000
* $p < 0.05$; ** $p < 0.01$

selected randomly from the same registers. Screening history during 5 years before the date of diagnosis of cases was ascertained from the files of the screening facilities, and 93 cases and 375 controls were eligible for analysis. The odds ratio for death from breast cancer was 0.93 (95% CI, 0.48–1.79) and 0.59 (95% CI, 0.31–1.14) after participation in screening at least once in the 1-year and 5-year intervals before diagno-

sis, respectively (Table 34). More cases than controls were symptomatic at screening. When women who had had symptoms in their breasts were classified as not screened, the odds ratio decreased to 0.56 (95% CI, 0.27–1.18) for the 1-year interval and 0.45 (0.22–0.89) for the 5-year interval.

It is likely that a careful protocol for clinical breast examination will be required if this technique is to be used

effectively. This will require standardized training of examiners (see Chapter 2). Furthermore, if clinical breast examination is used in a screening programme, there must be complete follow-up of all women with abnormal findings. This might be difficult to achieve in developing countries, as found in a randomized controlled trial of clinical breast examination in the Philippines (IARC, 1997): only 30% of women who were found to have

**Table 34. Odds ratios for death from breast cancer among women in Japan participating in screening at least once during the index interval**

| Interval[a] | Cases | | Controls | | Odds ratio | 95% CI |
|---|---|---|---|---|---|---|
| | No. | % participated[b] | No. | % participated[b] | | |
| 1 | 93 | 17 | 375 | 18 | 0.93 | 0.48–1.79 |
| 2 | 88 | 24 | 347 | 25 | 0.86 | 0.46–1.60 |
| 3 | 83 | 24 | 328 | 31 | 0.63 | 0.33–1.18 |
| 4 | 80 | 25 | 319 | 33 | 0.57 | 0.30–1.07 |
| 5 | 75 | 25 | 299 | 33 | 0.59 | 0.31–1.14 |

From Kanemura et al. (1999); CI, confidence interval
[a] Years before diagnosis of case
[b] Percentage of women who had ever participated in screening within each interval

abnormalities at screening received a definitive diagnosis after assessment.

Thus, cancers detected by clinical breast examination tend to be diagnosed at a slightly earlier stage than those not detected by screening, but this had only a minor impact on survival. One case–control study and one ecological study (both in Japan) suggested that clinical breast examination reduces mortality from breast cancer. In one randomized trial in Canada, mortality from breast cancer was similar among women who received combined screening (mammography and clinical breast examination) and those who had clinical breast examination screening alone.

## Efficacy of screening by breast self-examination

### Randomized trials
Two randomized trials of breast self-examination with mortality from breast cancer as the primary end-point have been conducted. The first, initiated in Moscow and St Petersburg, Russian Federation, were begun in 1985 (Semiglazov et al., 1993). Preliminary results on deaths due to breast cancer have been reported only from the St Petersburg portion of the study (Semiglazov et al., 1992, 1999). In that city, nine polyclinics and five enterprises were randomly selected as intervention facilities, and nine and five, respectively, as control facilities. Women aged 40–64 who received their care in the intervention facilities were invited to participate in the trial. Medical personnel in the clinics examined each woman's breasts, and the women in the intervention facilities were given detailed instruction in breast self-examination. They were also given a calendar to record their monthly practice and asked to return annually for reinforcement sessions. Women in the control clinics received clinical breast examinations alone. The results are summarized in Table 35. Significantly more women in the group given instruction than in the control group were referred for evaluation of a breast lump ($p < 0.05$), and more were found to have a benign lesion. Breast cancer was diagnosed in more women in the group given instruction than in the control group, but the difference could have been due to chance, and the malignant

**Table 35. Results of a randomized trial of breast self-examination in St Petersburg, Russian Federation**

| Feature of study | Group given instruction | Control group |
|---|---|---|
| No. of women | 57 712 | 64 759 |
| No. referred for evaluation | 4 300 (7.5%) | 2 438 (3.8%) |
| No. with breast cancer | 493 (0.9%) | 446 (0.7%) |
| No of deaths from breast cancer after about 10 years of follow-up | 157 (0.27%) | 167 (0.26%) |
| Survival 9 years after date of detection (%) | 65 | 55 |

From Semiglazov et al. (1999)

tumours in the two groups of women did not differ appreciably in size or percentage with axillary node involvement. Although the survival rate 9 years after diagnosis was somewhat more favourable for women who received instruction than in the control group (relative survival, 0.77 in log rank test), the difference was not statistically significant. After approximately 10 years of follow-up, almost equal percentages of women in the two groups had died with breast cancer (0.27% and 0.26%). One possible explanation for these results is poor compliance with the instructions for breast self-examination. In a sample of participants 1 year after training in the technique, 82% of the interviewed women reported practising breast self-examination more than five times per year, and 53% reported monthly practice. However, by year 4, these percentages had dropped to 56% and 18%, respectively. Another possible reason for the results is that breast self-examination is not effective in reducing mortality from breast cancer among women who are also screened by clinical breast examination.

The second randomized trial was conducted in Shanghai, China (Thomas et al., 1997, 2002). Between 1989 and 1991, over 266 000 current and retired 30–64-year-old female employees of the Shanghai Textile Industry Bureau, who worked in 519 different factories, were randomized by factory to receive instruction in breast self-examination or to a control group. Groups of about 10 women received initial instruction in breast self-examination, two reinforcement sessions 1 and 3 years later, consisting of videos and discussion groups, multiple reminders to practise breast self-examination and periodic practice sessions supervised by factory medical workers about every 6 months for 5 years. No breast cancer screening was offered to women in the control group. High levels of participation in the reinforcement and supervised breast

self-examination sessions were documented during the first 4–5 years of the trial, during which time the women practised breast self-examination under medical supervision an average of about once every 4–5 months. Women were encouraged to practise self-examination monthly, but the frequency of practice outside the clinic setting is unknown. Randomly selected women in the intervention group were more proficient in detecting lumps in silicone breast models than the control group. The results after 10–11 years of follow-up are summarized in Table 36. Benign breast lesions were diagnosed in more women in the group given instruction than in the control group (1.8% vs 1.0%). As expected, the numbers of women with breast cancer were similar in the two groups, and the breast cancers in the two groups did not differ appreciably in size (45% vs 42% were ≤ 2 cm) or stage (47% vs 48% had no axillary nodal involvement). Also, the proportion of deaths due to breast cancer (0.1% in each group; odds ratio for death, 1.04; 95% CI, 0.82–1.33) and the cumulative rates of mortality from breast cancer were nearly identical in the two groups, as were the survival rates of women with breast cancer, both from entry into the trial and from date of diagnosis. Evidence was presented that these results are not readily explicable

by an absence of statistical power, insufficient duration or completeness of follow-up, failure of the randomization procedure to select two groups at equal risk for breast cancer, selective exclusion of women after randomization, incomplete or differential ascertainment of breast cancer cases or deaths, screening in the control group or insufficient treatment for breast cancer.

Neither the trial in St Petersburg, where compliance was limited, nor the trial in Shanghai, where the level of compliance was probably as high as could be achieved in a public health programme to promote breast self-examination, showed a reduction in mortality from breast cancer among women taught breast self-examination.

## Cohort studies

Reports are available from three studies in which the rates of death from breast cancer were compared in women who did and did not practise breast self-examination. The results are summarized in Table 37.

As part of the trial for early detection of breast cancer in the United Kingdom (Ellman et al., 1993; UK Trial of Early Detection of Breast Cancer Group, 1999), women in the cities of Huddersfield and Nottingham were invited to attend educational sessions in breast self-examination, including a talk

## Table 36. Results of randomized trial of breast self-examination in Shanghai, China

| Feature of study | Group given instruction | Control group |
|---|---|---|
| No. of women | 132 979 | 133 085 |
| No. with benign breast lesions | 2 387 (1.8%) | 1 296 (1.0%) |
| No. with breast cancer | 864 (0.7%) | 896 (0.7%) |
| No. of deaths from breast cancer after 10–11 years of follow-up | 135 (0.1%) | 131 (0.1%) |

From Thomas et al. (2002)

**Table 37. Ratios of rates of mortality from breast cancer in relation to practice of breast self-examination (BSE) in prospective studies**

| Reference (country) | Years of follow-up | Practised BSE | No. of women | No. of breast cancer deaths | Rate ratio (95% CI) |
|---|---|---|---|---|---|
| Holmberg et al. (1997) (USA) | 13 | Yes | 177 602 | 925 | 1.03[a] (0.95–1.12) |
| | | No | 272 554 | 1375 | 1.00 (reference) |
| Gästrin et al. (1994) (Finland) | 14 | Yes | 29 004 | 95 | 0.71 (0.57-0.87) |
| | | No | General population | 34[b] | 1.00 (reference) |
| | | | | 134 | |
| UK Trial of Early Detection of Breast Cancer Group (1999) (United Kingdom) | 16 | Yes: | | | |
| | | Total | 63 373 | 661 | 0.99[c] (0.87-1.12) |
| | | Huddersfield | Not reported | 187 | 0.79[c] (0.65-0.96) |
| | | Nottingham | Not reported | 474 | 1.09[c] (0.95-1.26) |
| | | No | 127 123 | 1312 | 1.00 (reference) |

[a] Adjusted for age, parity, family history of breast cancer, ages at menarche and first pregnancy and body mass index
[b] Expected on basis of age-specific rates in general population of Finland
[c] Adjusted for age and pre-trial standardized mortality ratio

and a film. In Huddersfield, calendars were sent out annually as reminders and for women to record their monthly breast self-examination practice. The rates of breast cancer mortality among women invited to breast self-examination training (whether or not they attended) were compared with those in four centres in which women received no breast cancer screening or breast self-examination instruction. No overall difference in mortality rates from breast cancer was observed between the women in the two instruction centres combined and the women in the four comparison centres (Table 37). However, the rate ratio in Huddersfield was significantly lower than unity and similar to that observed in the Finnish Mama Program. As in that programme, it was the centre from which calendars were sent, suggesting that the difference might have been due to more intensive breast self-examination practice in Huddersfield. More women in Huddersfield than Nottingham also received breast-conserving surgery, chemotherapy and tamoxifen, whereas the participation rates in the breast

self-examination instruction were higher in Nottingham than in Huddersfield, suggesting that differences in treatment or other factors could explain the discrepant results.

In the Mama Program for Breast Screening (Gästrin et al., 1994), beginning in 1973, groups of 20–50 women in Finland were given detailed instruction in breast self-examination, followed by periodic reminders and annual mailings of calendars for the women to record their practice. Mortality among the participants was compared with that of the general population of Finland. As shown in Table 37, the rate of mortality from breast cancer among the participants was significantly lower than expected (rate ratio, 0.71; 95% CI, 0.57–0.87), in spite of a higher incidence of breast cancer than expected (incidence rate ratio = 1.2). Lower rates of death due to breast cancer were observed among women in most age groups and were most pronounced 3–6 years after entry into the study. However, the mortality rates from all causes were similarly significantly lower (observed

deaths, 2658; standardized mortality ratio = 0.67), suggesting that the participants were generally healthier than women in the general population, and that their lower rate of death from breast cancer was due to factors related to better survival, other than early diagnosis resulting from breast self-examination, which were not controlled for in the analysis.

Holmberg et al. (1997) calculated the rates of death from breast cancer in a cohort of women who, in 1959, were asked: "Many doctors recommend that women examine their breasts monthly. Do you do so?" A "Yes" answer presumably indicated that the woman practised breast self-examination monthly, and a "No" answer indicated she they did so less frequently or not at all. After a 13-year follow-up period, no association was found between breast cancer mortality and the answer to this question. The major strengths of this study are its large size, long follow-up, strong statistical power and control of multiple possible confounders. However, the absence of detailed information on the frequency or manner of breast self-examination practice by the women in the study reduces the usefulness of the negative findings, since many of the women who reported practising self-examination may not have done so adequately.

Two case–control studies nested within randomized trials, which did not rely on self-reported breast self-examination practice, provide additional evidence for a beneficial effect of this practice.

Locker et al. (1989b) performed a case–control analysis of data for women invited to enrol in the Trial of Early Detection of Breast Cancer in Nottingham. Death from from breast cancer more than 3 months after invitation was recorded for 68 of 180 women (38%) who had attended the breast self-examination instruction class and 258 (43%) of 603 age-matched control women at the Nottingham centre, for an estimated relative risk of 0.70 (0.50–0.97). The comparable relative risk estimates in pre- and post-menopausal women were 0.85 (0.45–1.6) and 0.66 (0.45–0.97), respectively. These estimates were not controlled for factors other than age and might be confounded by other risk factors for breast cancer that were also associated with a decision to attend the breast self-examination instruction class.

Harvey, B.J. et al. (1997) conducted a case–control study nested in the Canadian National Breast Screening Study on the basis of answers to questions on the frequency of breast self-examination before enrollment and during the trial and the results of annual assessments of breast self-examination proficiency. Thus, 220 women with fatal or mestastatic disease and 2200 age-matched controls were selected from those enrolled in the trial. Comparison of women who had practised breast self-examination before enrollment with those who had not gave a relative risk for fatal or advanced breast cancer of 1.27 (95% CI, 0.96–1.68). The relative risks

decreased with increasing frequency of breast self-examination practice prior to enrollment. The relative risk for advanced and fatal disease also increased slightly with decreasing frequency of breast self-examination during the trial, but none of the estimates or trends was statistically significant. A significant decrease in relative risk was found with increasing proficiency of breast self-examination, as observed in clinics by trained examiners 2 years before diagnosis of the cases. The level of proficiency was defined by exclusion of visual inspection, use of finger pads and systematic search, three key elements of proper self-examination. Similar but weaker trends in risk were observed in relation to level of proficiency 1 and 3 years before diagnosis, but none of the 95% confidence l imits excluded 1.0. The relative risk estimates were not confounded by family history of breast cancer, age at menarche or menopause, education or occupation.

## Case–control studies

The results of two additional case–control studies were also available.

Muscat and Huncharek (1991) compared 435 women in Connecticut, USA, with regional or distant breast cancer at diagnosis with 887 control women selected by random-digit dialling. Breast self-examination at least once a month was reported by 27% of the patients and 20% of the controls. After control for a family history of breast cancer, age at birth of first child, race and frequency of mammograms, a relative risk of 1.3 (95% CI, 0.77–2.1) was estimated, but it is not clear from the report whether this estimate was for women who practised breast self-examination monthly or also less frequently.

Newcomb et al. (1991) compared self-reported breast self-examination practice by 209 members of a prepaid health plan who developed late-stage (TNM III or IV) breast cancer during a

defined period and 433 age-matched controls selected randomly from members of the same plan. The relative risk for advanced disease in women who had ever practised breast self-examination was 1.15 (95% CI, 0.73–1.81), and, unexpectedly, the relative risk increased with frequency of self-examination.

Both of these studies relied on self-reported practice, and the frequency reported by the women might have been inflated by reports of self-palpation in response to symptoms of breast cancer. The finding in the study of Newcomb et al. (1991), that the relative risks decreased with increasing proficiency in breast self-examination, suggests that women who regularly practised the technique according to rigorous standards may have accrued some benefit. These estimates were controlled for age and frequency of clinical breast examination. Other risk factors for breast cancer were considered as possible confounders but found not to alter the estimates.

The results of these two case–control studies thus provide some additional evidence that breast self-examination may reduce the risk for fatal or advanced breast cancer if practised with a high degree of proficiency.

## Studies of survival

If breast self-examination is effective in preventing deaths from breast cancer, follow-up studies of women with breast cancer should show that those who examined their breasts lived longer than those who did not. In addition, the observed differences in survival should be sufficiently large that they cannot reasonably be attributed to enhanced lead time or length bias sampling. Table 38 summarizes the results of five studies in which the survival after diagnosis of women who either practised or received instruction in breast self-examination was compared with that of women who did not. In the first three studies shown, the observed difference in survival was

## Table 38. Survival from breast cancer in women who did and did not receive instruction in or practice breast self-examination (BSE)

| Reference | Years of follow-up | Definition of BSE practice | Practised BSE | No. of cases | % alive at follow-up |
|---|---|---|---|---|---|
| Foster & Costanza (1984) (USA) | 5<br>5 | History of BSE practice | Yes<br>No | 424<br>411 | 80<br>62 |
| Huguley et al. (1988) (USA) | 8<br>8 | History of BSE practice | Yes<br>No | 1400<br>683 | 70<br>51 |
| Locker et al. (1989a,b) (United Kingdom) | 6 | Accepted invitation to attend BSE instruction | Yes<br>No | 372<br>379 | ~61[a]<br>~40[a] |
| Le Geyte et al. (1992) (United Kingdom) | 6<br>6 | History of being taught BSE | Yes<br>No | 226<br>390 | 73<br>66 |
| Auvinen et al. (1996) (Finland) | 5<br>5 | Frequency of BSE practice | Monthly<br>None | 448<br>104 | 80[b]<br>78[b] |

[a] Estimated from graph
[b] Differences not statistically significant

large, and the authors of the first two studies estimated that a lead time of about 3 years would be necessary to explain their results completely. In the last two studies summarized in the table, the differences in survival were smaller. The results of the study by Le Geyte et al. (1992) could be explained by a lead time of about 18 months, and the differences in survival reported from the Finnish study (Auvinen et al., 1996) could readily have been due to chance. In another study (Senie et al., 1994), conducted in New York City, USA, survival was not associated with the frequency of breast self-examination, but no details were provided.

Three studies addressed the survival of women who detected their breast cancer while practising breast self-examination in comparison with that of women whose neoplasm was detected by other means (Kuroishi et al., 1992; McPherson et al., 1997; Koibuchi et al., 1998). Although all three studies showed a slight survival advantage in women who found their tumour while practising breast self-examination, the differences in the first two studies were small and not statistically significant; in the third study,

the difference could presumably be attributed to greater lead time.

The results of most of the studies of survival were inconsistent with a beneficial effect of breast self-examination on survival from breast cancer, and there are alternative explanations for most of the findings. These studies therefore do not provide strong evidence for the efficacy of breast self-examination in reducing deaths from breast cancer.

## Studies of extent of disease at diagnosis

Many studies have been conducted to determine whether the practice of breast self-examination is associated with breast cancers that are smaller or at less advanced stage at the time of diagnosis than expected in the absence of self-examination. Table 39 summarizes the results of studies in which the stage of breast cancer at diagnosis in women who found their tumour while practising breast self-examination was compared with the stage of diagnosis in women whose tumour came to their attention by means other than screening. In all the studies except one, the proportion of women whose tumour was diagnosed

when it was confined to the breast was slightly higher among those who found their tumour while practising self-examination than among those who did not. None of the comparison groups intentionally included women screened by mammography.

Tumour size at diagnosis was reported in five of the studies shown in Table 39, and in each the tumours detected by breast self-examination were slightly smaller than those in the comparison group. Smith et al. (1980) found that 23% of 57 tumours detected by self-examination and 22% of 35 tumours detected by accident were < 2 cm in diameter; in a second study, Smith and Burns (1985) found that 21% of 125 tumours detected by self-examination and 19% of 92 tumours detected incidentally were < 2 cm in diameter. In addition, the mean diameters of tumours detected by self-examination and in comparison groups of cases were 2.2 and 2.5 cm (Owen et al., 1985), 2.8 and 2.9 cm (McPherson et al., 1997) and 2.2 and 2.5 cm, respectively (Koibuchi et al., 1998).

Tumour size and stage at diagnosis were compared in women who reported

**Table 39. Stage of breast cancer at diagnosis in women who did and did not detect their cancer while practising breast self-examination (BSE)**

| Reference (country) | Defintion of early stage | Method of detection | | | | Definition of comparison group |
|---|---|---|---|---|---|---|
| | | Breast self-examination | | Comparison group | | |
| | | Total no. of cases | % at early stage | Total no. of cases | % at early stage | |
| Greenwald et al. (1978) (USA) | TNM clinical stage I | 53 | 38 | 178 | 27 | Accidental |
| Smith et al. (1980) (USA) | In situ or localized to breast | 107 | 59 | 57 | 58 | Not BSE or CBE |
| Gould-Martin et al. (1982) (USA) | Localized to breast | 60 | 48 | 169 | 59 | Accidental |
| Philip et al. (1984) (United Kingdom) | TNM N0 | 35 | 83 | 109 | 66 | Not BSE |
| Owen et al. (1985) (USA) | In situ plus localized | 189 | 58 | 1218 | 52 | Causal discovery |
| Smith & Burns (1985) (USA) | In situ plus localized | 185 | 60 | 134 | 50 | Not BSE |
| Kuroishi et al. (1992) (Japan) | TNM Tis or I | 355 | 37 | 1327 | 29 | Chance |
| Auvinen et al. (1966) (Finland) | Localized | 34 | 59 | 518 | 56 | Not BSE |
| McPherson et al. (1997) (USA) | Localized | 200 | 56 | 364 | 53 | Incidental |
| Koibuchi et al. (1998) (Japan) | TNM Tis or 0 or 1 | 68 | 47 | 178 | 44 | Not BSE |

CBE, clinical breast examination

practising breast self-examination at different frequencies. As shown in Table 40, eight of ten studies showed that a higher percentage of women who reported practising breast self-examination monthly had tumours confined to the breast than women who did not examine their breasts. In five of seven studies in which stage at diagnosis was reported in women who practised breast self-examination, the percentage of cases with no axillary node involvement was higher among women who practised self-examination monthly than in those who did so less than once a month. Similarly, studies have fairly consistently shown

tumour size at diagnosis to be inversely associated with the frequency of breast self-examination (Table 41). However, Gould-Martin et al. (1982) found that the risk for regional disease at diagnosis was not lower for women who practised breast self-examination routinely in comparison with women screened by clinical breast examination and was not lower for women who used techniques judged to be adequate than for women whose practice was considered not to be adequate. In addition, among women invited to attend classes in breast self-examination as part of a non-randomized trial of breast cancer screening in

Huddersfield, England (Philip et al., 1984), who developed breast cancer during the next 3 years, 45% of those who attended the classes and 31% of non-attenders had tumours that were ≤ 2 cm, but nearly equal proportions (53% of 32 attenders and 54% of 70 non-attenders) had no involvement of axillary nodes, as confirmed histologically.

Women who were taught breast self-examination more frequently reported having found their tumours themselves than women who had not been taught the technique (Philip et al., 1984). This is not surprising, as women who have not received instruction in breast self-exami-

## Table 40. Stage of breast cancer at diagnosis in relation to self-reported frequency of breast self-examination

| Reference (country) | Definition of early stage | Frequency of breast self-examination | | | | | |
|---|---|---|---|---|---|---|---|
| | | Never | | < 1/month | | ≥ 1/month | |
| | | Total no. of cases | % early stage | Total no. of cases | % early stage | Total no. of cases | % early stage |
| Feldman et al. (1981) (USA) | TNM stage 0 or I | 588[a] | 40 | 221 | 54 | 187 | 53 |
| Tamburini et al. (1981) (Italy) | Axillary nodes not involved | 330 | 49 | 170[b] | 59 | – | – |
| Hislop et al. (1984) (Canada) | No palpable lymph nodes | 104 | 78 | 264 | 85 | 36 | 86 |
| Foster & Costanza (1984) (USA) | Axillary nodes not involved | 292 | 15 | 192 | 29 | 177 | 37 |
| Mant et al. (1987) (United Kingdom) | No report of involved nodes | 294 | 54 | 82 | 64 | 144 | 68 |
| Ogawa et al. (1987) (Japan) | TNM N0 | 60 | 82 | 60 | 80 | 30 | 87 |
| GIVIO (1991) (Italy) | TNM N0 | 1307 | 52 | 480 | 53 | 329 | 56 |
| Gästrin et al. (1994) (Finland) | Localized | 1679 | 52 | – | – | 432 | 52[c] |
| Auvinen et al. (1996) (Finland) | Localized | 104 | 54 | 202 | 57 | 246 | 57 |
| Koibuchi et al. (1998) (Japan) | Axillary nodes not involved | 167 | 62 | – | – | 64[d] | 63 |

[a] Rarely or never practised breast self-examination
[b] Includes 56 women who practised breast self-examination monthly
[c] Includes an unknown number of women who practised breast self-examination less than monthly
[d] Monthly or every 2 months

nation may not even know what it is. However, it is of relevance for assessing the efficacy of this technique to determine whether women who practise it regularly and competently are more likely to find their breast tumours themselves than women who have received instruction but practise it less diligently. Results from three studies suggest that this is so. Gould-Martin et al. (1982) found that 7 (44%) of 16 women who practised breast self-examination regularly and adequately found their tumours, compared with 4 (29%) of 14 women who were judged to practise the examination less competently. Hislop et al. (1984) reported that 92% of 36 women in whom breast cancer was diagnosed when they were currently practising breast self-examination with techniques considered to be proper found their tumours, in comparison with 87% of 264 women who were currently practising breast self-examination but using improper techniques. Ogawa et al. (1987) observed that 70% of 21 women who had been practising breast self-examination monthly detected their tumours compared with 40% of 24 women who did so less frequently.

Most of the evidence from clinical and epidemiological studies therefore suggests that women who regularly and competently practise breast self-examination are more likely to detect their breast tumours themselves and to have tumours diagnosed when smaller and at a less advanced stage than women who do not practise breast self-examination.

## Efficacy of screening women at high risk

Women who are at high risk for breast cancer might benefit more from breast screening programmes than women at average risk. Although there are many proposed risk factors for breast cancer, only a few clearly define groups of women who are at high risk. Foremost are women with a family history of breast cancer and those who are found by

**Table 41. Percentage of cases of tumours < 2 cm in diameter by self-reported frequency of breast self-examination**

| Reference (country) | Frequency of breast self-examination | | | | | |
|---|---|---|---|---|---|---|
| | Never | | < 1/month | | ≥ 1/month | |
| | Total no. cases | % < 2 cm | Total no. cases | % < 2 cm | Total no. cases | % < 2 cm |
| Feldman et al. (1981) (USA) | 223[a] | 39 | 140[b] | 56 | – | – |
| Tamburini et al. (1981) (Italy) | 330 | 21 | 170[c] | 37 | – | – |
| Hislop et al. (1984) (Canada) | 98 | 14 | 254 | 13 | 34 | 21 |
| Foster & Costanza (1984) (USA) | 352 | 6.5 | 197 | 18 | 169 | 30 |
| Mant et al. (1987) (United Kingdom) | 294 | 33 | 82 | 44 | 144 | 45 |
| Ogawa et al. (1987) (Japan) | 60 | 15 | 60 | 23 | 30 | 33 |
| GIVIO (1991) (Italy) | 1307 | 43 | 480 | 48 | 329 | 52 |
| Koibuchi et al. (1998)[d] (Japan) | 178 | 44 | – | – | 68[e] | 47 |

[a] Rarely or never practised breast self-examination
[b] Monthly plus several times yearly
[c] Includes 56 women who practised breast self-examination monthly
[d] Tis + T0 + T1 in TNM classification
[e] Monthly or every 2 months

genetic testing to be carriers of deleterious mutations in the *BRCA1* or *BRCA2* gene. In the latter, the lifetime risk may exceed 80% (Ford et al., 1998). Women with a history of atypical hyperplasia, DCIS or LCIS are also at elevated risk. Several models have been developed for estimating individual breast cancer risk which combine family history with other risk factors, such as a history of benign breast disease and reproductive history. Women with a history of invasive breast cancer are also at high risk for a second cancer. A small group of women are at high risk for breast cancer because of a history of therapeutic radiation, in particular, young women who have been treated for Hodgkin disease (Bhatia et al., 1996) and also those who have undergone thymic irradiation (Hildreth et al., 1989) or chest fluoroscopy (Miller et al., 1989). There is emerging evidence that certain biomarkers, such as serum concentrations of insulin-like growth factor-1 (Hankinson et al., 1998a) or estradiol (Hankinson et al., 1998b), the presence of proliferative cells in a nipple aspirate (Wrensch et al., 2001) and breast density (Boyd et al., 1998) can be used to define high-risk groups, but it has not yet been proposed that these women are candidates for greater surveillance. Also, the majority of breast cancers occur among women without greater mammographic density (Tabár & Dean, 1982) or who belong to other high-risk groups, and it would be inappropriate to exclude them from screening programmes.

The relative risks and benefits of mammography may be different for different groups of women within a population. For example, the risk–benefit ratio may be favourable for women at high risk. As breast cancer is more prevalent in high-risk groups, this will affect the positive predictive value of the test used and the cost–benefit ratio. Conversely, women at high risk might benefit less from mammography than women at average risk. This would be the case if carriers of deleterious mutations were particularly radiosensitive or if the natural history of hereditary breast cancer were accelerated by radiation. It is therefore important to assess the efficacy of screening mammography for women at different levels of risk and with different risk profiles. It is also possible that the distribution of factors related to detectability by mammography might be different for women at high risk than for women at average risk. Such factors may include age and mammographic density. Hereditary breast cancers typically occur in young women, and tumours in women under 50 are more likely to be missed by mammography than tumours in women over the age of 50 (Ma *et al.*, 1992). To some extent, this reduction in sensitivity may be due to higher mammographic density, which is an established risk factor for breast cancer (Boyd *et al.*, 1998) and correlates with other known risk factors, such as parity and oophorectomy. Because density can obscure cancer, screening mammography is less sensitive in women with mammographically dense breasts than in women with mammographically lucent breasts (Mandelson *et al.*, 2000). Therefore, mammographic screening will be more difficult for a risk group with breasts of a greater than average mammographic density. To some extent, mammographic density is a heritable trait (Pankow *et al.*, 1997), but there is little evidence that mammographic density is greater among women at high genetic risk for breast cancer.

## Radiation sensitivity

It has been proposed that the benefits of screening mammography might be offset in predisposed women by their enhanced sensitivity to the carcinogenic effects of radiation. Radiation is an established risk factor for breast cancer (see Chapter 5). The groups at risk include women with previous therapeutic exposure (Hildreth *et al.,* 1989; Miller *et al.*, 1989; Bhatia *et al.*, 1996) and survivors of the atomic bombs (Tokunaga *et al.*, 1994). In a recent analysis of women who were exposed to the atomic bomb blasts, their risks for breast cancer were estimated separately for those exposed before and after the age of 35. The relative risk was much greater for the women who were younger at the time of exposure (Tokunaga *et al.*, 1994). Because of the strong association between age at onset and hereditary breast cancer, the authors suggested that radiation-induced breast cancer might be a form of hereditary breast cancer or, alternatively, that, among women with hereditary predisposition, radiation may be an important cofactor.

Several of the genes that have been implicated in susceptibility to breast cancer are involved in DNA repair, including *BRCA1* and *BRCA2* and the gene for ataxia telangiectasia (*ATM*). Both *BRCA1* and *BRCA2* participate in DNA repair through homologous recombination (Hoeijmakers, 2001). This mechanism is responsible for repair of double-strand breaks, which are typical of the damage induced by ionizing radiation. Concern has been expressed that women who carry a single mutant copy of the *ATM* gene are at increased risk for breast cancer and may be sensitive to the carcinogenic effects of ionizing radiation. Several recent studies support the hypothesis that heterozygous carriers of certain *ATM* mutations are at increased risk for breast cancer (Angèle & Hall, 2000; Dork *et al.*, 2001; Geoffroy-Perez *et al.*, 2001; Olsen *et al.*, 2001; Chenevix-Trench *et al.*, 2002). No epidemiological studies have been conducted to evaluate whether mammography (or other forms of ionizing radiation) poses a hazard to carriers of either *ATM* or *BRCA1* or *BRCA2* mutations.

## Tumour factors

Certain characteristics of the tumours typically found in high-risk women might complicate screening them. These characteristics include the growth rate or metastatic potential of the tumours (which reduces the preclinical latent period or sojourn period) and mammographic appearance (which reduces the sensitivity of screening). Fast-growing cancers are more likely to present as interval cancers than are slowly growing tumours. The histological features of a breast cancer may also be associated with mammographic detectability. Tumours with lobular or mucinous tissue are less likely to be detected by mammography than are ductal carcinomas (Ma *et al.*, 1992; Narod & Dubé, 2001). In contrast, tumours with tubular features or with extensive in situ components are particularly likely to be identified at screening (Ma *et al.*, 1992). Other features related to detectability on screening include low grade and the presence of estrogen receptors (ER). Although there is no consistent characteristic of hereditary breast cancer, several features are commonly seen. The majority of breast cancers in carriers of *BRCA1* mutations are high-grade ductal carcinomas, are ER-negative and have a high proliferative index (Lakhani *et al.*, 1998). Carriers of *BRCA1* mutations also show less DCIS in relationship to the invasive tumour (Breast Cancer Linkage Consortium, 1997), but the rate of DCIS in *BRCA2* carriers is similar to that of controls. The young age of the patients and the typical histological features can contribute to the difficulty of using mammography to detect hereditary breast cancer.

Women can be considered to be at increased risk for breast cancer on the basis of a family history, the results of a genetic test or both. In general, women at risk of familial cancer fall into one of three groups: those with a documented deleterious mutation in *BRCA1* or *BRCA2;* those with a strong family history of breast cancer and a history of breast cancer; and those with a strong family history of breast cancer but no personal history of breast cancer. The lifetime risk of women in the third group is much lower than that of the first two groups, because, even if a susceptibility gene is present in the family, the chance that a healthy relative will have inherited the predisposing mutation is less than 50%. In contrast, almost all affected women in the family will be carriers. Screening programmes for high-risk women may include any or all of the groups listed above.

## Family history

A family history of breast cancer is a consistent risk factor for the disease. In a large meta-analysis, the cumulative risk for breast cancer up to the age of 80 was 7.8% for women with no affected first-degree relative, 13% for women with one affected first-degree relative and 21% for women with two affected first-degree relatives (Collaborative Group on Hormonal Factors in Breast Cancer, 2001). The risk also depends on the age at diagnosis of the cancer. One factor in favour of screening high-risk populations is that the prevalence of breast cancer is greater than expected among women with a family history of breast cancer. In a screening study in San Francisco, USA (Kerlikowske *et al.*, 1993), a family history of cancer was strongly related to both the prevalence of breast cancer and the positive predictive value of the test. In the age group 50–59, the positive predictive value of mammography was 0.22 for those with a positive family history and 0.09 for those with a negative family history. In the age group 40–49, the positive predictive value was 0.13 for those with a positive family history and 0.04 for those with a negative family history.

Many centres have now developed screening programmes for high-risk women. Lalloo *et al.* (1998) screened 1259 women under the age of 50 who had a family history of breast cancer. Twelve invasive cancers were detected, with 8.45 expected (relative risk, 1.42). Kollias and colleagues (1998) followed a high-risk cohort of 1371 women under the age of 50 for a mean of 22 months and detected 23 invasive and six in situ cancers. They estimated this rate to be five times higher than expected.

### BRCA1 and BRCA2

Only a small proportion of women with a family history of breast cancer carry a mutation in one of the breast cancer genes. Among women with a *BRCA1* or *BRCA2* mutation, the risk for breast cancer is estimated to be approximately 80% up to the age of 70 (Ford *et al.*, 1998; Figure 30). In general, in the presence of a mutation, the estimated cancer

risk is due to the mutation alone, i.e. it is not established that the family history adds additional predictive power. However, both genetic and non-genetic factors have been shown to modify the risk for breast cancer in carriers of *BRCA* mutations (Narod, 2002). Several studies are consistent in reporting the poor performance of mammography as a screening tool for *BRCA* carriers. Goffin *et al.* (2001) reviewed the mammography records of 161 Ashkenazi Jewish women with breast cancer and classified them according to mutation status. Tumours < 2 cm in diameter were less likely to be detected by mammography among carriers than non-carriers (46% versus 89%; p < 0.001). In a small study in Asia, four of nine *BRCA1*-associated breast tumours were not mammographically visible, despite an average tumour size of 4.1 cm (Chang *et al.*, 1999). In this study, the mammographic density of the *BRCA1* carriers was reported to be higher than that of non-carrier controls.

In a prospective screening study, Brekelmans *et al.* (2001) found four

cases of DCIS and 31 cases of invasive breast cancer in 1198 women with a high familial risk for breast cancer. Nine interval cancers occurred between 8 weeks and 10 months after the last negative screen. The detection rates were 33 per 1000 per year in the *BRCA* mutation carriers, 8.4 per 1000 per year in the high-risk familial group and 3.3 per 1000 per year in the moderate-risk group. Of the 29 tumours of known size, 10 were < 1 cm, eight were 1–1.5 cm and 11 were > 1.5 cm. Eleven (35%) had node involvement, and five of nine of the cancers in mutation carriers had node involvement at diagnosis. Four of nine cancers detected in *BRCA1* carriers were interval cancers. This study clearly demonstrates the high risk associated with a *BRCA* mutation but presents little evidence to support the benefit of mammographic screening. A large proportion of the cancers among carriers were missed by mammography, and many women had involved lymph nodes at diagnosis.

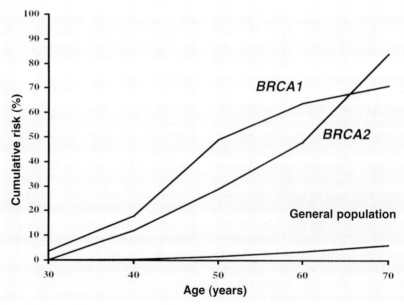

**Figure 30** Cumulative breast cancer risk in carriers of *BRCA* mutations
From Ford *et al.* (1998)

Scheuer *et al.* (2002) followed 165 women with *BRCA* mutations for a mean of 25 months and diagnosed nine incident, invasive, primary breast cancers. Three of these were detected by mammography, and six were detected in the interval between mammograms: five by self-examination and one by clinical examination. The women with interval cancers were younger than those with screen-detected cancers (41 years versus 57 years; *p* = 0.05).

## Magnetic resonance imaging

Because of the limitations of screening mammography (illustrated in the study of Brekelmans *et al.*, 2001), there has been much interest in evaluating more sensitive techniques of detecting breast cancer, including magnetic resonance imaging (MRI). MRI has been compared with mammography in screening of high-risk women in four studies. In none were

mortality rates compared, and in none were women assigned to screening at random, but all four studies found MRI to be more sensitive than mammography. Kuhl *et al.* (2000) screened 192 asymptomatic high-risk women with MRI and found invasive or in situ cancers in six women at the first screening round (3.1%) and in three of 101 women (3.0%) at the second round. Of the nine MRI-detected cancers, only three were apparent on mammography. In a similar study, Warner *et al.* (2001) compared mammography with MRI in 196 high-risk women in Ontario, Canada. Six invasive breast cancers were diagnosed; all were identified by MRI, but only two were identified by mammography. All the cancers were in women with either a *BRCA* mutation or a history of breast cancer. The six invasive cancers showed no node involvement, and each was < 1 cm in diameter. In this study, the specificity

of MRI examination was lower than that of other screening modalities. Meijers-Heijboer *et al.* (2001) followed a cohort of 63 women with *BRCA* mutations for a mean of 3 years, the women being screened annually with MRI, mammography or both. Eight incident cases of breast cancer were identified in the cohort. Examination by MRI allowed detection of six of eight breast cancers, but mammography allowed detection of only two of eight breast cancers. In a study from The Netherlands, Stoudjesdijk *et al.* (2001) studied a cohort of 179 women at high risk for breast cancer and also found that the sensitivity of MRI was significantly greater than that of mammography. Each of these studies was small, but, taken together, they provide evidence that the sensitivity of MRI is superior to that of mammography in screening women at high hereditary risk.

# Chapter 5
# Effectiveness of screening

## Has screening been implemented in accordance with the results of screening trials?

National screening programmes were introduced in a number of countries, including Sweden, The Netherlands and the United Kingdom, following randomized controlled trials, and the experience from the trials was used to decide how screening should be implemented. A number of trials conducted after the start of those programmes concentrated on more specific issues and also influenced national programmes.

There are now many national and regional population-based screening programmes, with various characteristics (see Tables 9–11, pp. 49–53). Ballard-Barbash et al. (1999) reviewed breast cancer screening programmes in 21 countries and divided them into three groups:

- those with national, government-supported, centrally organized health care systems, which have highly organized screening programmes that are distinct from the delivery of general medical care;
- those with government-supported programmes that are organized more locally; and
- those with government-supported programmes, where breast cancer screening is conducted within the context of general medical care.

These distinctions were used to focus the discussion below, although examples from the first group were used mainly.

The screening process can be a continuum, from organized national programmes through to opportunistic screening in which no 'programme' as

such effectively exists (see Chapter 3). Organized programmes cover a defined population, and women in a specific age range are invited at regular intervals. These programmes are based on information on all women in a geographical area, which allows tracking of both those who attend and those who do not. Organized programmes can be evaluated by the techniques described below. Opportunistic screening is that conducted after a request by a physician or a woman rather than by specified routine call and recall. In practice, many programmes have elements of both organized and opportunistic screening. By its nature, opportunistic screening is less amenable to quality control and the detailed evaluation specified for organized screening programmes; the evaluation may therefore be limited to technical considerations.

### Methods of invitation

For the majority of the randomized trials, population registers were obtained or compiled before randomization, from electoral or health authority registers (Tabár et al., 1985; Roberts et al., 1990) or from private health plan membership lists (Shapiro et al., 1967), and women in the intervention group were sent personal invitations. An exception is the Canadian trials (Miller et al., 1991b), in which women volunteered after media publicity. The advantages of a population-based approach with individual invitations is that the whole eligible population and range of socioeconomic groups are identified. In most countries where this is feasible, such an approach was adopted for national screening programmes. In many countries, existing

population registers were used, whereas in others (e.g. Ireland) registers had to be compiled from various sources. In a survey of screening in 21 countries, personal invitation was used as the only means for recruitment in five, and this was the commonest method in a further nine (Ballard-Barbash et al., 1999). In the USA, referral by a physician was the commonest method of recruitment. Media publicity was used in a number of countries, but it was the commonest method of recruitment in only two.

In countries or regions where recruitment is not organized by invitation, it may be difficult to encourage certain groups to attend for screening, and specific interventions may be needed (Whitman et al., 1991; Paskett et al., 1999). In addition, it may prove more difficult to ensure that such women attend for further investigation when recommended or return for routine re-screening (Segura et al., 2000). In the province of Florence, Italy, a self-referral policy resulted in only 10.2% of the target population having a mammogram (Giorgi et al., 1994).

### Screening processes

The screening process is described comprehensively in Chapter 3. It should be emphasized that screening comprises a series of elements, starting from identification of the target population, through invitation of the woman and the point at which a women has a negative screening result or breast cancer is detected and treated, and the outcome is evaluated. Detailed information on the screening trials that have been performed is given in Chapters 1 and 4, including those with conventional mammography. This chapter addresses how the trials have influenced the implementation of screening. In most of the randomized trials, the further assessment of women with abnormalities detected on screening mammograms was also described. The extent to which this is done in population screening programmes depends partly on the health care system.

## Age range

The most convincing evidence from randomized controlled trials of the benefit of screening was for women aged 50–69 at entry to the trial. Few results are available for women aged ≥ 70. With further results and increased follow-up, a benefit is becoming apparent from some trials for women younger than 50 at entry, although it remains unclear to what extent this is due to screening after the age of 50 (de Koning et al., 1995b; Fletcher, 1997; National Institutes of Health, 1997; see also Chapter 4).

All countries in which population screening is conducted (either nationally or sub-nationally) include women aged 50–64, and a number include women up to the age of 69. Concern about lower attendance of older women led to an initial upper limit for invitation of 64 in the United Kingdom, but on the basis of the results of recent studies (Moss et al., 2001), the upper limit is to be increased to 70, and that in The Netherlands has been increased to 74. In some countries, including the USA, there is no recommended upper limit. As stated above, little evidence is available from the trials about the benefit of screening women > 70.

If screening women younger than 50 is to be effective, the interval will probably need to be < 2 years. A randomized controlled trial of women aged 40–41 at entry given annual mammography is being conducted in the United Kingdom, and a report will become available within the next few years

(Moss, 1999). Breast cancer is less common among younger women, and, while more life-years will potentially be gained, cost–effectiveness will be a key consideration for this age group. At present, in most countries with screening programmes, routine screening of women under 50 is not recommended (National Institutes of Health, 1997; Ballard-Barbash et al., 1999).

## Screening interval

Most of the randomized controlled trials involved a 1- or 2-year screening interval. In the Swedish Two-county study, a 24-month interval was used for women aged 40–49 and a 33-month interval for those aged 50–75 at entry. Tabár et al. (1989) recommended that the interval should be no more than 18 months for women aged 40–49 and no more than 2 years for women aged ≥ 50, on the basis of the results of randomized controlled trials.

Many countries have adopted a 2-yearly screening interval because of the high interval cancer rates seen in the third year in trials. The United Kingdom is unusual in opting for a 3-year interval for women aged 50–64, but the programme is restricted by budget. The Microsimulation Screening Analysis (MISCAN) model (see p. 128) predicts that substantial reductions in mortality would follow from extending the age range of women screened to 69 or reducing the screening interval to 2 years and suggests that the difference between these two policies would be so small that, depending on the outcome measure considered, either could be used (Boer et al., 1998). The results of Markov-chain models of breast tumour progression to determine the optimal screening interval (Duffy et al., 1997), with the data from the Swedish trials, suggest that the screening interval is critical for women aged 40–49 but less so for older women. For women aged

40–49, a 3-year interval would result in little reduction in mortality (4%), but annual screening would result in a 36% reduction. For women aged 60–69, the predicted reductions in mortality with 3-yearly, 2-yearly and annual screening are predicted to be 34%, 39% and 44%, respectively.

## Mammography

### Number of mammographic views

In mammography, a single mediolateral–oblique view with or without a second cranio-caudal view is usually used. Single-view mammography was used in the Swedish Two-county and Stockholm trials, while two-view mammography was used in the Malmö, Göteborg, Health Insurance Plan and Canadian trials and in the first screen in Edinburgh. The results of a meta-analysis of these trials (Kerlikowske et al., 1995) suggested that there was no difference in the reduction in breast cancer mortality between screening with one view or two views; however, the trials were not designed to answer this question.

In most national screening programmes, two views are used for the prevalence screen; in some, two views are used for all screens. In The Netherlands, two views are used for prevalence screens and about 20% of all subsequent screens if indicated (Fracheboud et al., 1998). In the United Kingdom, a single view was recommended for all screens; in 1995, however, on the basis of the results of the randomized controlled trial (Wald et al., 1995), the country changed its policy to two views for prevalence screens. It recently changed the policy again, to recommend two views for all screens by 2003. In a national screening programme, film readers will, at least initially, be less skilled than the experts involved in randomized controlled trials. Experience in the United Kingdom showed a 32% increase in the detection of small invasive cancers when the programme changed from one view to two views at prevalence screens (Blanks et al., 1998) and also showed that two views were beneficial at incidence screens (Given-Wilson & Blanks, 1999).

### Double reading

Deciding how many film readers to use is complicated by the number of ways in which film reading can be undertaken (see box).

No randomized controlled trials have been conducted to examine this question specifically; a systematic review of 10 cohort studies showed that double reading increased the rate of cancer detection (Dinnes et al., 2001), but cost–effectiveness remains an open issue (see Chapters 2 and 6). The policies of national screening programmes vary, but two readers are used in most. For example, in The Netherlands, all films are read independently at a central unit by two radiologists. Consensus between the two readers is required for a referral, which may contribute towards the low referral rate in that country.

## Number of readings and readers

| Technique | No. of readers |
|---|---|
| Single reading | 2 |
| Double reading with recall if necessary | 2 |
| Double reading by censensus | 2 |
| Double reading with arbitration | 3 |

In the United Kingdom, the policy is for single reading, although, in practice, some kind of double reading is used in most programmes. Radiographers (technicians trained to take radiographs) may also be trained as film readers, particularly where too few radiologists are available. While issues such as screening interval, number of mammographic views and the lower age limit for screening have been further evaluated in specific trials, the issue of double reading has not, and it is likely to remain an open question. Studies will probably be undertaken to evaluate film reading by non-radiologists and with use of computer-aided detection (see Chapter 2).

## Clinical breast examination

In most population-based screening programmes, mammography is the only method used for detection, although clinical breast examination is added in some countries or regions (see Chapter 2 and Shapiro et al., 1998). No randomized trials of clinical breast examination versus no screening have been completed (see Chapter 4).

Some form of clinical breast examination was used in the Health Insurance Plan, Edinburgh and Canadian trials. In the Health Insurance Plan study, 67% of cases were detected by clinical examination (with or without mammography), but in the UK Trial of Early Detection of Breast Cancer, which included the intervention arm of the Edinburgh trial, the relative sensitivity of clinical breast examination was only 70% at first screens and 44% at subsequent screens (Moss et al., 1993). As shown in Chapter 4, no difference in the reduction in mortality was found in trials with clinical breast examination and those with mammography alone.

The Canadian trial of women aged 50–59 was specifically designed to compare annual mammography plus clinical examination with clinical examination only (Miller et al., 1992b). No difference

was found in the rate of death from breast cancer between the two arms of the trial after 13 years of follow-up, although more small tumours without node involvement were detected with mammography, and the confidence interval of the relative risk for breast cancer mortality was wide (RR, 1.02; 95% CI, 0.78–1.33) (Miller et al., 2000).

Clinical examination is used alone in Japan, where annual screening is carried out by medical practitioners. Recent evidence suggested that this can reduce mortality rates (Kuroishi et al., 2000). Screening by clinical breast examination alone has also been proposed for developing countries with limited resources (Mittra et al., 2000).

## Breast self-examination

There is no evidence from randomized trials that breast self-examination is effective in reducing breast cancer mortality (see Chapter 4). A study in Shanghai, China, in which women employed in factories were assigned randomly to a self-examination instruction group or to a control group on the basis of factory, showed no difference in cumulative breast cancer mortality at 10–11 years (Thomas et al., 2002). Nevertheless, a number of countries or programmes include it in their recommendations.

## Indicators for monitoring and evaluating the effectiveness of screening programmes

An organized screening programme should have access to an information system that covers the programme and the entire target population. The background measures of coverage and attendance relate to the target populations and the women in it, whereas performance indicators, such as predictive value and detection rate, are related directly to the mammography unit and other diagnostic facilities. Mortality from

## Why the reduction in mortality due to screening takes longer to become evident in national mortality statistics than in randomized controlled trials

| Reason for delay in mortality reduction from national screening programme compared with trials | Comments and comparison with trials |
|---|---|
| Dilution due to breast cancer deaths in cases diagnosed before any invitation to screening | Pre-exisiting cases are excluded from both arms of trials. |
| Long time to cover national population, e.g., in the United Kingdom, the first invitations were sent between 1988 (start of programme) and 1995 (completion of prevalence round), depending on area of residence. | Women enter trials at time of first invitation, which is time zero. |
| Learning time for many staff new to screening | Trials usually have highly experienced staff. |

breast cancer, excess mortality and total mortality are the indicators that cover the entire process. As they are related directly to the purpose of screening, mortality is the necessary and sufficient indicator of effectiveness. All other measures are necessary, and may be early indicators that the programme is operating as expected, but they are not sufficient and cannot as such be taken as proof of effectiveness.

The aim of any breast cancer screening programme is to reduce breast cancer mortality. However, such a reduction will take many years to emerge in a population-based screening programme, starting from a few years after introduction of the programme but taking decades to show a full effect. The effect is much slower than in randomized controlled trials, for the reasons shown in the box below. Implementation of national screening programmes has tended to be slow: the United Kingdom and The Netherlands started screening in 1988 and 1990, respectively, but all

women were not screened until 1995 and 1997.

The reduction in breast cancer mortality rates due to screening at a given time after the start of the programme is complex to measure because, in the absence of screening, breast cancer mortality in a defined age group is affected by a number of factors. These include cohort effects, improvements in treatment, presentation at an earlier stage as a direct result of the introduction of the programme and the attendant publicity (Stockton et al., 1997) and changes in death certificate coding. Furthermore, the effect of screening in reducing breast cancer mortality, as seen in national statistics, will be diluted by deaths among women in whom breast cancer is diagnosed before an invitation to screening. If record linkage to a cancer registry is available, 'refined breast cancer mortality' can be used, which excludes deaths among women in whom cancer was diagnosed before the start of screening (Hakama et al., 1999).

A further complexity is that, although the reduction in breast cancer mortality seen in trials is related to the age of the women at entry into the trial, national breast cancer mortality statistics are a measure of the decrease in breast cancer mortality rates of women at the age at which they die. Therefore, some effect is seen in increasingly older women with time since the start of screening. Useful information is derived by comparing breast cancer mortality among women invited to screening with that of women who were not invited and that among invited women who participate with that of non-participants. However, these comparisons can be biased by differential access to treatment by uninvited women and by a differential cancer risk of non-attenders, unless proper controls are found.

Therefore, early indicators are needed to ascertain whether adjustments are required to a screening programme in the early stages. These indicators of performance can be used to predict the final reduction in breast cancer mortality that is likely to be achieved with the current level of screening performance. National screening programmes in countries with relatively small populations, and therefore large statistical uncertainty in breast cancer mortality rates by 5-year age band, and in which no control group is included are unlikely to allow a reliable estimate of the effect of screening unless indicators of performance are used.

### Origins of indicators of effectiveness of screening

Nearly all measures of the performance of breast cancer screening programmes are compared with target or expected values, which are derived, either explicitly or implicitly, from information from randomized controlled trials. Use of the results of such trials is essential, as they have produced well-defined reductions in breast cancer mortality. Application of the parameters of these trials, adjusted for local conditions, allows prediction of the eventual reduction in breast cancer mortality likely to be achieved in a national programme. In general, the targets or standards for measures such as cancer and interval cancer detection rates in a particular population-based screening programme should take into account age range, background incidence and screening interval. Accordingly, separate calculations are required for each population-based screening programme.

Some of the first suggestions were made by Day *et al.* (1989) on the basis of experience from the Swedish Two-county trial. In the latest follow-up, there was a 32% (95% CI, 20–41%) reduction in breast cancer mortality in the invited compared with the control group (Tabár *et al.*, 2000b). Table 42 lists these indicators of performance in chronological order of availability of data. Proactive evaluation of breast cancer screening requires evaluation of data on an annual basis, even after the first year of screening, to determine whether corrective action is required. The European guidelines for performance are given as examples in Tables 43 and 44.

## Performance indicators
### Participation
The first important indicator of performance is attendance to screening (also called participation, compliance or uptake). Determination of this indicator can be deceptively complicated. For example, in a programme in which women aged 50–69 are screened every 2 years, 10 possible screening invitations can lead to $2^{10}$, or 1024, different possible attendance patterns, all attending and all not attending being the extremes. If a woman attends only two screens at the ages of 50 and 52, the potential benefit will be clearly different from that of a woman who attends at the ages of 66 and 68. This is true for all variations in attendance pattern. The indicators used currently

## Table 42. Measures of monitoring

| Measure | Type of evaluation provided |
|---|---|
| Participation (or compliance) rate | Indicates potential for effectiveness of the overall programme |
| Prevalence rate at initial screening test and rate of interval cancers | Provides estimates of sensitivity, lead time, sojourn time and predictive value |
| Stage (or size) distribution of screen-detected cancers | Indicates potential for reduction in absolute rate of advanced cancers |
| Rate of advanced cancers | Early surrogate of mortality |
| Breast cancer death rate | Final evaluation |

From Day *et al.* (1989)

## Table 43. Indicators for assessing the performance of a breast cancer screening programme for women aged 50–64

| Performance indicator | Acceptable level | Desirable level |
|---|---|---|
| Participation rate | > 70% | > 75% |
| Technical repeat rate | < 3% | < 1% |
| Recall rate | | |
|     Initial screening | < 7% | < 5% |
|     Subsequent regular screening | < 5% | < 3% |
| Additional imaging rate at time of screening | < 5% | < 1% |
| Pre-treatment diagnosis of malignant lesions | > 70% | > 90% |
| Image-guided fine-needle aspiration cytology procedures with insufficient result | < 25% | < 15% |
| Benign:malignant biopsy ratio | | |
|     Initial screening | ≤ 1:1 | ≤ 1:1 |
|     Subsequent regular screening | ≤ 0.5:1 | ≤ 0.2:1 |
| Re-invitation within the specified screening interval | > 95% | 100% |

From Commission of the European Communities (2001)

**Table 44. Early surrogate indicators for assessing the effectiveness of a breast cancer screening programme for women aged 50–64**

| Surrogate indicator | Acceptable level | Desirable level |
|---|---|---|
| Interval cancer rate/background incidence | | |
| 0–11 months | 30% | < 30% |
| 12–23 months | 50% | < 50% |
| Breast cancer detection rate | | |
| Initial screening | 3 x incidence rate | > 3 x incidence rate |
| Subsequent regular screening | 1.5 x incidence rate | > 1.5 x incidence rate |
| Stage ≥ II/total cancers detected at screening | | |
| Initial screening | 25% | < 25% |
| Subsequent regular screening | 20% | < 20% |
| Invasive cancers ≤ 10 mm/total invasive cancers detected at screening | | |
| Initial screening | ≥ 20% | ≥ 25% |
| Subsequent regular screening | ≥ 25% | ≥ 30% |
| Invasive cancers/total cancers detected at screening | 90% | 80–90% |
| Node-negative cancers/total cancers detected at screening | | |
| Initial screening | 70% | > 70% |
| Subsequent regular screening | 75% | > 75% |

From Commission of the European Communities (2001)

tend to be simplified measures of attendance, although they are likely to be reasonably accurate within the context of their use.

When participation in screening is used to predict reduction in breast cancer mortality, the participation rate is compared with the target measure. For example, in the United Kingdom National Health Service Breast Screening Programme, the percentage of invited women who attended for screening was about 70% (Blanks et al., 2002), while in the Swedish Two-county trial it was about 90%; the relative attendance is therefore 0.78. If equivalent rates of detection of invasive cancer, or interval cancers, are assumed after allowing for differences in background incidence between the United Kingdom and Sweden, then the estimated reduction in the United Kingdom would simply be 0.78 x 30% = 23%. This calculation is based on the assumption that there is no major effect of selection bias. Calculation of selection bias requires information on breast cancer incidence rates among non-attenders.

## Estimated reduction in breast cancer mortality based on cancer detection and participation rates

Cancer detection rates are the first indicator of screening performance and, if monitored and evaluated on an annual basis, give the earliest information on achievable mortality reduction. They are subject to overdiagnosis bias (see later in this chapter), but participation and cancer detection rates can give the earliest indication of possible under-performance of a regional or national programme. Corrective action can then be taken early, rather than waiting for other indicators, such as interval cancer rates, which can be measured only several years later. It is important to distinguish invasive from non-invasive cancers, as a high rate of detection of invasive cancers is the principal measure of interest. Cancer detection rate targets should take into account age range, background incidence and screening interval, and separate targets are required for prevalence and incidence screens.

Detailed evaluations were made of the screening programme in the United Kingdom in 1995 by using the background rates in England and Wales to estimate the expected rates of detection of invasive cancers and interval cancers (Blanks et al., 1996; Moss & Blanks, 1998). The standardized detection ratio was introduced, in which indirect age standardization was used to calculate the expected number of invasive cancers that would indicate parity with the Swedish Two-county study. The ratio was used to evaluate the performance of regional screening programmes among the 95 programmes in the United Kingdom, after adjustment of the expected number of invasive cancers by local background incidence (Blanks & Moss, 1996). In practice, the standardized detection ratio was found to be a good quality assurance measure for detecting under-performing programmes. A standardized detection ratio of < 0.75

(the lowest recorded statistically stable ratio being 0.5) was taken to indicate possible under-performance and the need for a visit by quality assurance staff. On its own, a low standardized detection ratio merely suggests under-performance and might be misleading if screened women have a different distribution of risk from the target population. In the United Kingdom, this appears rarely to be the case, but it might hold in other countries.

Table 45 shows the observed and expected numbers of invasive cancers in the United Kingdom annually between 1 April 1993 and 31 March 2000 for women aged 50–64 (Blanks et al., 2000a). The participation rate in the United Kingdom was about 70%, and the final reduction in mortality was estimated from the relative uptake x standardized detection ratio x 30%. In 1993–94, this was (70/90) x 0.83 x 30% = 19.4%; by 1999–2000, it had risen to (70/90) x 1.14 x 30% = 26.6%. Previous work showed that, over the range 0.8–1.3, the standardized detection ratio and interval cancer rates are strongly correlated (Given-Wilson et al., 1999), which justifies these calculations. The reduction in mortality is that which would have been achieved in a comparable randomized controlled trial, given similar diagnosis and treatment.

Table 45 shows that, in the United Kingdom, the rate of detection of invasive cancers was inadequate in the early years of the programme, as confirmed by the high rates of interval cancers. This low rate was not observed earlier partly because of a high rate of detection of DCIS, which contributed to achievement of what was considered to be an adequate cancer detection rate. In fact, the high DCIS detection rate 'masked' a poor rate of detection of small invasive cancers. This example illustrates why the rates of detection of invasive cancers and small invasive cancers should be considered separately (Day et al., 1995) and cautiously because of overdiagnosis. Overdiagnosis is commonly associated with DCIS but is also likely to occur in the case of some invasive cancers and strongly correlates with stage of disease. A further measure used in the United Kingdom is the standardized detection ratio (< 15 mm), which is the ratio of the observed number of invasive cancers < 15 mm to that expected from the Swedish Two-county study. Alternatively, a standardized detection ratio for invasive cancers < 10 mm can be used.

### Estimated reduction in mortality based on interval cancer rates and participation

Interval cancers are those which present in the interval between screens after a negative screen. The rate can be expressed either as that of interval cancers or as a proportion of the expected incidence rate (had screening not been undertaken). These estimates assume the existence of cancer registration. Poor quality cancer registration and/or record linkage can lead to underestimation of interval cancer rates and therefore overestimation of programme performance. If it is assumed that the data are of sufficient quality, the expected reduction in mortality can be calculated from participation and the combined proportionate incidence of interval cancers. If the proportionate incidence is x% in the first year, y% in the second and z% in the third, the combined proportionate incidence is (x + y + z)/3.

Table 46 shows data for the Anglia region of the United Kingdom on interval cancer rates during the early years of screening (Day et al., 1995). The background incidence in the absence of screening was estimated as 2.2 per 1000. The combined proportionate incidence was (0.24 + 0.59 + 0.79)/3 = 0.54, indicating that 54% of the incidence expected in the absence of screening was observed. The Dutch screening programme, with a 2-year interval, gave similar estimates for the early years of screening, with proportional incidences of 27% and 52% in the first and second years (Fracheboud et al., 1999). The combined proportionate incidence can be used to estimate the expected reduction in mortality in conjunction with the participation rate.

Day et al. (1995) were then able to calculate the expected reduction in mortality in the early years of screening

### Table 45. Observed and expected numbers of invasive cancers in women aged 50–64 in United Kingdom National Health Service breast screening programme

| Screening year | Observed | Expected | SDR | Modelled mortality reduction (%)[a] |
|---|---|---|---|---|
| 1993–94 | 4447 | 5344.6 | 0.83 | 19.4 |
| 1994–95 | 4452 | 4952.5 | 0.90 | 21.0 |
| 1995–96 | 4486 | 4725.5 | 0.95 | 22.2 |
| 1996–97 | 4833 | 4799.7 | 1.01 | 23.6 |
| 1997–98 | 5187 | 4964.2 | 1.04 | 24.3 |
| 1998–99 | 5744 | 5064.2 | 1.13 | 26.4 |
| 1999–2000 | 5795 | 5076.6 | 1.14 | 26.6 |

From Blanks et al. (2000a); data for 1999–2000 are unpublished
SDR, standardized detection ratio
a Estimated on the basis of 70% participation

**Table 46. Interval cancer rates during early years of screening in the United Kingdom (Anglia region)**

| | Time since last negative screen (months) | | |
| --- | --- | --- | --- |
| | 0–11 | 12–23 | 24–35 |
| Interval cancer rate per 10 000 women–years | 5.2 | 12.8 | 18.9 |
| Proportionate incidence | 0.24 | 0.59 | 0.79 |

From Day *et al.* (1995)

by inference to the Swedish Two-county study, as shown in Table 47. The participation rate in Anglia was 80%, which gave an estimated reduction in mortality of 21% at a combined proportionate incidence of 54%. As 70% participation is achieved in the United Kingdom as a whole, an 18% reduction can be expected, with a combined proportionate incidence of 54%. This reduction is closely in line with the estimate of 19% from screening in 1993–94 by use of the standardized detection ratio and participation rate (see Table 45). This is to be expected, as the standardized detection ratio and interval cancer rates are highly inversely correlated (Given-Wilson *et al.*, 1999).

### Estimated reduction in breast cancer mortality on the basis of prognostic factors

*Reduction in incidence of advanced cancer*

If screening programmes are successful in allowing earlier diagnosis of cancer, an overall reduction in the rates of advanced cancer should be observed in the target population. This should result in reduced mortality from advanced disease. Day *et al.* (1989) suggested that differences in stage distribution by mode of detection would appear immediately,

an effect on advanced cancer rates at diagnosis would appear only about 4 years after initiation of screening, and an effect on mortality some 2 years later, i.e. 6–7 years after the onset of screening. On the basis of observations in the Swedish Two-county trial, they suggested that screening should decrease the rate of advanced (stages II–IV) tumours by at least 30% after 4 years.

*Obtaining information on stage*

Stage has major prognostic implications. It is based on several factors: size of the tumour mass, its degree of spread both locally and to distant (metastatic) sites and involvement of regional lymph nodes; it is recorded according to the TNM system (UICC, 2002), American Joint Committee on Cancer (2002) stage (I–IV) or the summary 'extent of disease' (local, regional, distant). In the last scheme, tumours classified as TNM T2N0M0 or stage IIA of the American Joint Committee on Cancer (2 < 5 cm, localized to the breast) are considered 'localized'. Thus, in different studies, advanced disease may correspond to stage II–IV or IIB–IV.

Cancer registries do not always include information on stage of cancer. Registries may vary in the quality of information on stage and its completeness (proportion of 'unstaged' cases)

(Berrino *et al.*, 1995) and over time. This must be taken into account in comparative studies of incidence by stage, including time trends. Comparisons over time may be also be biased by the increasing availability of techniques for staging, so that cancers that might have been described as localized with less sophisticated diagnostic techniques are now described as advanced. This phenomenon is known as 'stage migration'. As the size of a primary tumour is less subject to this type of bias, it is the measure preferred by many workers for evaluating stage, with corresponding prognostic implications for the patient. Size is ideally assessed from resected pathological specimens, as described in Chapter 1.

*Rates, not proportions*

Comparisons of prognostic factors (size, stage) should be presented as rates per population screened, as opposed to percentages. Rates allow consideration of changes in the proportions of cancers detected by screening. In the early phase of a screening programme, when most examinations are prevalence screens, a high proportion of small or early-stage cancers will be detected (and, in consequence, a decreased percentage of advanced cancers). Similarly, significant 'overdiagnosis'

**Table 47. Expected reduction in mortality from screening in the United Kingdom (Anglia region) on the basis of participation and interval cancer rates**

| Interval cancers (combined proportionate incidence) | Mortality reduction with 70% participation | Mortality reduction with 80% participation |
| --- | --- | --- |
| 0.34 | 24 | 29 |
| 0.40 | 22 | 26 |
| 0.50 | 19 | 22 |
| 0.54 | 18 | 21 |
| 0.60 | 15 | 18 |
| 0.66 | 13 | 15 |

From Day *et al.* (1995)

of small lesions would lead to a decreased percentage of advanced tumours, altough the absolute rates may be unchanged. Expression of results as the percentage reduction in the incidence of advanced cancers requires an estimate of the incidence of advanced cancers that would have been observed in the absence of the screening programme.

*Time trends in the incidence of breast cancer by stage of disease*

In an analysis of data from the Surveillance, Epidemiology and End Results (SEER) programme in the USA for 1973–93, significant decreases in mortality were seen after 1989 in all age groups (a slight increase in rates had preceded this). The possibility that screening may have been partly responsible was suggested by the increased incidence of localized disease and a subsequent decline in the incidence of regional disease in women in each age group over 40. By 1990, more than 40% of women had received a mammogram in the previous year, mainly for screening purposes (Chu *et al.*, 1996).

In Limburg, The Netherlands, the annual number of breast cancers diagnosed increased by almost 50% immediately after the introduction of screening and then decreased to previous levels after completion of the first screening round. There was a 10% decrease in the incidence of stage II–IV tumours and a 15% decrease in tumours with node involvement over those seen in the period directly before screening began (1987–90). The incidence of tumours with node involvement was 1% lower in 1994 and 15% lower in 1995 (Schouten *et al.*, 1998).

In the study in East Anglia, United Kingdom, the increase in the incidence of small cancers in the early years of screening was much greater than the subsequent decrease in the incidence of advanced cancer, suggesting that the reduction in mortality might have been

somewhat lower than that targeted (McCann *et al.*, 1998; Table 48). The authors used three methods to estimate the 'expected' incidence of advanced cancer in the absence of screening. The first was a projection from the incidence observed in 1976–86 to that in 1995. For the second, they took the average rate of advanced cancers observed in 1987–88, immediately before the onset of screening, and compared it with the 1995 rate. Finally, they took the ratio of advanced to early cancers in 1989–94 in women who had not yet received an invitation to screening, generated an expected incidence rate of advanced cancers, and multiplied this by the actual number of cases in order to obtain the number of cases expected. The predicted rates of advanced cancers from data for 1987 and 1988 suggested a reduction of about 20%, while the predicted rate with exclusion of 1987 and 1988 indicated a much smaller reduction (5.3%).

The screening programme in New South Wales (Australia) was started in 1989. Between 1984 and the end of 1995, an estimated 72% of women in

their 50s and 67% of women in their 60s had had at least one mammogram in the organized screening programme or in the private health system (Kricker *et al.*, 1999). Before 1989, the incidence of breast cancer increased only slightly (+1.3% annually), but between 1990 and 1995 it increased more rapidly (+3.1% annually). Between 1986 and 1995, the rates of small cancers (< 1 cm) increased steeply, by 2.7 times in women aged 40–49 and by 5.6 times in women aged 50–69. The incidence of large breast cancers (≥ 3 cm) up to 1995, after little apparent change up to 1992, fell by 17% in women aged 40–49 and by 20% in those aged 50–69 years. Mortality from breast cancer increased slightly between 1972 and 1989 (+0.5% annually) but then fell (−2.3% annually) between 1990 and 1995 (Kricker *et al.*, 1999). The decline in the incidence of advanced cancer was not, however, seen overall in 1995–97 (Coates *et al.*, 1999).

For countries without organized screening programmes, monitoring and evaluation have certain requirements and limitations. The minimum level of information needed to make some

**Table 48. Incidence rates per 100 000 of invasive breast cancer by TNM stage in women aged 50–69 years, East Anglia region, United Kingdom**

| Stage | Year of diagnosis | | | | | | | | |
|---|---|---|---|---|---|---|---|---|---|
| | 1981–86 | 1987–88 | 1989 | 1990 | 1991 | 1992 | 1993 | 1994 | 1995 |
| Early stage (stage I) | 55.5 | 76.1 | 89.1 | 141 | 160 | 142 | 123 | 141 | 119 |
| Advanced (stages II, III, IV) | 131 | 162 | 159 | 140 | 129 | 110 | 134 | 135 | 132 |
| Total (including unknown stage) | 196 | 245 | 256 | 289 | 297 | 257 | 263 | 282 | 253 |
| Proportion of advanced (%) | 70 | 68 | 64 | 50 | 45 | 44 | 48 | 49 | 53 |

From McCann *et al.* (1998)

estimate of performance is an indication of routine attendance for mammography (every 3 years or less), obtained from sample surveys with questionnaires, if no other source of information is available. Cancer registration provides some indication of screening activity. Trends in rates of advanced disease, as shown in the SEER programme in the USA (Chu et al., 1996) are informative.

The screening programme in Tuscany, Italy (1970–97), showed a small decline in the rate of advanced cancers, but the timing and the fact that it occurred throughout the Province and not just where the organized screening programme had been introduced, suggested that the changes were the result of widespread 'spontaneous' early detection activities (Barchielli & Paci, 2001).

*Estimation of reduction in mortality from observed distributions of tumour grade, size and nodal status (surrogate measures)*

With the availability of detailed information on tumour size, grade and node status, a more sophisticated estimate can be made of the reduction in mortality. The technique requires, however, an uninvited comparison group as well as detailed information on survival in relation to size, grade and nodal status. This technique was used by McCann et al. (2001) with results from the Anglia region of the United Kingdom, where the introduction of screening was staggered by district and by year of birth. There were thus sufficient numbers of women in the region and in the age group targeted for screening who did not receive a first invitation until well after the start of screening in the region in 1989. The technique is more complex than estimates based on interval cancer rates and detection rates. The results suggested that screening in Anglia would reduce mortality by around 7% in women aged 50–54 at diagnosis and by 19% in those aged 55–64 at diagnosis. Overall,

for women aged 50–64 at diagnosis, the reduction would be 15%. However, the technique is sensitive to the lead time for the screen-detected cases: using a 3-year lead time rather than 2 years gave an overall reduction in mortality of 19% in women aged 50–64 at diagnosis. The method is also dependent on assumptions about long-term survival, improved diagnostic classification (stage migration) and confounding by treatment.

Table 49 summarizes the estimates of mortality reduction with the three techniques described above. For Anglia, the techniques result in a range of estimates, from 15% to 21%. In the United Kingdom as a whole, the two simple estimates are 19% and 18%. The broad conclusions are similar in all cases: that

the programme in the United Kingdom was less effective in the early years of screening than in the Swedish Two-county study. The performance of the United Kingdom programme has increased markedly in recent years for a number of reasons. First, use of two views and double reading has increased; secondly, standardization of film density has improved image quality; thirdly, under-performing programmes have been identified with the standardized detection ratio method and have been improved; fourthly, radiologists have become more experienced at both film reading and assessment during the decade since the start of the programme (Tabár et al., 1995; Blanks & Moss, 1999).

## Table 49. Estimated final reduction in mortality from breast cancer for women aged 50–64 at diagnosis, with three techniques, from the early screening data in the United Kingdom

| Technique (reference) | Population | Mortality reduction (%) |
|---|---|---|
| Standardized detection ratio plus participation (Blanks et al., 2000a) | United Kingdom | 19 |
| Interval cancer rate plus participation (Day et al., 1995) | Anglia | 21 |
| Interval cancer rates plus participation (Day et al., 1995) | United Kingdom | 18 |
| Grade, size and nodal status (2-year adjusted lead time) (McCann et al., 2001) | Anglia | 19 |
| Grade, size and nodal status (3-year adjusted lead time) (McCann et al., 2001) | Anglia | 15 |
| MISCAN model[a] (van den Akker-van Marle et al., 1999) | United Kingdom<br>Netherlands | 24<br>29 |

From Tabár et al. (1995); Blanks & Moss (1999)

[a] The estimates of mortality reduction from the MISCAN model are based on the estimated sensitivity of the screening test and the screening interval and age range of the invited women. The estimate for the United Kingdom is higher than that with the other techniques because of the poor sensitivity of the screening programme in the early years.

Any of these methods could be used to estimate mortality reduction, and, ideally, all the methods would be used sequentially as the data became available. The standardized detection ratio method is useful for timely estimates of screening performance and can result in rapid implementation of quality assurance checks if the ratio is too low. It has the further advantage that the calculations are very simple once the target rates for each age range and type of screen have been calculated. Use of interval cancer rates as a performance indicator takes longer but is in theory a better method, provided the data are of sufficient quality. Finally, surrogate measures represent the most sophisticated method for estimating the likely reduction in breast cancer mortality that will be achieved.

### MISCAN model

In The Netherlands, the effectiveness of screening has often been estimated with the MISCAN approach (van den Akker-van Marle et al., 1999), in which a simulated population is used which represents the demographic characteristics and the breast cancer incidence and mortality of the population under study. The natural history of breast cancer is modelled as a progression through successive disease states. Indicators of screening programme performance (e.g. attendance and sensitivity) are added to the model, and the effects on breast cancer mortality with and without screening are estimated. It has been estimated with the MISCAN model that breast cancer mortality in The Netherlands would decrease in women aged 55–74 by 5% in 1996, by 18% in 1999 and by 29% in the long term.

Many of the above conclusions were reached by comparing performance with that in the Swedish randomized trials (as the gold standard) and modelling experience with intermediate indicators to the expected mortality reduction (de Koning et al., 1995b).

## Mortality from and screening for breast cancer in different countries

Screening for breast cancer with mammography is based on the evidence from several randomized trials (see Chapter 4) that showed reductions in mortality from breast cancer of about 20–30% for women aged $\geq$ 50. The important question is whether these results are reproducible as a public health policy, by applying mammography in routine screening. It is likely that the organization, the quality of the technique and the devotion and skills of the persons running a routine programme are different from those in a scientific trial.

Routine screening programmes can be evaluated most readily by time trends and differential mortality from the disease for which screening is being performed. Probably the best known is screening for cervical cancer. The substantial differences among the Nordic countries in the extent of organized screening were closely matched by the mortality rates from cervical cancer (Läärä et al., 1987).

Screening for breast cancer is done either as an organized public health policy or by more spontaneous activity. The International Breast Cancer Screening Network (Shapiro et al., 1998; Klabunde et al., 2001b) comprises 22 countries with national, regional or pilot programmes for screening with mammography. The best known are those in the Nordic countries, The Netherlands and the United Kingdom. Regional efforts are being made in Italy and other southern European countries, and spontaneous activity is widespread, e.g. in Germany and the USA. The implementation period of these programmes is described in Chapter 3.

One of the first papers to report the correlation between routine screening and breast cancer mortality was that of Quinn and Allen (1995) in England and Wales. A change in the trend of mortality was found at the time screening was introduced, whereas there should have been a lag between screening and death if the prolongation of life was due to screening. Hence, the change in trend was too early and probably due to a change in the national treatment policy. Up to the late 1990s, the trend in mortality from breast cancer was linear, with no major indication of an effect of mammography (Figure 31). However, in a detailed analysis, Blanks et al. (2000b) estimated a 6% reduction in breast cancer mortality due to screening among women aged 55–69 in 1998, in a programme which covered the population between 1988 and 1995. This estimate is likely to represent the beginning of the effect of screening in the United Kingdom.

In Sweden, the screening programme started as a cluster-randomized trial in two counties (Tabár et al., 1985); individually randomized trials in various parts of Sweden soon followed (Nyström et al., 1993). A study based on geographical differences in mortality rates in Sweden and a comparison of the results of the original trials showed an estimated reduction in breast cancer mortality of 19%, i.e. somewhat less than those reported in the original trials (Törnberg et al., 1994).

Jonsson et al. (2001) compared counties in Sweden and estimated a 20% reduction in breast cancer mortality due to screening in women aged $\geq$ 50. The estimate was based on deaths only among women in whom breast cancer was diagnosed after the start of the programme. This refined mortality rate is not readily available in routine statistics and, furthermore, assumes the availability of a cancer registry and data protection legislation that allow linkage of the two data sources. As only 27% of all deaths from breast cancer occurred among women in whom breast cancer was diagnosed after the start of the programme, the effect on overall breast cancer mortality can be estimated to be 5–6%, which is clearly too small an effect to be readily identifiable in routine statistics (Figure 32). It is close to the 6% arrived at in the United Kingdom by Blanks *et al.* (2000b). Sjonell and Stahle (1999) found no reduction in mortality in Swedish national data. Given the smaller population and therefore greater

due to these data. Depending on the comparison group (Arnhem or The Netherlands) and the assumptions used in the model, a nonsignificant 6–16% reduction in mortality was estimated.

The acceptability of using a whole country as the control implies that the

effect of the national programme on the risk for death from breast cancer is small; this is confirmed in Figure 33. In 2001, the National Evaluation Team for Breast Cancer Screening reported that the first significant reduction in breast cancer mortality had occurred in 1997–99, among women aged 55–74, of 7–13% in comparison with the pre-screening period of 1986–88. This effect was, however, less than the estimate arrived at with the MISCAN model (Fracheboud *et al.*, 2001a).

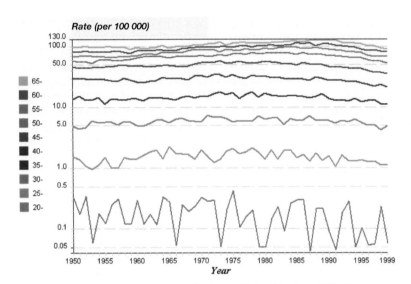

**Figure 31** Trends in breast cancer mortality by age, United Kingdom, 1950–99
From WHO (1999b)

As mentioned earlier, a substantial fall in mortality from breast cancer was seen in Australia (Kricker *et al.*, 1999), which was not totally attributable to screening. The difficulty of evaluating effectiveness can be exemplified by the situation in Finland, where overall breast cancer mortality can be specified for those populations first subjected to screening, then by mortality refined for prescreening diagnosis and finally for those women first invited to screening, with preselected (i.e. unbiased) controls at each stage. A nationwide population-based screening programme for breast cancer was started in 1987 and gradually

instability of breast cancer mortality rates in Sweden, an early effect of breast cancer screening is unlikely to be seen.

The effect of routine screening on mortality from breast cancer was also difficult to estimate in The Netherlands (van den Akker-van Marle *et al.*, 1999). In a recent study, Broeders *et al.* (2001) evaluated the effect of the screening programme that started in Nijmegen a quarter of a century ago. Mortality from breast cancer between 1969 and 1997 was analysed and compared with data for Arnhem, with no such programme, and for The Netherlands as a whole. Data were not available on deaths among patients in whom breast cancer was diagnosed before screening started, but the long follow-up and use of elegant modelling techniques reduced the bias

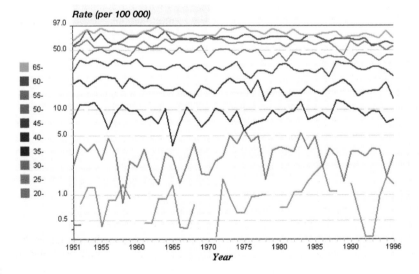

**Figure 32** Trends in breast cancer mortality by age, Sweden, 1951–96
From WHO (1999b)

extended to cover all women aged 50–64 (Hakama *et al.*, 1991). Women in 1-year birth cohorts recommended by the National Board of Health were identified individually and invited for screening, and the same women were re-screened every 2 years. In 1987, it was recommended that women born in 1928, 1932 and 1936 should be screened, and the programme was expanded to cover all the other even-year birth cohorts. More age cohorts were included in the programme during the implementation phase.

A centralized, comprehensive information system is provided by the Mass Screening Registry within the nationwide Finnish Cancer Registry for identification, invitation and follow-up of women and for evaluation of the effectiveness of the programme. Cancer registration is virtually complete (Teppo *et al.*, 1994). The National Population Registry, the National Register of Deaths and the Cancer Registry are linked with the screening results via the Mass Screening Registry. Intermediate indicators derived from this programme, such as attendance, specificity and sensitivity, show good quality (Pamilo *et al.*, 1990; Saarenmaa *et al.*, 1999).

National figures are appropriate for evaluating the Finnish programme because the policy is nationwide and the programme was implemented for a relatively short time. No obvious change in national trends in mortality from breast cancer corresponding to the screening programme was seen (Figure 34) in the crude data, but a more refined analysis is needed.

Any change in mortality rates should first be seen in women born in 1928, 1932 and 1936—that is, in the cohorts that were screened first, in 1987, the first year of the public health policy. As screening was delayed for several years and for a minimum of 2 years among women born in the adjacent cohorts of odd birth years, they were selected as controls. It was assumed that any effect

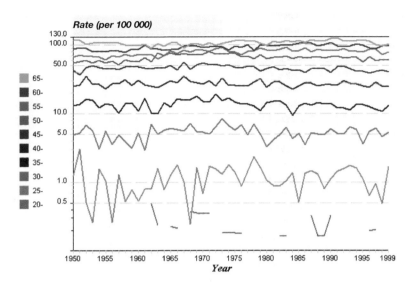

**Figure 33** Trends in breast cancer mortality by age, The Netherlands, 1950–99
From WHO (1999b)

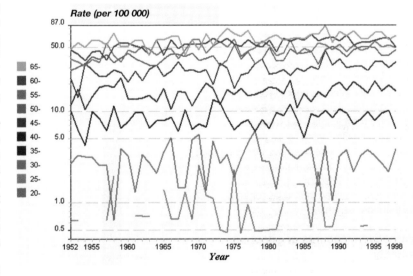

**Figure 34** Trends in breast cancer mortality by age, Finland, 1952–98
From WHO (1999b)

would be seen some years after screening but before the controls benefitted from screening. As the mortality rates by birth cohort were similar (Figure 35), the cohort-specific deaths did not indicate any effect of screening.

Screening will affect only deaths from breast cancer among women in whom breast cancer was diagnosed after the start of screening. There was no substantial difference in mortality between the target and the control populations when incident cases diagnosed before 1987 were excluded (refined mortality rate) (Figure 36).

The design of the Finnish programme allowed identification of individual women by screening status and by date of invitation to screening (Hakama et al., 1997). The participants in the programme were women born between 1927 and 1939. Invitations to screening were given in 1987–89, and the invited women were classified as screened or non-responders. The controls were women in the same municipalities, matched for age with those screened and individually identified at the same time as women invited for screening. By the end of 1992, 64 women invited for screening and 63 controls had died from breast cancer diagnosed after the start of follow-up. The refined breast cancer mortality rate was lower for those invited to screening than for the controls (RR = 0.76), indicating a 24% protective effect of screening. This was not statistically significant (95% CI, 0.53–1.09). For the cohorts born in 1932 and after, the effect was larger (RR = 0.56) and statistically significant (95% CI, 0.33–0.95). The protective effect appeared relatively early, from the third year of follow-up. More details of this trial-like evaluation of the public health policy are given in Chapter 4. The effect could not be demonstrated by routine statistics owing to dilution and selection. A study with randomized, matched individual controls was therefore essential.

## Alternative measures of effect on mortality

A number of alternative measures derived from the estimated reduction in mortality due to screening may be useful in decision-making (Hakama et al., 1999). These were calculated for the Finnish population, in which mammographic screening has been estimated to have achieved a 24% reduction in breast cancer mortality among women aged 50–64 years who were invited to

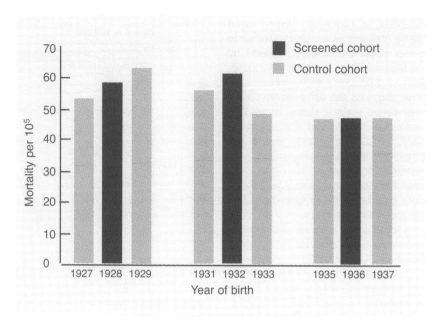

**Figure 35** Birth cohort-specific mortality rates from breast cancer (per 100 000 woman–years) in Finland, 1990–95
From Hakama et al. (1999)

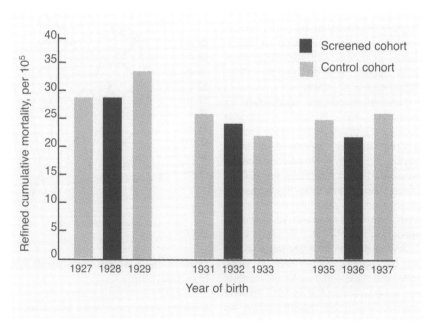

**Figure 36** Cumulative (refined) mortality rates from breast cancer (per 100 000 woman–years) in Finland by birth cohort during 1987–95 after exclusion of incidence cases diagnosed before 1987.
From Hakama et al. (1999)

screening (Hakama *et al.*, 1997). These measures include: the number of cancer deaths prevented per screen (estimated to be four deaths per 10 000 screens), life span gained per breast cancer death prevented (estimated to be 15 years), life span gained per patient with breast cancer detected by screening (estimated to be 1.5 years); life span gained per screen (estimated to be 2.2 days, which can be compared with the estimated half day spent by a woman attending for screening) and life span gained per invitation to screening, i.e. per member of the target population of women (estimated to be 1.9 days).

## Balance between false-positive and false-negative results

Screening quality must be evaluated in parallel with estimates of breast cancer mortality reduction. While the emphasis in the United Kingdom screening programme tended to be on detection rates of invasive cancers, the screening programme in The Netherlands focused on prevention of too many false-positive results. Verbeek *et al.* (1991) suggested that the "first measure to pay attention to is the specificity. If the specificity does not meet the reference value, improvements have to be made irrespective of the other control outcomes [positive predictive value and detection rate]. In such a screening set up [a high] proportion of healthy women with a positive screening test is not acceptable." They therefore introduced simultaneous evaluation of performance and quality.

The screening programme in The Netherlands started in 1988, around the same time as that in the United Kingdom, and is notable for its very low recall rate for assessment (de Koning *et al.*, 1995b). Verbeek *et al.* (1991) suggested a target recall rate of < 1%, while the Forrest (1986) report indicated that the acceptable recall rate in the United Kingdom could be as high as 10%. In the United Kingdom, variations in positive predictive value, referral rates for diag-

nostic confirmation (also called recall rate) and cancer detection rates from individual programmes were studied with charts showing positive predictive value of referral against referral rate, with the cancer detection rate expressed as isobars (Blanks *et al.*, 2001). The variation in individual programmes for both measures was shown to be very high, the positive predictive value ranging from 26% to 6% and the recall rate from 2% to 9%. Programmes tended to have similar results each year. The diagrams suggest that, in the United Kingdom, a positive predictive value of 25% is too high and results in a marginally lower detection rate. Programmes with recall rates of about 4%, positive predictive values of 15–20% and standardized detection ratios of around 1.3 achieved the highest quality of screening. It is clear that some individual programmes have better quality screening. In many cases, it is possible to suggest how detection rates could be improved. Like the standardized detection ratio, the positive predictive value–referral diagram is useful as an internal quality control measure for centres with similar risk distributions in their target populations. In the United Kingdom, the emphasis has been on detection rates and then on improving

screening quality once those rates have been achieved. This was true particularly after the high interval cancer rates reported in the early years of screening.

It is interesting to compare the screening programmes in The Netherlands and the United Kingdom in terms of quality. It should be noted that the procedures used in the two countries are different, and some caution should be exercised in comparing the percentages of women referred and positive predictive value. Nevertheless, in The Netherlands, there has been a strong effort to maintain high specificity (Verbeek *et al.*, 1991) and, as a consequence, a high positive predictive value and a low referral rate. The low referral rates are based partly on the low rates in the pilot study and the Nijmegen study and show the influence of those studies on national screening programmes.

Table 50 shows the results of The Netherlands screening programme between 1990 and 1995. The referral rates are very low indeed, particularly at subsequent screens, and this is acknowledged as a feature of the national programme. However, the cancer detection rate at subsequent screens was 20% lower than expected, and the low referral rates at subsequent

---

**Table 50. Comparison of observed and expected results of The Netherlands screening programme, 1990–95, for women aged 50–69**

|  | Initial screens | | Subsequent screens | |
|---|---|---|---|---|
|  | Observed | Expected | Observed | Expected |
| Referrals (% of screened women) | 1.4 | 1.6 | 0.7 | 0.6 |
| Positive predictive value of referral (%) | 48 | 41 | 51 | 57 |
| Detection rate per 1000 women screened | 6.6 | 6.5 | 3.4 | 4.3 |

From Fracheboud *et al.* (1998). Expected values estimated from MISCAN model

screening rounds have been postulated as a possible explanation (Fracheboud *et al.*, 1998).

The screening programme in the United Kingdom provides an interesting contrast. Table 51 shows the data on subsequent screening in The Netherlands and the equivalent data for the United Kingdom in 1994–95. The comparison is interesting, although it also illustrates that great care should be taken in in interpreting performance data among countries, as women are referred differently in The Netherlands and the United Kingdom. Nevertheless, the dramatic difference is surprising, as is the difference in cancer detection rates. Further work is required to enable a more useful comparison. It is debatable whether screening performance measures, particularly those related to quality, can be adequately compared across countries.

Factors such as screening quality vary not only among countries but also dramatically within countries. In the United Kingdom, referral rates can vary by 2–9% and positive predictive value by 6–26% (Blanks *et al.*, 2001). Giordano *et al.* (1996) reported data derived by applying the performance measures in the European guidelines (Commission of the European Communities, 2001) to the Italian breast screening programmes and found that most have attained 'acceptable' or 'desirable' levels for many indicators. The differences in indicators of screening quality show that the interpretation of the measures is to some extent subjective. How many false-positive referrals should be tolerated for each cancer detected? In The Netherlands, the number is very low, but in the United Kingdom it depends on the clinician in charge of the screening centre. Setting screening quality targets is much more subjective than setting targets for screening effectiveness in reducing breast cancer mortality. Furthermore, measurement of screening quality is complicated by differences in the screening protocols among countries. Comparison of referral rates is complex, even when the national organized programmes are superficially not very different, as in The Netherlands and the United Kingdom. Any comparison with, for example, the USA, which does not have a national organized screening programme, would therefore be invidious.

In contrast, measures of screening effectiveness in terms of reducing mortality, e.g. participation, cancer detection rates (standardized detection ratios), interval cancer rates (as a proportional incidence measure) and stage distribution of screen-detected cancers, can be compared across countries more readily.

## Conclusion

Screening programmes should ultimately be monitored in terms of deaths, the measure directly related to the purpose of screening. The effect of screening is real but small at present, the estimates of change in national overall breast cancer mortality rates being 5–10% in countries with the longest experience. The estimates were larger in a few studies of sub-populations and after removal of bias due to deaths in cases diagnosed before the start of screening. The gain in life years per screen is nevertheless likely to remain small. Small reductions in breast cancer mortality, usually < 10%, will increase with length of follow-up and may ultimately approach the estimates found in randomized trials, of 20–30%. As such results will take a long time to achieve, the change will be very gradual and probably not immediately visible in national trends. Prolongation of follow-up will not affect the small estimated time gained in comparison with time spent, as screening is usually repeated every 2 years.

Although screening for breast cancer may thus appear to be insufficiently effective for use as a public health policy, that conclusion is probably not justified. Screening for breast cancer also has a humanitarian value, in addition to the prolongation of life. Screening, in principle, offers a greater chance to select the type of intervention, including breast-conserving and less invasive treatment. Most recalls are due to false-positive results, which cause unnecessary anxiety and invasive or otherwise unpleasant investigations. A decision on whether to screen should depend on a

**Table 51. Observed and expected values for subsequent screens: Netherlands (1990–95, age 50–69) and United Kingdom (1994–95, age 50–64)**

|  | United Kingdom | | Netherlands | |
|---|---|---|---|---|
|  | Observed | Expected[a] | Observed | Expected[b] |
| Referrals (% of screened women) | 3.4 | ≤ 7 | 0.7 | 0.6 |
| Positive predictive value of referral (%) | 13 | – | 51 | 57 |
| Detection rate per 1000 | 4.3 | > 3.5 | 3.4 | 4.3 |

From Fracheboud *et al.* (1998); Blanks *et al.* (2000a)
[a] In early years
[b] Based on MISCAN model

weighting of all the effects and how they compare with other health services. Many other health activities have not been properly evaluated and may be even less effective.

Reliable monitoring of a screening programme should be based on death as the outcome indicator and on measures derived from deaths. When such an approach is not possible, surrogate outcome indicators should be used, although favourable results based on established standards do not necessarily imply a reduction in breast cancer mortality. Only in special circumstances will it be possible to distinguish the component of the reduction in mortality that can be attributed to screening from other effects, such as treatment. Screening with mammography prevents some deaths from breast cancer. The effect is certain but small. In terms of prolongation of life, the effect is about 2 days per woman per screen. In terms of standardized mortality ratios, the effect may approach that seen in trials and ultimately a reduction in breast cancer mortality of about 20%.

## Hazards (risks) of screening

The underlying rationale for breast cancer screening is to promote health by identifying women with breast cancer at an early enough stage that treatment will cure the disease. However, the vast majority of women undergoing screening do not have breast cancer at the time of the examination, and these women cannot derive a direct health benefit from screening; they can only be harmed. The following sections address the two major categories of possible harm that are relevant to any programme of early detection: false-positive results and overdiagnosis. In addition, although a diagnosis of breast cancer earlier than its clinical presentation is part of the pathway to potential benefit, it also

implies that women have to live longer knowing that they have a potentially serious disease. For some women, this is balanced by more conserving surgery and improved survival or cure, but for the majority is represents only a disadvantage. The effect of an earlier diagnosis of disease on the quality of life is an immediate negative aspect of screening, against which any prolongation of life should be weighed (Figure 37).

Two possible harms specific to mammography are also considered: an early increase in mortality from breast cancer and radiation-induced cancer.

## Occurrence and consequences of false-positive results in mammography
### False-positives and overdiagnosis
The term 'false-positive' refers to an abnormal mammogram (one requiring further assessment) in a woman ultimately found to have no evidence of cancer. 'Overdiagnosis' refers to the diagnosis and treatment of cancers that would never have caused symptoms. Thus, a false-positive result can be found only in a woman without cancer, while

overdiagnosis can be made only for women with cancer. While an individual woman can readily be identified as having had a false-positive result, overdiagnosis can never be identified reliably for an individual, as virtually all abnormalities labelled 'cancer' are treated.

The 'harm' of false-positive mammograms relates to the additional testing, invasive procedures and anxiety that would never have happened in the absence of screening. The 'harm' of overdiagnosis relates to unnecessary anxiety (associated with a diagnosis of potentially fatal disease) and unnecessary treatment. Both harms are inevitable if a screening programme is to be effective (Morrison, 1992). The challenge is to minimize both while still detecting those cancers for which early diagnosis and treatment can alter the clinical course of disease.

### Definition of a false-positive rate
Two definitions have been used to define a false-positive screening result. The broad definition includes all mammograms that are accompanied by a recommendation for further assessment (e.g. repeat examination, clinical exami-

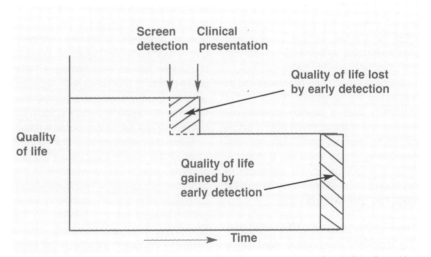

**Figure 37** Quality of life over time for women whose breast cancers are found clinically and by screening

nation, diagnostic mammogram, ultrasound or breast biopsy) for women who are found ultimately not to have cancer. A narrower approach is to count only those recommendations that ultimately lead to a breast biopsy in these women (Kopans, 1992). While breast biopsies are arguably the most important adverse effect of a false-positive mammogram, the broader definition is used here, both because it is commoner and because it more completely captures all subsequent events.

The frequency of false-positive mammograms is conceptually measured only among women ultimately found not to have cancer and is defined as:

$$\frac{\text{Number of exams with a recommendation for further assessment among women known not to have cancer}}{\text{Number of exams among women known not to have cancer}}$$

In practical terms, however, the same number is well estimated as a product:

$$\text{\% of all mammograms requiring further assessment} \times (1 - \text{PPV})$$

where PPV is the positive predictive value or the percentage of mammograms requiring further assessment that are ultimately found to be cancer.

Either approach can be interpreted as answering the question: 'What is the probability that a healthy woman will require further assessment after a single screening mammogram?' Although this measure is, strictly speaking, a probability or a proportion, in the remainder of this chapter it is referred to by its familiar label: the 'false-positive rate'.

*False-positive rates observed in practice*
The reported false-positive rates range from < 1% to > 10% (Table 52). Two broad observations can be made from these data. First, false-positives are more frequent at a woman's first screening examination than at subsequent examinations. This observation probably reflects the value of having a previous film for comparison and, in national programmes, cumulative experience in mammography.

Secondly, different groups of radiographers perform differently. In particular, false-positive rates are an order of magnitude higher in community practice in the USA than in The Netherlands screening programme. This difference may reflect different thresholds for recommending further evaluation of specific mammographic abnormalities, such as calcifications and well-circumscribed nodules. For example, the false-positive rate will increase if further evaluation is suggested for smaller, less characteristic clusters of calcifications. These differences may, in turn, be explained by the distinct medico-legal climate in the USA, where a missed diagnosis of breast cancer is now the commonest and second most costly basis for malpractice suits (Black *et al.*, 1995; Mitnick *et al.*, 1995; Physician Insurers Association of America, 1995).

*Cumulative risk*
Most false-positive results are reported from a single mammogram. However, as women undergo screening mammograms repeatedly, an individual woman's cumulative risk of ever having a false-positive results increases with repeated screens. From the woman's perspective, therefore, it may be important to know the cumulative risk for a false-positive result.

Some data are available. During the 4 years of the Health Insurance Plan programme, about 5% of women in the screened group had a recommendation for biopsy after a false-positive mammogram (Shapiro *et al.*, 1988a). In the Stockholm trial, approximately 1% of biopsies conducted as a result of false-positive mammograms were performed in women invited for two annual rounds of screening (Lidbrink *et al.*, 1996). This low rate was seen after only two screens, but there was also a low rate of abnormal mammogram readings (0.8–1.8%) in the Stockholm study. In the Screening Mammography Program of British Columbia, Canada, the cumulative risk for a false-positive mammogram after 10 screens was estimated to be 38% for women aged 40–49, 35% for women aged 50–59 and 29% for those aged 60–69 (Olivotto *et al.*, 1998).

In the USA, Elmore *et al.* (1998) studied the experience of 2400 women screened in a health plan in Massachusetts. After a 10-year follow-up, 23.8% of the women had had at least one false-positive result and 5.1% had had an invasive procedure as a result of a false-positive result. Using a Bayesian version of a product or an estimate of the Kaplan-Meier type, in which mammographic screening events were used instead of time, the authors estimated that, after 10 mammograms, 49% (95% CI, 40–64%) of the women would have had a false-positive result. When the definition of a false-positive result was limited to women without cancer who underwent a breast biopsy, the cumulative risk over 10 mammograms was estimated to be 19% (95% CI, 10–41%).

The same general approach was used to estimate the cumulative risk of ever having a false-positive result as a function of the two most relevant inputs: the false-positive rate (in which first and subsequent screens are distinguished) and the number of times screening is repeated (a function of the screening interval; Table 53). The effects of various conditions on the cumulative risk for a false-positive result are clear.

*Adverse consequences of false-positive results*
The adverse effects reported after false-positive results include increased use of health care and increased patient anxiety.

**Table 52. Chance that a women without breast cancer will require further assessment after a single mammogram**

| Setting | Proportion of | | False-positive rate (% abnormal x (1–PPV)) (%) |
|---|---|---|---|
| | Mammograms requiring further assessment (% abnormal) | Abnormal examinations in which cancer is diagnosed (PPV) (%) | |
| *National programmes* | | | |
| Netherlands (de Koning *et al.*, 1995b) | | | |
| First screen | 1.4 | 48–51 | 0.7 |
| Subsequent screens | 0.9 | 36–54 | 0.5 |
| United Kingdom (Blanks *et al.*, 2000a) | | | |
| First screen | 7–8 | 6–8 | 7.0 |
| Subsequent screens | 3–4 | 12–14 | 3.0 |
| US National Breast and Cervical Cancer Detection Program (May *et al.*, 1998) | | | |
| First screen | 5 | 9.5 | 4.5 |
| Subsequent screens | 4 | 5.6 | 3.8 |
| *Other* | | | |
| US academic practice (Kerlikowske *et al.*, 1993) | | | |
| First screen (age 50–59) | 7 | 9 | 6.4 |
| First screen (age 60–69) | 8 | 17 | 6.6 |
| Subsequent screens (age 50–59) | 2 | 16 | 1.7 |
| Subsequent screens (age 60–69) | 2 | 7 | 1.9 |
| US Medicare (age 65–69) (Welch & Fisher, 1998) | | | |
| Mixture of first and subsequent screens | 8.5 | 8 | 7.8 |
| US community practice (Brown *et al.*, 1995) | | | |
| Mixture of first and subsequent screens | 11 | 3.5 | 10.6 |

PPV, positive predictive value

*Increased cost and health-care use*
False-positive results are associated with increased numbers of office visits, diagnostic mammograms, ultrasounds and breast biopsies. Lidbrink *et al.* (1996) reported that 502 women with false-positive results in the Stockholm trial made 1539 visits to a physician and had 542 fine-needle aspiration biopsies, 257 diagnostic mammograms and 118 surgical biopsies. The cost of evaluating the false-positive results was 26.5% that of screening. In the study of Elmore and colleagues (1998), 631 false-positive results generated 601 office visits, 384 diagnostic mammograms, 176 breast ultrasounds, 100 open or core biopsies, 28 fine-needle aspirations and one hospitalization. In the same study, it was estimated that about US$ 33 would be spent on follow-up procedures to evaluate false-positive results for every US$ 100 spent on screening mammography. May *et al.* (1998) found that abnormal mammogram results generated additional mammographic views in 56%, sonography in 31%, clinical examinations in 30%, fine-needle aspirations in 8.7% and breast biopsy in 28% of cases. These percentages were not broken down according to true- and false-positive results, and no costs were included.

None of these studies included the costs of increased health-care use by patients. Barton and colleagues (2001) found that, in the 12 months after recommended follow-up, false-positive results were associated with more patient-initiated visits for both breast-related (incidence ratio, 4.03; 95% CI, 2.97–5.47) and non-breast-related (incidence ratio, 1.18; 95% CI, 1.09–1.28) reasons, including mental health services. Extrapolating to women

## Table 53. Estimated cumulative risk of ever having a false-positive result on mammography under various conditions

| First screen | Subsequent screens | False-positive results (%) 20-year programme of screening with examination every: | | |
|---|---|---|---|---|
| | | 3 years | 2 years | 1 year |
| 0.7 | 0.5 | 3.2 | 5 | 10 |
| 2.0 | 1.0 | 7 | 10 | 19 |
| 4.0 | 2.0 | 13 | 20 | 35 |
| 6.0 | 3.0 | 19 | 29 | 47 |
| 8.0 | 4.0 | 25 | 36 | 58 |
| 10.0 | 5.0 | 30 | 43 | 66 |
| 10.6 | 10.6 | 49 | 67 | 89 |

The cumulative risk is calculated as 1 minus the chance of never having a false-positive result (which, in turn, is the product of the probabilities of having a normal result in multiple examinations). For example, consider the upper left-hand cell — the probability of ever having a false-positive result of a women screened every 3 years for 20 years in a programme with a false-positive rate of 0.7% on the first screen and 0.5% on subsequent screens. The chance of not having a false-positive result is 99.3% on the first examation and 99.5% on each subsequent screen. The cumulative risk over 20 years in which six examinations are performed is 1 − (0.993 × 0.995 × 0.995 × 0.995 × 0.995 × 0.995) or 3.2%.

eligible for screening in the population of the USA, the authors estimated that false-positive results could generate as many as 14.4 million non-breast-related physician visits over a decade.

*Emotional and psychological effects* Rimer and Bluman (1997) reviewed nine studies conducted before 1997 which specifically addressed the psychological impact of false-positive results of mammography. Using the same search strategy, the Working Group identified nine more studies (Table 54). The studies vary by country, the type of patients studied, when in relation to the mammogram they were studied and the instruments used to determine their psychological state. Nonetheless, all but one showed transient negative psychological effects associated with a false-positive result.

Most of the studies showed that the increase in anxiety was moderate. Although the increase was short-lived in most women (e.g. Brett *et al.*, 1998; Gilbert *et al.*, 1998; Olsson *et al.*, 1999), some experienced longer-term consequences of a false-positive result. In one study, an increased anxiety score was reported 3 months after an abnormal mammogram, and in another the score was still increased 18 months after the test (Gram *et al.*, 1990; Lerman *et al.*, 1991).

Few studies have addressed the impact of a false-positive result on behavioural measures. One study showed that women who were recalled were more likely to continue practising breast self-examination (Bull & Campbell, 1991). Barton *et al.* (2001) reported that physicians were more likely to record breast-related concern for women who had had a false-positive result and that

these women were more likely to use health-care services, for both breast and non-breast-related problems.

Three studies have been conducted of the effect of a false-positive result on future screening behaviour. Burman and colleagues (1999) compared the subsequent adherence to screening mammography of 813 women who had had false-positive results and 4246 women who had had normal mammograms. After adjustment for multiple risk factors, the women who had had a false-positive result were slightly more likely to attend for their next screening mammogram than women with a normal result (odds ratio, 1.21; 95% CI, 1.01 1.45). Pisano *et al.* (1998) surveyed 43 women who had undergone excisional breast biopsy after receiving a false-positive result 3 years earlier. When compared with 53 randomly selected women with normal mammograms and 83 women with 6-month recall, the women who had had a biopsy were slightly more likely to attend for subsequent screening mammography. Lerman *et al.* (1991) also found that more women who had had a false-positive result than those with normal screens attended for their next scheduled screening mammogram (74–78% versus 68%, *p* > 0.05). No studies were found of screening behaviour after repeated false-positive results.

Clearly, substantial proportions of women who have a false-positive result become anxious about breast cancer. This was true in several countries and cultures. Anxiety tends to be greatest at the time of notification of an abnormality and less (or resolved) when the work-up is completed without breast cancer being found. There is no evidence that false-positive results decrease future adherence to screening recommendations and in fact may increase it slightly. Women may therefore understand that false-positive results are a part of mammography. Schwartz *et al.* (2000) found that 99% of 479 women were

## Table 54. Studies of psychological status and health behaviour after a false-positive result on a screening

| Reference and country | Type and time of measurement | Groups and numbers of women and response | Response rate (%) | Results |
|---|---|---|---|---|
| Ellmann et al. (1989) United Kingdom | General health questionnaire in person. At visit and 3 months later | Normal mammogram: 295<br>False-positive result: 271<br>Breast cancer: 134 | Overall, 98 | % anxious:<br>Normal / False-positive result<br>At visit: 35 / 44<br>3 months later: 26 / 29<br>$p < 0.02$–$0.02$ at visit |
| Bull & Campbell (1991) United Kingdom | Mailed self-administered questionnaire. Before screening. 6 weeks after screening | Invited to screening: 750<br>Normal mammogram: 420<br>False-positive result, no invasive test: 240<br>False-positive result, biopsy: | 72<br>79<br>72<br>68 | % anxious about breast cancer / % practising self-examination<br>5 / 10<br>4 / 10<br>2 / 24<br>6 / 35<br>Not significant / $p < 0.00$ |
| Sutton et al. (1995) United Kingdom | Mailed general health questionnaire with 7-item anxiety subscale. Before screening. At screening. 9 months after screening | 1021<br>795<br>795 | 68<br>78<br>78 | Retrospecitive anxiety score:<br>False-positive result / Normal<br>1.6 / 1.6<br>1.7 / 1.3<br>1.1 / 1.1 |
| Swanson et al. (1996) United Kingdom | Psychological consequences questionnaire, mailed and on-site. At invitation. At screening. At recall | False-positive result: 33 | 49<br>68<br>100 | Mean psychological score<br>Invited / Screened / Recalled<br>Physical 0.7 / 0.2 / 3.0<br>Emotional 1.3 / 0.5 / 4.1<br>Somatic 1.1 / 0.5 / 3.3<br>* All recall scores significantly differ from earlier scores |
| Ong et al. (1997) United Kingdom | Mailed psychological conseqences questionnaire. 1 month after final visit | Regular recall: 130<br>after assessment: 128<br>after fine-needle aspiration: 106<br>Early recall after assessment: 130<br>Regular recall after biopsy: 30 | Overall, 75 | % psychological consequences<br>29<br>50<br>58   $p < 0.0005$<br>63<br>87 |

**Table 54 (contd)**

| Reference and country | Type and time of measurement | Groups and numbers of women and response | | Response rate (%) | Results | |
|---|---|---|---|---|---|---|
| Brett et al. (1998) United Kingdom | Mailed psychological consequences questionnaire 5 months after screening | Normal mammogram<br>False-positive result, non-non-invasive work-up:<br>False-positive result, fine-needle aspirate cytology:<br>False-positive result, biopsy:<br>False-positive result, 6-month recall: | 52<br>51<br><br>41<br>45<br>23 | Overall, 76% | % psychological consequences<br>10<br>45<br><br>44<br>59<br>61 | $p < 0.0001$ |
| Gilbert et al. (1998) United Kindom | Mailed and (on-site hospital) anxiety and depression scale and health questionnaire<br>Before screening<br>At screening<br>At recall<br>5 weeks after recall<br>4 months after recall | <br><br>2110<br>1463<br>122<br>90<br>90 | | <br><br>90<br>70<br>98<br>74<br>74 | % anxious:<br>39<br>31<br>47<br>34<br>33<br>$p < 0.02–0.001$ for recall vs others | |
| Gram et al. (1990) Norway | Mailed self-administered questionnaire 18 months after screening | Normal mammogram:<br>False-positive result: | 152<br>126 | 73<br>79 | % anxious about breast cancer:<br>13<br>29<br>$p = 0.001$ | |
| Gram & Slenker (1992) Norway | Mailed self-administered questionnaire 1 year after screening | Normal mammogram:<br>False-positive result: | 209<br>160 | 84<br>89 | % anxious about breast cancer<br>22<br>40<br>$p < 0.05$ | |
| Lidbrink et al. (1995) Sweden | Self-administered questionnaire: and blood tests on site At follow-up test 3 weeks after completed work-up | False-positive result: | 48 | 98 | Mood score:<br>Time I: 2.3<br>Time 2: 3.4<br>$p < 0.05$<br>No difference in cortisol or prolactic concentration or in lymphycytic stimulation | |

## Table 54 (contd)

| Reference and country | Type and time of measurement | Groups and numbers of women and response | Response rate (%) | Results |
|---|---|---|---|---|
| Olssen et al. (1999) Sweden | Mailed psychological consequences questionnaire 1 and 6 months after final visit | False-positive result: Normal mammogram: | 93 89 | Mean psychological score<br>         1 month  6 month<br>~0.75  ~0.3<br>~0.19  ~0.17<br>$p < 0.001$ between false-positive result and normal mammogram |
| Lerman et al. (1991) USA | Anxiety questionnaire by telephone interview Mammography adherence by telephone interview 3 months after false-positive result: All work-up completed 15 months later | Normal mammogram: False-positive result, low suspicion: False-positive result, high suspicion: | Not reported | % anxious about  % attendance at mammography  next screen<br>48  68<br>61  78<br>70  74<br>$p = 0.008$  $p < 0.05$ |
| Pisano et al. (1998) USA | Record of intention for screening mammogram, by telephone interview 3–4 years after index screening | False-positive result and excisional biopsy: False-positive result and 6-month recall: Normal mammogram: | Overall, 75 | % intended  % attended regular future  screen x 3 years screens<br>72  98<br>58  82<br>66  90<br>$p = 0.26$  $p = 0.036$ |
| Burman et al. (1999) USA | Screening mammogram, by computerized record review Up to 6 months after next recommended screening | False-positive result: Normal mammogram: | Overall 85 | % returned for recommended screen:<br>73<br>74<br><br>% medical records with anxiety about breast cancer noted |
| Barton et al. (2001) USA | Office visits by medical record reviewer For 12 months after screening | Normal mammogram: False-positive result: | 100 (medical records) | 0.2<br>10.0<br>$p = 0.001$ |
| Cockburn et al. (1994), USA | Mailed and on-site psychological consequences questionnaire At screening Before results At recall clinic 1 week after 'all clear' 8 months later | False-positive result: Normal mammogram: 'Community': | 70 68 72 | Mean emotional and physical dysfunction scores significantly increased in group with false-positive results at recall and 1 week after 'all-clear'. Otherwise, scores in 3 groups similar |

**Table 54 (contd)**

| Reference and country | Type and time of measurement | Groups and numbers of women and response | Response rate (%) | Results |
|---|---|---|---|---|
| Lowe et al. (1999) Australia | Mailed, self-administered questionnaire, general health questionnaire, psychological consequences questionnaire<br>At appointment<br>At recall<br><br>1 month after recall | 3158<br>False-positive result:  182<br>Normal mammogram:  182<br>False-positive result:  182<br>Normal mammogram:  182 | 95<br>94<br>81<br>81<br>81 | Women with false-positive results more concerned about breast cancer and more so than for normal mammogram after 1 month (p < 0.05) |
| Scaf-Klomp et al. (1997) Netherlands | Psychological consequences questionnaire for false-positive result<br>Self-administered questionnaire for normal mammogram<br>8–10 weeks after first mammogram<br>6 months after first mammogram | False-positive result  74<br>Normal mammogram:  113<br>Randomly selected women without mammogram:  238 | 78<br>59<br><br>59 | Women with false-positive result scored higher on psychological consequences questionnaire than those with normal mammogram but no higher than randomly selected women without mammogram |

aware that false-positive results occur, and most accepted them as a consequence of screening. This was true regardless of whether the respondent had actually experienced a false-positive result.

### Decreasing the adverse effects of false-positive results

As false-positive results cannot be totally eliminated, strategies to reduce the occurrence and severity of the adverse psychological effects and behaviour should be developed. Lindfors et al. (2001) compared stress in women who had undergone immediate work-up and received a false-positive result and women who returned for later work-ups and reports. The mean overall stress rating on a five-point scale was 2.3 for women who had undergone immediate work-up and 2.8 for women who returned later for work-up. The response rate to the survey was 40%, but the two groups of women who did respond were similar in terms of demographic variables. Women receiving immediate follow-up evaluation after an abnormal result may not have time to become anxious before the result is clarified, and some may be unaware that an extra view or ultrasound is conducted because an abnormality was found on their screening mammogram. Immediate follow-up requires the presence of a radiographer, and the cost implications of this strategy should be assessed if the finding that immediate follow-up reduces anxiety is repeated.

Ong and Austoker (1997) studied the effect of discussion of results with nurses when patients were recalled for further evaluation after an abnormal mammogram. Fewer women who had a chance to talk with a nurse wanted to talk later about why the assessment was needed (4%) than women who did not talk to a nurse (30%), and fewer wanted additional information. The result was similar when an information leaflet was added to the recall letter (Austoker & Ong, 1994).

When information was given in the leaflet, women perceived less need for more information. Whether educating women about false-positive results in general or making counselling services available prevents or lowers anxiety is not known and should be studied.

### Decreasing the rate of false-positive results

Although the literature on strategies for lowering the false-positive rate is sparse, and no formal trials of strategies were found, it would appear reasonable to address the risk factors for false-positive results. The literature suggests that characteristics relating to both the subject and the mammography process are involved.

*Factors related to women that affect the false-positive rate*

Age is inversely related to the false-positive rate (Kerlikowske et al., 1993; Kopans et al., 1996; Lidbrink et al., 1996), at least partly because dense breasts are more difficult to read radiographically (Fajardo et al., 1988). However, it was found in one study (van Gils et al., 1998) that no such difficulty was apparent for mammograms read after 1983, when compared with those read between 1975 and 1982. No stratification by age was reported, which could be important, because average breast density decreases slightly as women age and epithelial tissue is replaced with fatty tissue (Tabár & Dean, 1982). White et al. (1998) demonstrated that the breast density of premenopausal women was greater during the luteal (2 weeks before onset of menses) than the follicular (2 weeks after onset of menses) phase of menses.

Several studies have shown that postmenopausal hormonal replacement therapy also increases breast density (Berkowitz et al., 1990; Stomper et al., 1990; Kaufman et al., 1991; McNicholas et al., 1994; Laya et al., 1995; Greendale et al., 1999). Four studies documented an increased frequency of false-positive readings in postmenopausal women on hormone replacement therapy. Laya and colleagues (1996) found a relative risk for a false-positive mammogram reading of 1.71 (95% CI, 1.37–2.14) in current users and 1.16 (95% CI, 0.93–1.45) in former users, versus never users of estrogen replacement therapy. Christiansen et al. (2000) found similar effects, while Kavanagh et al. (2000) found that, in comparison with non-users, users of hormone replacement therapy had an adjusted odds ratio of 1.12 (95% CI, 1.05–1.19) for a false-positive result. Thurfjell et al. 1997 found decreased mammographic specificity, especially in women treated with both estrogen and progesterone replacement.

Having had a breast biopsy was associated with a higher risk for a false-positive result (Brenner & Pfaff, 1996), although one prospective study of recall rates among women with and without a history of breast biopsy showed no difference (Slanetz et al., 1998). Christiansen et al. (2000) found a risk for a false-positive result of 20% for women with a history of three or more breast biopsies, 13% for women with two, 11% for women with one and 6.1% for women with no history of a breast biopsy ($p < 0.01$).

*Factors related to mammography that affect the false-positive rate*

Perhaps the most important effects on the risk for a false-positive result are related to the diagnostic ability of the radiographer. Brown et al. (1995) found that the frequency of reading screening mammograms in 50 individual practices in a representative national sample in the USA ranged from a low of 3% to a high of 57%. Using a model with adjustment for multiple variables relating to the woman, Christiansen et al. (2000) studied 35 community radiologists and estimated that the odds of a woman having a false-positive result was 11-fold higher (95% CI, 2–17) if the film was read by the radiologist with the highest false-positive rate than when it was read by the radiologist with the lowest rate. While some of this variation undoubtedly reflects the small sample studied (mean of 35 films per radiologist in both studies), the variation is nonetheless substantial.

The availability of previous mammogram films for comparison when reading mammograms has been shown to decrease the frequency of false-positive results. Christiansen and colleagues (2000) found that the false-positive rate was halved when previous films were available. Frankel et al. (1995) found that the frequency of abnormal results dropped from 7% at initial examination to 3% on subsequent examinations at which previous films were available.

Only one report (Christiansen et al., 2000) was available of the combined effect of patients' risk profile and radiological variables on a woman's risk for a false-positive result in multiple screens. The characteristics examined included the age, history of previous breast biopsy, family history of breast cancer, menopausal status, estrogen use, body mass index, race and median household income of the patient and comparison with previous mammogram, time since last mammogram and radiologist's recall rate. In a multivariable model, four patient variables emerged as independent risk factors. The risk decreased with the patient's age and increased with the number of breast biopsies, family history of breast cancer and estrogen use. In addition, all three radiological variables were independent risk factors. A woman with average risk factors had a 15% chance of having a false-positive result by the ninth mammogram if her films were read by a radiologist with a low recall rate, and an 86% chance if her mammograms were read by a radiologist with a high recall rate. This study was of one setting and may not be generalizable to others. Also, breast density was not included as a variable. Although many of these features are immutable, all three radiological variables associated with false-positive readings are modifiable.

Banks et al. (2002b) predicted the recall rate after a false-positive result for 60 000 women in the United Kingdom who were not using hormone replacement therapy. Premenopausal and perimenopausal women were more likely than postmenopausal women to be recalled for false-positive results, and the variation in recall rate by age was accounted for by the menopausal status of the women. Furthermore, women were more likely to be recalled if they had had breast surgery in the past, and less likely to be recalled if a comparison mammogram was available. There were also weak associations with parity and weight, but other factors, including educational level, family history of breast cancer, tobacco and alcohol consumption, height, age at birth of first child, breastfeeding history and past use of hormonal contraceptives had no effect on the recall rate.

*Possible strategies for decreasing false-positive rates*

It may be reasonable to alter estrogen use in the short term, thereby decreasing the false-positive rates for women on hormonal replacement therapy. In a preliminary study, Harvey et al. (1997) found that stopping hormone replacement therapy for 10–30 days before a repeat mammogram resulted in resolution of or a decrease in mammographic abnormalities in 35 of 47 patients.

Changing mammographic practices in settings with high false-positive rates is probably a more relevant option. One way of lowering the frequency of false-positive results is to set explicit goals for lowering recall rates. In the USA, the Agency for Health Care Policy and Research has recommended that the recall rate be no more than 10% of screening mammograms (Bassett et al., 1994a). In Europe, the Europe Against Cancer Programme suggested that the 'acceptable' level of recall after the first screen should be < 7%, and the 'desirable' level should be < 5% (Commission of the European Communities, 1996). Lowering recall rates may be easier in Europe than in North America because of the tendency for malpractice suits in the latter.

It has been suggested that more experienced radiologists with a higher volume of mammographs have lower false-positive rates (Sickles et al., 1990), but this requires confirmation. There is evidence that the availability of previous mammograms and interpretation of the image by two radiographers (see above) can decrease the false-positive rate. Both of these ideas should be weighed against increased costs, the feasibility of obtaining previous mammograms (Bassett et al., 1994b) and the costs of more professional input.

## Overdiagnosis

An obvious source of harm associated with any screening programme is unnecessary treatment of cancers that were not destined to cause death or symptoms. This section describes the concept of overdiagnosis and reviews the evidence for overdiagnosis of breast cancer after screening mammography. The section concludes with a description of autopsy series in which there was a reservoir of undetected breast cancers, which might be diagnosed as imaging techniques become capable of detecting progressively smaller lesions. The following section describes mammographic detection of DCIS, for which overdiagnosis may be particularly common.

### The concept of overdiagnosis

Overdiagnosis refers to the detection of cancers that would never have been found were it not for the screening test (Prorok et al., 1999). Patients in whom such indolent cancers are detected do not benefit from screening and can only experience harm: the worry associated with a 'cancer' diagnosis and the complications of therapy. For most prospective screenees (and many clinicians), overdiagnosis is a foreign concept. This is understandable, given the widespread perception of cancer as a relentlessly progressive disease which, if left untreated, leads to death.

In fact, lesions called 'cancer' by pathologists can have very different growth rates. The concept of overdiagnosis is probably best understood by collapsing this spectrum of growth rates into four discrete categories, fast, slow, very slow and non-progressive, as depicted in Figure 38. Fast-growing cancers metastasize rapidly, produce symptoms and cause death. While they are potentially detectable by screening, they are easily missed and instead become evident in the interval between screening tests (so-called 'interval cancers'). Slowly growing cancers are destined to cause symptoms and death but can be detected by routine screening. It is on deaths from these cancers that screening is likely to have its greatest impact.

The two other growth rates represent cancers that never result in symptoms or death—cancers that Morrison (1992) and others have referred to as 'pseudodisease'. Some cancers progress so slowly that they are interrupted by death from unrelated causes before symptoms develop. The existence of this type of pseudodisease is therefore a function not only of the cancer's growth rate but also of the patient's competing risks for death. Although, in principle, screening will always lead to its detection (simply because some patients with screen-detected cancers will die of other causes), the problem is most relevant for cancer screening in the elderly, prostate cancer serving as the best example. Furthermore, some cellular abnormalities that are labelled 'cancer' never grow (or may even get smaller), and these non-progressive cancers will never cause symptoms, no matter how long

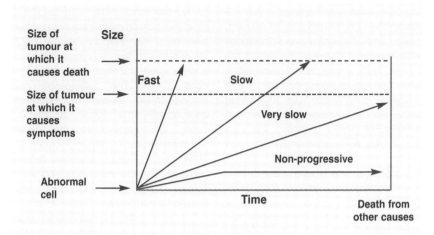

**Figure 38** Growth rates of cancers

the patient lives. One can postulate a number of mechanisms for this type of pseudodisease: some cancers may outgrow their blood supply (and be starved), others may be recognized by the host's immune system (and be successfully contained), and some may never have been that aggressive. In the case of breast cancer screening, this second type of pseudodisease is probably the most relevant.

While the foregoing theoretical framework is a simplification of a wide spectrum of growth rates, it does serve as a basis for a straightforward definition of overdiagnosis. If pseudodisease is detected, then overdiagnosis has occurred. Practically, however, it is extraordinarily difficult to determine overdiagnosis, because virtually all detected cancers are treated, making it impossible to distinguish their natural history from the effect of treatment. Nonetheless, there are two sources of data from which some inferences about overdiagnosis can be made: randomized trials of mammography and population-based incidence rates.

### Overdiagnosis in randomized trials of mammography

No screening test has been as thoroughly studied as screening mammogra-

phy: over 500 000 women have been entered into eight randomized trials (see Chapter 4). As in each trial a group of women undergoing regular mammography (with or without clinical breast examination) is compared with those who are not, these studies provide some indica-

tion of the effect of mammography on the observed incidence of cancer, and the relative incidences in the screened and control groups can shed some light on the question of overdiagnosis.

The trials differ, however, in ways that potentially affect the rate of overdiagnosis. The screening intensity was greatest in the Canadian trials both because of the intervention (two-view mammography performed annually) and because of the high participation rate (nearly 100% at the first screening). If mammography resulted in overdiagnosis, it would be expected to be most obvious in these two trials. In trials with less intense interventions (single-view mammography every 2 or 3 years) or lower participation rates, overdiagnosis would be expected to be less evident.

Figure 39 shows the incidence of breast cancer in each of the trials at the end of the intervention period, 5–8 years after randomization. This figure highlights another characteristic that affects the relative incidence in the screened

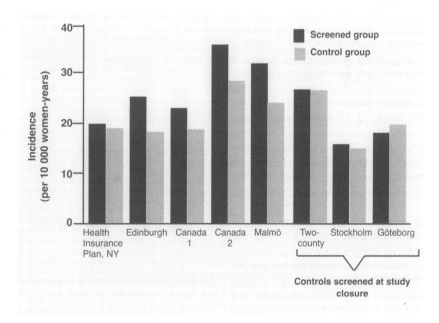

**Figure 39** Breast cancer incidence among women invited to screening versus those who were not (controls) in eight randomized trials of screening mammography

and control group: whether or not the control group was screened at the close of the intervention period.

In the three Swedish trials in which the control group was screened at the end of the study, the relative incidence was essentially 1. This suggests either that there was no overdiagnosis or that it was confined to prevalent cases detected during the initial screening (their counterparts in the control group being detected during screening at closure). If there was overdiagnosis during subsequent screening, the control group would be expected never to catch up to a relative incidence of 1. The Two-county trial showed directly that the number of cancers detected after the prevalence round is no greater in the screened population than among controls.

In the five other trials, the relative incidence (screened versus control) ranged from 1.07 in the Health Insurance Plan trial to 1.38 in the study in Edinburgh. Because the Health Insurance Plan trial was performed in the 1960s, with mammographic equipment with much lower resolution than is available today, it does not provide relevant information on the problem of overdiagnosis. If the control groups in the remaining four trials are taken as representing the underlying 'true' incidence, then mammographic screening initially increases the observed incidence of breast cancer by 24–38%, suggesting potential overdiagnosis. Furthermore, long-term follow-up of women in the Canadian trials showed that this excess persists (Miller *et al.*, 2000, 2002).

### Overdiagnosis in population-based incidence rates

#### Matched communities
Population-based data from two communities in The Netherlands point to over-diagnosis of similar magnitude and support the notion that the problem is largely confined to the initial screening (Peeters *et al.*, 1989b). In 1975, the City of Nijmegen started population-wide

screening with mammography every 2 years. The neighbouring city of Arnhem, which had had a similar overall incidence in the preceding 5 years, served as the control. In the 4-year period immediately after initiation of screening, the overall incidence in Nijmegen was 30% higher than that in Arnhem. In the two subsequent 4-year periods, the incidence rates were again similar.

#### National screening programmes
Another means for investigating over-diagnosis is to examine breast cancer incidence rates in countries before and after initiation of national screening programmes. As other factors may influence incidence trends, inferences based on these data are less sure than those from randomized trials. Nevertheless, they offer the advantage of external validity; they offer, in fact, the best opportunity to see what happens in the real world. To make the inferences more secure, candidate countries should have initiated screening at a defined time, have programmes that are truly national in scope and have mature

tumour registries. Two countries that meet these three criteria are Finland and the United Kingdom. In January 1987, Finland started two-view mammography screening every 2 years among women aged 50–59. The participation rate among those invited to screening approached 90% (Dean & Pamilo, 1999). One year later, the United Kingdom (Breast Screening Programme, 1999) began 3-yearly one-view (with a subsequent single view) mammographic screening of women aged 50–64 and reported a participation rate of > 70%.

In both countries, the incidence of breast cancer among women in the target age group rose after the introduction of screening (Figure 40). It should be emphasized that a temporary rise is not only expected but is necessary for screening to be successful, as the time of diagnosis is advanced for pre-existing cases (Morrison, 1992). While the rise may be temporary, it is nonetheless substantial: both countries experienced roughly a 50% increase in incidence in the target age group during 5 years after introduction of screening. Current data

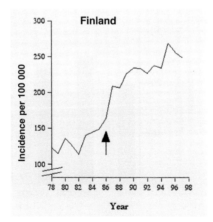 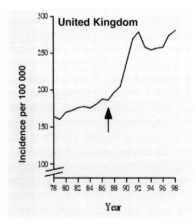

**Figure 40** Trends in incidence of invasive breast cancer among women of screening age in Finland (50–59) and the United Kingdom (50–64)

Data from European Network of Cancer Registries (2001). The Finnish data are nationwide; data for the United Kingdom are from eight registries that have been collecting data since 1978 (East Anglia, Merseyside and Cheshire, North-western, South Thames, Trent, Yorkshire, Scotland and Wales). The arrow denotes the last data point before initiation of the national screening programme in each country.

from both countries suggest that the rise may be persisting.

Because incidence rises with age, one plausible explanation for the continuing rise in age-specific incidence is that the rates among women of screening age are 'shifted up' to the higher rates of older women. In other words, 60–64-year-old women assume the incidence rates of women aged 65–69 as their time of diagnosis is advanced. Were this to be the case, some fall in incidence would be expected in older, unscreened women. As shown in Figure 41, the breast cancer incidence in women aged 65–69 has in fact fallen slightly since 1991. Thus, to some extent, the increase in incidence simply reflects an advance in the time of diagnosis. However, the observed incidence rate among women aged 60–64 now exceeds that of women aged 65–69 and exceeds that which would be predicted in women aged 65–69 if the underlying 1.5% increase incidence had persisted. These data suggest that overdiagnosis is occurring in the United Kingdom. Early modelling indicated that

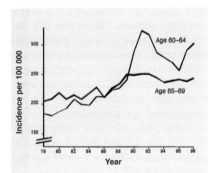

**Figure 41** Age-specific breast cancer incidence trends in the United Kingdom for the oldest women invited to screening (60–64) and the next oldest unscreened group (65–69). Screening started between 1988 and 1995

overdiagnosis represents about 6% of detected cancers (Boer et al., 1994).

## Reservoir of potentially detectable breast cancer

In this section, we report on the 'disease reservoir' of breast cancer, which is the term given to the prevalence of disease observed at autopsy but undetected during life (McFarlane et al., 1987).

Although the evidence for this reservoir is derived from data on cancers detected after death, a proportion of those cancers could be detected during life, given enhanced imaging (e.g. computed tomography or magnetic resonance imaging) and/or more frequent biopsy. In other words, these data provide some sense of the upper limit of the problem of overdiagnosis of breast cancer.

A number of careful autopsy studies of the breast have been conducted (Table 55; Welch & Black, 1997). The series fall into two broad categories: hospital-based and forensic autopsies. The latter are consecutive cases presented to a coroner's office (e.g. deaths in which homicide is suspected). Each series was restricted to women not known to have breast cancer during life. Although the level of scrutiny varied from study to study (e.g. in terms of how many tissue sections were made and whether post-mortem mammography was used), the same fundamental approach was used in each study, comprising systematic pathological examination of the breast.

## Table 55. Studies of the prevalence of breast cancer in women not known to have had breast cancer during life, from autopsy series

| Reference | Location | No. (autopsy type) | Mean no. of slides per breast | Invasive cancer (%) | DCIS (%) | Proportion of middle-aged women with any breast cancer (%) |
|---|---|---|---|---|---|---|
| Kramer & Rush (1973) | USA | 70 (hospital) | 40 | 1.4 | 4.3 | ND |
| Wellings et al. (1975) | USA | 67[a] (hospital) | ND | 0 | 4.5 | 10 (age 50–70) |
| Nielsen et al. (1984) | Denmark | 77 (hospital) | 95 | 1.3 | 14.3 | ND |
| Alpers & Wellings (1985) | USA | 101 (hospital) | ND | 0 | 8.9 | 13 (age 40–70) |
| Bhathal et al. (1985) | Australia | 207 (forensic) | 11 | 1.4 | 12.1 | ND |
| Bartow et al. (1987) | USA | 221 (forensic) | 9 | 1.8 | 0 | 7 (age 45–54) |
| Nielsen et al. (1987) | Denmark | 109 (forensic) | 275 | 0.9 | 14.7 | 39 (age 40–49) |

DCIS, ductal carcinoma in situ; ND, not described
[a] Reported as number of breasts, not number of women; prevalences are therefore percentages of breasts, not of women.

The median observed prevalence of invasive breast cancer among women not known to have breast cancer was 1.3% (range, 0–1.8%). The median prevalence of DCIS was 8.9%, but this varied widely: one series found none, while in three DCIS was found in over 10% of women undergoing autopsy. The observed prevalences were higher among women most likely to have been screened — middle-aged women — as much as one-third of whom showed some evidence of cancer. By comparison, the lifetime risk of dying from breast cancer was less than 4%. Consequently, many more breast cancers can be found than will ultimately matter to women.

## Ductal carcinoma *in situ*

Aspects of the pathology and molecular biology of DCIS are described in Chapter 1. Clinical follow-up of women found to have DCIS has shown that it is a pre-invasive neoplastic lesion and that the histological grade is related to prognosis (recurrence rates). Atypical ductal hyperplasia shows molecular genetic changes similar to those in DCIS and is also associated with an increased risk for the development of invasive cancer.

In the past, DCIS was a rare diagnosis, but the introduction of screening programmes for breast cancer resulted in the diagnosis of large numbers of cases of DCIS. High-grade DCIS more frequently shows abnormal mammographic features than low-grade DCIS, as the calcification present is more obvious, and the high-grade form is more specific for malignancy (see Chapter 1, Figure 42).

In screening programmes in Europe, the proportion of DCIS diagnosed ranged from 9 to 21% (Giordano *et al.*,

1996; Fracheboud *et al.*, 1998; Blanks *et al.*, 2000a). In the USA, about one-third of all mammographically detected cancers are DCIS (Kerlikowske *et al.*, 1993; Beam *et al.*, 1996a; Poplack *et al.*, 2000). With increased screening by mammography and increased sensitivity, perhaps combined with readier use of biopsy and diagnosis, the incidence (or, more correctly, the diagnosis) rates have increased dramatically. For example, the age-adjusted incidence of DCIS in the registries of the SEER programme in the USA have increased almost 10-fold over the past 20 years (from 2.7 to 25 per 100 000) (National Cancer Institute, 2001b).

Some researchers consider that detection of DCIS is one of the benefits derived from breast cancer screening. Indeed, aggressive screening for what was then called 'minimal breast cancer' was strongly advocated in the belief that only by detecting such lesions would mortality from breast cancer be reduced (Moskowitz *et al.*, 1976). Minimal breast cancer as then defined consisted of two components: invasive breast cancers < 10 mm in size and DCIS.

Until recently, the usual treatment for DCIS was mastectomy. This probably explains the excess rate of mastectomy in the groups receiving mammography in the Canadian trials, for example (Miller, 1994), and the increased rate of mastectomy associated with increased detection of DCIS in the SEER programme (Ernster *et al.*, 1996). With the advent of large numbers of mammographically detected DCIS, breast-conserving therapy has been used more widely. The two approaches have not been compared in a randomized controlled trial; however, when DCIS was treated by local excision, local recurrence was observed in 16% of cases within 4 years (Julien *et al.*, 2000), and the percentage was significantly lower (9%) when radiotherapy was given. The risk for invasive recurrence was not related to the histological type of DCIS,

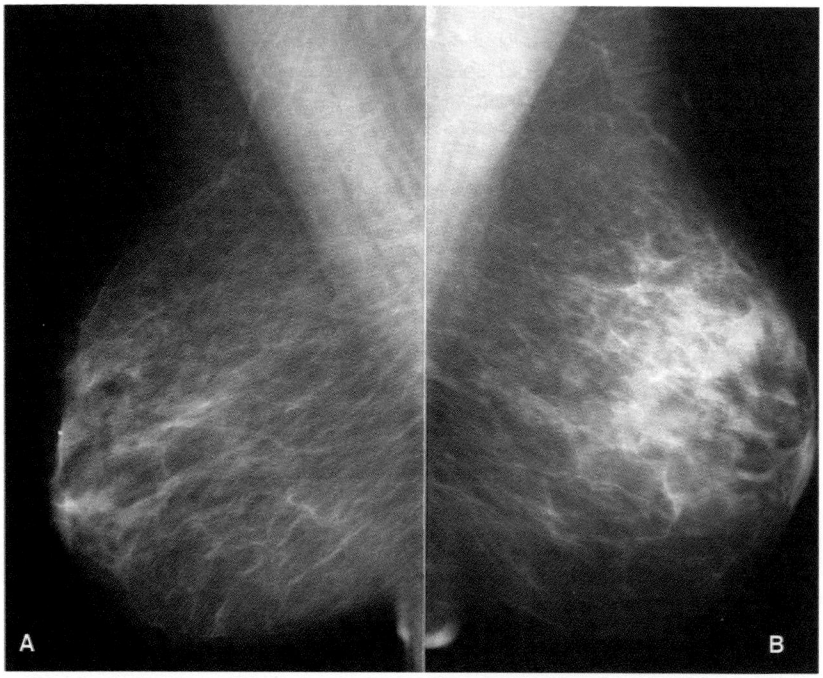

**Figure 42** Mammograms of a patient who presented with a striking nonpalpable breast asymmetry. The structure of the tissue of the right breast (A) imitates glandular tissue. Magnetic resonance imaging (MRI) was performed, which showed intense enhancement with contrast medium of the patient's left breast (B). A histological diagnosis of high grade papillary ductal carcinoma in situ (DCIS) was made.

although distant metastasis was significantly more common in poorly differentiated DCIS (Bijker *et al*., 2001b). About 20% of the DCIS lesions in these studies were palpable; the natural history of DCIS detected solely by mammography is less clear. Holland *et al*. (1990) found no association between the mode of detection of DCIS and the size of the resected lesion. Frequently, DCIS extends over more than one quadrant of the breast, making breast-conserving surgery impossible.

The important issue is what proportion of cases of DCIS detected at screening would have progressed to invasive cancer if they had not been detected, and how many represent 'over-diagnosis'. If a substantial proportion of cases of DCIS were destined to progress to invasive breast cancer, some decrement in the rate of invasive breast cancer would be expected as DCIS was increasingly diagnosed (a 'new case of cancer' can occur only once). In other words, as DCIS becomes an increasingly common diagnosis, women destined to get invasive cancer are counted as new cases of DCIS, not as new cases of invasive breast cancer. One diagnosis is substituted for the other.

Information on the extent to which the incidence of invasive breast cancer might be reduced by detection of DCIS is available from the long-term follow-up in the Canadian National Breast Screening Study of women aged 50–59 on entry (Miller *et al*., 2000). Of the 267 invasive breast cancers detected at annual mammography, 48 were < 10 mm in size, whereas only 6 of 148 found by clinical breast examination were this size. In addition, 71 in situ breast cancers were detected in the women receiving annual mammography and 16 in those examined physically. However, there was no evidence that the detection of in situ cancers resulted in a reduction in breast cancer incidence: the cumulative numbers of invasive breast cancers (including those ascertained after the

end of the 4–5-year screening period) were 622 in women with annual mammography and 610 in those given clinical breast examination. The data for the 50 000 women aged 40–49 on entry to the Canadian trial are similar (Miller *et al*., 2002). Once again, more in situ cancers were diagnosed in women given mammographic screening (71 cancers) than in those receiving usual care (29 cancers). However, no indication was found of a reduction in breast cancer incidence over the 11-year follow-up, the cumulative numbers of invasive cancers as determined by linkage to the national cancer registry being 592 and 552, respectively.

Similar follow-up data have not been published from the other breast cancer screening trials. However, many have reported the proportion of DCIS among the cancers detected, ranging from 8.4% in the Two-county trial to 16% in the Malmö trial (Fletcher *et al.*, 1993).

Studies of populations in which breast cancer screening has been implemented provide no evidence that the rising rates of incidence (diagnosis) of DCIS have been accompanied by a decrease in the incidence of invasive cancer. Data from the SEER programme in the USA (Figure 43) indicate that detection of DCIS simply

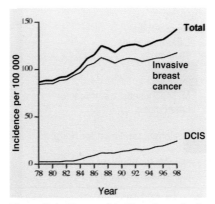

**Figure 43** Incidences of ductal carcinoma *in situ*, (DCIS), invasive breast cancer and the two combined, USA, 1978–98

From National Cancer Institute (2001b)

adds to the total number of cancers detected (although, of course, the increase in incidence of invasive cancer might have been even greater in the absence of DCIS detection and treatment).

DCIS does not always progress to invasive breast cancer, as shown by two lines of evidence. The first derives from studies of cases of DCIS followed only by biopsy (without treatment). Of 28 cases of non-palpable, low-grade (non-comedo) DCIS, seven (25%) developed into invasive cancer within 10 years and a further two within the next 20 years (Page *et al.*, 1995). In Bologna, Italy, only 3/28 cases (11%) of DCIS developed into invasive cancer during an average follow-up period of 17 years (Eusebi *et al.*, 1989). The second type of evidence derives from studies of the outcome (survival) of registered DCIS cases. The SEER data for 7072 cases of DCIS registered in 1978–89 showed a low risk for death from breast cancer during the 10-year follow-up. In cases diagnosed in 1978–83 (mainly before mammographic screening), the risk for death from breast cancer was 3.1 times (at 5 years) and 3.4 times (at 10 years) that of the general population. In cases diagnosed in 1984–89 (mainly detected by mammography), the relative risk for death was much lower: 1.6 (95% CI, 1.1–2.1) at 5 years and 1.9 (95% CI, 1.5–2.3) at 10 years. Some of the excess risk may be due to 'missed' invasive disease among the DCIS cases. The women with DCIS had an overall mortality rate that was 20–30% lower than that of the general population, as they represented a group with higher socioeconomic status, who undergo frequent mammography (Ernster *et al.*, 2000).

Part of the difficulty in determining the role of DCIS in screening is the fact that mammography has revealed a new spectrum of disease that would have been largely undiagnosed in the absence of screening, although the presence of a 'reservoir' of DCIS was evident from studies of autopsy series (see above).

This has contributed to confusion as to what these lesions truly represent and even whether it is appropriate to use the term 'carcinoma' when no precise guidance can be provided on eventual prognosis (Foucar, 1996). Miller and Borges (2001) suggested that true precursors of invasive cancer, with atypical epithelial hyperplasia and incipient invasion, are not detectable with current screening methods. Some high-grade cancers may have a transitory in situ phase, with rapid progression to invasion, thus not allowing time for their detection as DCIS (Barnes et al., 1992).

## Early mortality from breast cancer

A possible, nonsignificant excess of early mortality from breast cancer was noted among groups invited to screening, especially women under the age of 50, in some screening trials (Tabár et al., 1985; Andersson et al., 1988; Miller et al., 1992a, 2002). In a meta-analysis of all screening trials with data on women under the age of 50, Cox (1997) noted that the rate ratio for mortality at 3 years was 2.4 (95% CI, 1.1–5.4), although all the rate ratios computed earlier or up to 11 years after entry were approximately 1.0. Miettinen et al. (2002), in an analysis of the data on women aged 55–84 on entry to the Malmö trial, noted a 3-year average rate ratio of 1.5 3–4 years after entry, although the lower 95% CI was approximately 0.6 (data derived from a figure). Retsky et al. (2001a,b) suggested that the surgical removal of a primary breast tumour from premenopausal women with involved lymph nodes triggers the growth of temporarily dormant disease in approximately 20% of cases. This suggestion is in line with the results of tests in experimental animals (Fisher & Saffer, 1989).

## Risk for breast cancer induced by radiation

Several epidemiological studies have addressed the risk for breast cancer induced by radiation and provided quantitative estimates of the level of risk after different doses of radiation. Age-related risk estimates are needed for calculating the risk of a patient undergoing mammography, as the risk for radiation-induced breast cancer decreases with age at exposure. Additionally, information about the time between exposure and diagnosis is essential for risk evaluation, as there is a latency of 5–10 years between irradiation and the appearance of any excess cancer risk, with further increases over the next 5–10 years. The risk then probably persists for the remainder of the lifespan. The latency may be longer with lower doses. Although the data are not fully consistent, dose fractionation does not appear to reduce the risk. In other words, the effect of low doses seems to be additive, and low-dose fractions appear to be as effective in inducing breast cancer as a single large dose.

### Age-specific risk estimates from large epidemiological studies

Sixteen epidemiological studies have provided relative risk estimates for breast cancer associated with exposure to radiation: 12 for incidence and four for mortality (for overviews, see Boice, 2001; Little, 2001). Only eight of the studies of incidence and three of those of mortality provide estimates for women aged ≥ 20 at the time of exposure. Age-specific excess relative risks (ERRs) were summarized by UNSCEAR (1994, Annex A) and are presented in Table 56.

**Table 56. Excess relative risks for death from breast cancer associated with exposure to radiation by age at time of exposure**

| Study | Age at exposure (years) | | | |
|---|---|---|---|---|
| | 20–29 | 30–39 | 40–49 | > 50 |
| Japan, 1950–85 | | | | |
|   Incidence | 1.27 | 1.23 | 0.54 | 0.31 |
|   Mortality | 0.96 | 1.09 | | |
| Sweden, treatment for benign breast disease | 1.9 | 0.4 | 0.1 | 0.1 |
| Canada, treatment for tuberculosis, 1950–80 | | | | |
|   Nova Scotia | 1.6 | 0.8 | 0 | 0 |
|   Other provinces | 0.4 | 0.2 | 0 | 0 |
|   Canada | 0.22 | 0.04 | −0.01 | −0.03 |
| USA | | | | |
|   Massachusetts, treatment for tuberculosis | 0.5 | 0.2[a] | 0.2[a] | 0.2[a] |
|   California, treatment for Hodgkin disease | 0.4[b] | 0.4[b] | 0.1[b] | 0.1[b] |
|   New York, treatment for mastitis | 0.4 | 0.6 | | |
|   Contralateral breast | – | 0.2[c] | 0.2[c] | 0.0 |

From UNSCEAR (1994; Tables 11 and 20)
[a] One risk coefficient reported for women aged ≥ 30 at exposure
[b] One risk coefficient reported for women aged 20–39 and one for women aged ≥ 40 at exposure

The two largest cohort studies are the Life Span Study cohort of survivors of the atomic bombs in Japan and a cohort study of women who were examined frequently by X-ray fluoroscopy during therapy for tuberculosis in Massachusetts, USA. Age-specific risks were also reported in a Canadian study of women with tuberculosis and a Swedish study of benign breast disease. Other studies carried out on women irradiated for diagnostic, therapeutic or occupational reasons are summarized in *IARC Monographs* Volume 75 (IARC, 2000).

*Risk models for dose–response analysis*
The linearity of the dose–response curve for the ERR (or RR = 1 + ERR) is widely accepted for the relationship between exposure to radiation and risk for breast cancer. Two models, an 'age-at-exposure' model and an 'age-attained' model have been described. The 'age-at-exposure' model is often presented as a function of the form:

$$\text{ERR } (D) = D \times \alpha \times \exp(-\beta (e - 30)),$$

where $e$ is the age at time of exposure, $D$, the dose of radiation and $\alpha$ can be interpreted as the excess relative risk (ERR per Sv) of a women exposed at the age of 30. The model for the 'age-attained' model is often given in the form:

$$\text{ERR } (D) = D \times \alpha \times \exp(-\beta (a - 50)),$$

where $a$ is the age at diagnosis and $\alpha$ can be interpreted as the excess relative risk (per Sv) of a woman aged 50.

In models fitted with data from the Life Span Study, the ERR increased by 3.7% per year with the 'age-at-exposure' model, whereas the ERR increased by 4.6% per year with the 'age-attained' model. No significantly increased risk was seen for women aged ≥ 50 at the time of exposure (Thompson *et al.,* 1994; Tokunaga *et al.,* 1994).

The Committee on the Biological Effects of Ionizing Radiation (BEIR; 1990), the International Commission for Radiation Protection (ICRP, 1982, 1987, 1991) and the National Council on Radiation Protection and Measurements (USA; 1986) have reported risk coefficients for various organs, but the values are difficult to compare. The BEIR Committee reported age-specific coefficients for breast cancer separately. The lifetime risks for death due to radiation-induced breast cancer were given as 0.43% per Sv for women aged 30–40 at the time of exposure, 0.2% per Sv for women aged 40–50 and 0.06% for women aged 50–60. The risk coefficient for women > 60 at the time of exposure was 0. Most predictions of radiation-induced breast cancer are based on the age-specific risks reported by the BEIR Committee. Jung (2001) presented the risk coefficients reported by the three committees in a comparable way and showed that they differed substantially, particularly for exposure after the age of 50.

*Dose of radiation from mammography*
Considerable effort has been expended in estimating and measuring the dose of radiation to the breast during mammography (Hammerstein *et al.,* 1979; Stanton *et al.,* 1984; Wu *et al.,* 1994; Young *et al.,* 1996; Young & Burch, 2000). As it is now generally assumed that glandular tissue is the most vulnerable of the tissues making up the breast, some authors consider that the average dose to the glandular tissue is the most appropriate dosimetric quantity for predicting the risk for cancer. This quantity is also recommended by the ICRP (1987) and others. The average glandular tissue dose is calculated by multiplying the measured 'entrance surface air kerma free in air' by $g$, a conversion factor, which depends mainly on the radiation quality and the thickness and tissue composition of the breast.

The exposure of two groups of women who underwent mammography at a gynaecological clinic during two different periods was compared. The first group comprised 1678 women who were examined between February 1992 and July 1992 with a tungsten and wolfram anode tube, and the second comprised 945 women who were treated 1 year later (July 1993–November 1993) with a dual-track molybdenum–wolfram anode mammographic unit. The mean average glandular tissue doses were 1.6 and 2.1 mGy, with an average of 3.4 and 3.6 exposures per women, respectively (Klein *et al.,* 1997).

The doses to other organs were considered by the ICRP (1982) and were assumed to be negligible. Since then, few measurements of doses to other organs have been undertaken. In a report on thyroid doses due to mammo-graphy in 91 women, the average dose to the skin overlying the thyroid was 0.39 mGy per mammographic examination, the values ranging from background levels to 1.2 mGy. The authors estimated that this value corresponds to an average dose to the thyroid during mammography of 0.04 mGy, with an average dose to the breast of 4 mGy (Whelan *et al.,* 1999)

In a study of the dose absorbed by seven organs other than the breast during mammography, the absorbed dose was measured with an anthropomorphic phantom containing thermoluminescent dosimeters. Doses to the red bone marrow of the sternum and the thyroid, lung, liver, colon, oesophagus and stomach were considered. The mean dose to the red bone marrow was 0.40–1.3 $\mu$Gy/mAs, and that to the thyroid was 0.05–0.17 $\mu$Gy/mAs. The doses to the other five organs were considered negligible. When the effective dose of radiation was calculated, the dose to the breast contributed > 98% (Hatziioannou *et al.,* 2000).

*Estimated numbers of cases of or deaths from breast cancer due to mammography*
The risks and benefits of specific screening policies that include mammog-

## Table 57. Estimates of numbers of cases of breast cancer induced by screening mammography, with assumptions about screening policy, radiation dose and age at screening

| Reference, country | Dose, view | Total dose per exami-nation (both sides) | Total dose per length of observa-tion | Screening policy, age at screening | Breast can-cer incidence per $10^6$ women/mGy | Breast can-cer deaths per $10^6$ women/mGy | Lifetime risk per $10^6$ women | Comments |
|---|---|---|---|---|---|---|---|---|
| Howe et al. (1981), Canada | 0.7 mGy; max, 2.5 mGy | | 10 mGy 25 mGy 5 examina-tions | Age 40–59, annually for 5 years | 0.66 0.87 | | | Two values are for linear additive model and linear multiplicative model plus term for cell killing Latency, 10 years Mortality reduc-tion, 40% |
| Feig (1984), USA | | 1–8 mGy | | Age at expo-sure: 40 45 50 55 60 65 70 | 0.35 | 0.175 | 10 9 7 6 4 3 2 | Latency, 10 years National Cancer Institute model |
| Zuur & Broerse (1985), Netherlands | | 1 mGy | 30 mGy/30 examinations | Age 35–75, annually | 20 | 8 | 600 cases and 240 deaths 1071 cases and 428 deaths | Absolute risk model Relative risk model Latency, 10 years |
| Gohagan et al. (1986), USA | 0.6 mGy 4 mGy | 2–3 views, 1.2–1.8 mGy 2–3 views, 8–12 mGy | | Age 35 at baseline examination; age 40–80 annually | 2–3 | | 150 cases with 1.2 mGy/exami-nation; 1000 cases with 12 mGy/exami-nation | Low-dose film–screen sys-tem vs 4-mGy system; breast com-pressed to 6 cm |
| Law (1987), United Kingdom | 1 mGy 10 mGy | 2 mGy 20 mGy | | Age at expo-sure: 35 65 Single exami-nation at each age | | | 18.6 3.6 | Breast com-pressed to 5 or 8 cm at 2 doses Latency, 10 years |
| Hasert (1988), Germany | | 10 mGy 1 mGy | | Age ≥ 35, annually | 0.35 0.35 | 0.18 0.17 | | Not screen–film Screen–film Latency, 10 years |

## Table 57 (contd)

| Reference, country | Dose, view | Total dose per examination (both sides) | Total dose per length of observation | Screening policy, age at screening | Breast cancer incidence per $10^6$ women/mGy | Breast cancer deaths per $10^6$ women/mGy | Lifetime risk per $10^6$ women | Comments |
|---|---|---|---|---|---|---|---|---|
| Mettler et al. (1996), USA | 1.38 mGy | 2.8 mGy | 112 mGy/40 examinations 98 mGy/35 examinations 70 mGy/25 examinations | Age 35–75 Age 40–75 Age 50–75 Annually | | | 15 10 5 | Mortality reduction: 35–39, 5% 40–49, 15% 50–75, 25% Mortality, 40% Average lifespan, 75 years Latency, 10 years |
| Andersson & Janzon (1997), Sweden | 2 mGy | 4 mGy | 36 mGy/9 examinations 20 mGy/5 examinations | Age, < 50 Every 2 years | 5 | | | Mortality reduction, 36% (adjusted for fatal radiation-induced breast cancer) |
| Feig & Hendrick (1997), USA | 2.5 mGy 5.5–6.5 mGy | 4 mGy | | Age 40 Annual screening for 10 years Screening every 2 years for 10 years | | 0.05 0.05 | 8 deaths 4 deaths | Breast compressed to: 4.2 cm 5–5.7 cm |
| Beemsterboer et al. (1998a), Netherlands | 2 mGy | 1 view, 2 mGy 2 views, 4 mGy | 2 views at first screening, 1 view subsequently: 22 mGy 32 mGy 42 mGy 62 mGy | Age 50–69, every 2 years Age 40–69, every 2 years Age 40–49 annually and 50–69 every 2 years Age 40–69 annually | | | | Dose measured on phantom Attendance rates: 40–49, 75% 50–69, 70% |
| Mattson et al. (2000), Sweden | 1.5 mGy | Average, 2.25 mGy 1.5 views/ examination | 13 mGy/7 examinations 33 mGy/17 examinations | Age 40–49, every 18 months Age 50–69, every 2 years | | | Incidence: 530 with assumption of higher risk 120 with assumption of lower risk Deaths: 240 (higher risk) 50 (lower risk) | Annual mortality reduction beginning 7 years after examination: 40–49, 25% 50–69, 30% Latency, 10 years Attendance rate, 80% Recall rate, 5%, with 3 views at recall examination |

## Table 55 (contd)

| Reference, country | Dose, view | Total dose per examination (both sides) | Total dose per length of observation | Screening policy, age at screening | Breast cancer incidence per $10^6$ women/mGy | Breast cancer deaths per $10^6$ women/mGy | Lifetime risk per $10^6$ women | Comments |
|---|---|---|---|---|---|---|---|---|
| Young & Burch (2000), United Kingdom | Average mean glandular tissue dose: 2.03 mGy (oblique view) 1.65 mGy (cranial-caudal view) | 3.68 mGy | 2 views at first visit: 18.4 mGy; 1 view (oblique) at subsequent 4 visits: 11.8 mGy | | | | | Breast compressed to 4–4.5 cm |
| Jung (2001), Germany | Mean parenchymal dose/-view, 2 mGy | 4 mGy | 24 mgGy/6 examinations | Age at first exposure: 37.5 42.5 52.5 57.5 62.5 Every 2 years | 13 7.1 4.8 1.8 0.95 | 5.5 3.1 2.1 0.79 0.42 | Deaths: 133 74 51 19 10 | Breast compressed to 5.0–5.5 cm Relative biological effectiveness, 2 Equivalence dose, 8 mSv Latency, 12 years |
| Säbel et al. (2001), Germany | | | 2 mGy | Age 40–49 Age 50–59 | 4.5 1.5 | 2.0 0.65 | | Relative biological effectiveness, 1 Morbidity:mortality, 2.3 |

raphy have been estimated in a number of publications, sometimes with estimates of the numbers of cases of or deaths from radiation-induced breast cancer. However, different values for radiation dose, different risk models and different assumptions about age range and screening interval in the mammography programmes were used in the various papers. Some provided only risk–benefit ratios under an assumption for the effect of mammography screening and did not provide the numbers of radiation-induced breast cancer cases or deaths. Others calculated various indices for possible harm due to radiation and estimated, e.g., the lifetime risk of 1 million women. The model-based calculations are difficult to compare, as the results are presented differently. The assumptions used and the estimates made are summarized in Table 57.

Howe et al. (1981) assumed that women aged 40–59 were screened five times with a dose of 0.7–2.5mGy per view and used various models to calculate the number of induced cancers. A mortality reduction factor of 40% was taken to calculate the number of deaths from breast cancer; however, the estimated number of deaths was not given, as only the combination of induced and 'saved' deaths was calculated. In the model, 553 deaths from breast cancer would have occurred among unscreened women 20 years after entry into the study, while 487 (additive model) or 490 (multiplicative model) women in the screened group would have had breast cancer. The corresponding numbers after 30 years were 892 deaths in the unscreened group and 825 (additive model) or 831 (multiplicative model) in the screened group. It was concluded that the number of radiation-induced cancers is negligible in comparison with the spontaneous incidence.

Zuur and Broerse (1985) calculated the risk for breast cancer of women aged 35 who were screened with 1 mGy per examination every year until the age of 75, that is, 40 times. A latency of 10 years was assumed. Models for absolute and relative risk were used. With the absolute risk model, the estimated lifetime risk for 1 million screened women was 600 induced cases of breast cancer (incidence) and 240 deaths. The relative risk model resulted in somewhat larger numbers: 1071 additional breast cancer cases and 428 deaths from breast cancer.

Gohagan et al. (1986) estimated the number of deaths from breast cancer induced by a screening policy that included one baseline examination at the age of 35 and an annual examination between the ages of 40 and 80. Two mammographic techniques were assumed: a low-dose film–screen system emitting 0.6 mGy dose per view and a system emitting 4–mGy per view. Two to three views were assumed at each examination, resulting in typical absorbed doses of 0.12 and 0.18 mGy, or 8–12 mGy. In a linear dose–response model, the lifetime radiogenic risk in a population of 1 million women screened was 150 (low-dose film) or 1000 breast cancer cases (4-mGy system), compared with 93 000 'spontaneous' cases.

Law (1987) investigated the effect of a programme in which women were screened between the ages of 35 and 65 in three risk models. Screening at the age of 35 resulted in 18.6 additional cases (per examination), while screening at the age of 65 gave 3.6 induced cases per million screened women. The author concluded that screening from the age of 35 with current techniques was not recommendable.

Hasert (1988) compared the numbers of radiation-induced breast cancer cases that would be induced with a dose of 10 mGy per examination in conventional techniques and 1 mGy with a new screen–film combination. For women over 35, he estimated that there would be 3.5 additional cases of breast cancer per million women exposed to 10 mGy and 0.35 additional cases with the lower dose.

Mettler et al. (1996) assumed annual mammography beginning at 35, 40 and 50 years and continuing until the age of 75. The dose at each examination was assumed to be 2.8 mGy, resulting in a total dose of 112 mGy if screening began at the age of 35, 98 mGy with screening from the age of 40 and 70 mGy with screening from the age of 50. A linear model from the Life Span Study and a latent period of 10 years were used. If mammography was started at the age of

35, 15 fatal induced breast cancer cases per million women were predicted, 10 if screening started at the age of 40 and five if screening started at the age of 50. The authors also calculated risk–benefit ratios for breast cancer screening, arguing that the benefit to a woman beginning annual screening at the age of 35 and continuing until 75 would be 25 times greater than the potential risk. If screening began at the age of 50, the risk–benefit ratio would be about 100.

Andersson and Janzon (1997) assumed a dose of 4 mGy for each examination (both sides), resulting in a total dose of 36 mGy for women undergoing nine examinations and 20 mGy for women undergoing only five examinations. They assumed that screening every 2 years started at the age of < 50 but with incomplete participation rates. The calculations are based on a linear dose–response model with age-dependent risk coefficients. Ten radiation-induced breast cancer deaths were estimated per million women screened.

Feig and Hendrick (1997) assumed screening annually or every 2 years, beginning at the age of 40 or 50, and estimated the numbers of radiation-induced breast cancer with a dose of 4 mGy at a two-view examination. Three models were used to determine the dose–response relationship, with assumptions of a 10-year latency and age-specific factors from the BEIR Committee (BEIR, 1990). Annual screening for 10 years from the age of 40 was estimated to result in eight deaths from breast cancer per million women (lifetime risk), while screening every 2 years resulted in four induced breast cancer deaths. In an earlier paper, Feig (1984) compared linear, linear–quadratic and quadratic dose–response models, with an assumed latency of 10 years. In their worst-case scenario (assuming a dose of 100 mGy), 20 excess deaths from breast cancer would be induced during a lifetime. Fewer induced breast cancer cases were estimated with the other models.

Beemsterboer et al. (1998a) estimated the number of breast cancer deaths among 1 million screened women induced by various mammography programmes. The latency was taken to be 10 years, and models based on age at exposure and attained age were used with coefficients calculated by the BEIR Committee. It was further assumed that the ratio of incidence to mortality rates is 2.6. The total exposure of women screened every 2 years between the ages of 50 and 69 was estimated to be 22 mGy. With these assumptions, 5.1 deaths from breast cancer were estimated to be induced. With screening every 2 years between the ages of 40 and 69, for a total of 30 examinations, 7.3 deaths were estimated to be induced per 1 million women. For screening every 2 years between the ages of 50 and 69, the baseline scenario, the ratio of induced:prevented breast cancer cases was estimated to be 1:242, whereas the ratio was 1:97 when screening was performed for women aged 40–49 at a 2-year interval and 1:66 at a 1-year interval.

Mattsson et al. (2000) compared the risk–benefit relationship for a reduction in breast cancer mortality in various models and with various assumptions. Two polices were compared: screening of women aged 40–49 at an 18-month interval and screening of women aged 50–69 every 2 years, which would result in lifetime doses of 13 and 33 mGy, respectively. Risk models from various epidemiological studies were used. In a hypothetical cohort of 100 000 women aged 40 who were followed-up until the age of 100, the number of induced deaths ranged from 5 to 24 and the number of years lost from 71 to 325.

Jung (2001) investigated the risk of mammography in two models of screening: screening every 2 years and screening starting at different ages but continuing for 10 years for a total of six examinations. He assumed a mean parenchymal dose per view of 2 mGy, resulting in 4 mGy per examination and thus 24 mGy from the six examinations of the screening programme. He also assumed a relative biological effectiveness of 2, and consequently a dose of 8 mSv per examination, and a linear dose–response model based on BEIR Committee coefficients (BEIR, 1990). The risk–benefit ratio for women first screened in their 40s was about 6, and that for women first screened in their 50s was about 25. The risk for developing breast cancer increased from 9 for unscreened women to 9.036, and the risk for dying from breast cancer increased from 3.96 to 3.961. He concluded that the risk for death from breast cancer is negligible if screening starts at 50 but should be taken into consideration in screening women aged 40–50.

Säbel et al. (2001) calculated the risk associated with a single examination at 2 mGy for women aged 40–49 or 50–59. In the younger women, 4.5 cases of breast cancer would be induced per 1 million women, while for the group aged 50–59 only 1.5 additional cases would be induced. The incidence:mortality ratio was taken as 2.3, resulting in 1.96 and 0.65 breast cancer deaths, respectively.

Although the authors of these studies use different assumption for the screening programmes, such as different age groups, screening intervals, doses of radiation at each mammography and models to estimate the numbers of radiation-induced breast cancer cases, the  results are consistent in showing that few breast cancer cases are induced by radiation during mammography. If screening was begun at the age of 50, the number of deaths from breast cancer during the remaining lifespan was estimated to be 10–50 per million regularly screened women (10–20 screens, 2–5 mGy per screen), while if regular screening was begun at the age of 40, the number of radiation-induced deaths from breast cancer would be 100–200. These numbers can be compared with the tens of thousands of breast cancer deaths in un-screened populations (cumulative mortality). The low additional risk is due to the fact that exposure to radiation after the menopause is associated with a low risk, as observed in many epidemiological studies.

# Chapter 6

# Cost–effectiveness of population-based breast cancer screening

## Cost–effectiveness analysis: What and why ?

As resources are limited, more and more decisions about health care interventions are based on cost–effectiveness analyses, so that health care is spread as equitably and efficiently as possible. In many countries, it has become routine policy to assess the costs of new (promising) health care interventions in relation to their expected benefits before actually implementing them. Interventions have a price, and most do not save total expenditure, but a minor change to an intervention strategy can lower the cost without a substantial loss of benefit, or, on the contrary, more benefit can be expected for similar cost (van den Akker-van Marle et al., 2002). The most accurate instrument for comparing different strategies is a cost–effectiveness analysis, to calculate outcome measures of effectiveness, such as a decrease in mortality and/or morbidity, as economic costs. Usually, a cost–effectiveness analysis is used to compare alternative health care interventions, including current or proposed policy, with no intervention, taking future costs and benefits into account and estimating the cost per life–year gained with the different policies (Brown & Fintor, 1993). Preferably, the costs per life–year gained are adjusted for quality of life, but quality of life is not always measured in practice.

## Published analyses

International studies of the cost–effectiveness of breast cancer screening show substantial differences in cost per life–years gained (Brown & Fintor, 1993; de Koning, 2000b). The cost–effectiveness ratio appears to be more favourable for most well-organized screening programmes, often European ones, than for spontaneous screening. The probable explanation is that having a special organization only for screening helps keep costs low, promotes more efficient use of resources, with high attendance of invited women and good quality screening leading to a health benefit. Moreover, as the direct cost for the screening examination is probably the most important single factor in total costs (Brown, 1992), organized large-scale screening may reduce the average cost per screen.

Comparisons of cost–effectiveness ratios between programmes in different countries is complex. Even with similar quality of mammographic screening (e.g. sensitivity), differences are found in almost all the factors that affect both effectiveness and cost. Thus, not only the epidemiology of breast cancer but also the organization and the costs of health care in general may differ. It is therefore surprising that one of the lower (and therefore favourable) estimated cost–effectiveness ratios (2650 euros per year of life gained; 5% discount rate) is seen in Navarra, Spain, where the breast cancer incidence is substantially lower than in northern countries (de

Koning, 2000b; Table 58). The Navarra programme had a very high participation rate of invited women (90%), a high breast cancer detection rate, indicating a high-quality programme, and a relatively unfavourable clinical stage distribution of breast tumours before the introduction of screening (van den Akker-van Marle et al., 1997). Conversely, in Germany, the estimated cost–effectiveness ratio was high—9600 euros per life–year gained—which must be attributed to the decentralized health care system, the lack of centralized screening settings and of personal invitations to screening and lower breast cancer incidence and mortality rates than in, for example, the Netherlands (Beemsterboer et al., 1994).

The estimated cost–effectiveness ratios for the Netherlands and the United Kingdom were similar and relatively low (de Koning et al., 1991). Both countries have nationally organized health care systems, high rates of breast cancer incidence and mortality and strictly nationally coordinated screening programmes with clear quality assurance and evaluation criteria. During the 1990s, a reduction in breast cancer mortality was observed among women aged 55–74 in both countries. The reduction is likely to be due partly to the screening activities, but other components of breast cancer control may also have played a role (Quinn & Allen, 1995; van den Akker-van Marle et al., 1999; Blanks et al., 2000b), particularly in the United Kingdom, where breast cancer mortality had already decreased in the early 1990s.

**Table 58. Estimated effects, costs and cost–effectiveness of breast cancer screening every 2 years (unless stated otherwise) for women aged 50–69 in various countries**

| Country (age range) | Breast cancer deaths prevented (if 27 years of screening) | Life-years gained | Difference in life-years gained, 5% discounting | Difference in costs (euros)[a], 5% discounting | Cost-effectiveness ratio (euros/life-year gained)[a], 5% discounting |
|---|---|---|---|---|---|
| Spain, Navarra (45–65) | 1 100 | 22 000 | Not reported | 60 | 2650 |
| Germany | 54 300 | 860 000 | 206 500 | 2000 | 9600 |
| Spain, Catalonia | 195 per year | Not reported | 19 450 | 90 | 4475 |
| United Kingdom, north-west (50–64)[b] | 4 880 | 81 000 | 15 000 | 60 | 3950 |
| Australia | Not reported | 250 000 | 53 500 | 450 | 8300 |
| Spain | 22 000 | 316 000 | 79 000 | 560 | 7125 |
| France | 42 000 | 649 000 | 155 000 | 765 | 4950 |
| United Kingdom (50–69) | 72 000 | 1 046 000 | 252 000 | 730 | 2900 |
| Netherlands | 17 000 | 260 000 | 61 000 | 210 | 3400 |

From de Koning (2000b)
[a] www.exact.nl
[b] 6% discount rate

Improvements in clinical care may be favoured by implementation of a screening programme, because of improved diagnostic assessment and treatment, and this can be regarded as a positive side-effect of screening programmes. For this reason, it is important that cost–effectiveness analyses also take into account possible changes in treatment patterns.

## Application of strict rules

A major problem in comparing the cost–effectiveness ratios of different screening programmes is differences in the analyses. Brown and Fintor (1993) presented a good example of how differences in screening modality, in the assumptions made with respect to the expected effects and in the assessment result in very different cost–effectiveness ratios (see box below). They used a report from the Office of Technology Assessment (US Congress, Office of Technology Assessment, 1987) in the USA and the Dutch study (de Koning et al., 1991). After adjusting the data for the differences, the outcome of the Office of Technology Assessment study was very similar to the alternative described in the study of de Koning et al. The cost–effectiveness ratios for different studies cannot be compared unless such adjustments are made. Therefore, an overview of cost–effectiveness ratios based on the same method of analysis provides a better insight into how a screening programme can be ranked internationally. The cost–effectiveness ratios for Navarra, Spain, and for Germany were derived from studies in which the 'Dutch model' was applied (de Koning, 2000b).

## Elements of cost–effectiveness

The outcomes of a cost–effectiveness analysis are standard, in the following hierarchical order:
- number of prevented breast cancer deaths and life–years gained in absolute terms;
- discounted effects (see below); and
- discounted cost and cost–effectiveness ratio, adjusted for quality of life.

### Effectiveness

The most important benefit of an effective breast cancer screening programme is a reduction in breast cancer mortality, together with life–years of relatively good quality gained. In a cost–effectiveness analysis, this is the most important element. Screening conducted in the 1970s and 1980s was shown to be

## Example of revision and recalculation of cost–effectiveness ratios: reconciling calculations from the USA and from de Koning *et al.* (1991)

**Report from the Office of Technology Assessment, USA, 1987**

Cost–effectiveness = US$ 34 600 / life–year saved

*Adjustment for lag effects*

↘ Cost–effectiveness = US$ 26 183 / life–year saved

*Adjustment for screening price, US$ 50 → US$ 20*

↘ Cost–effectiveness = US$ 11 267 / life–year saved

*Adjustment for biopsy, costs → saving*

↘ Cost–effectiveness = US$ 8931 / life–year saved

*Adjustment for effectiveness, 13% → 16%*

↘ Cost–effectiveness = US$ 7256 / life– year saved

**de Koning *et al.* (1991)**

**Cost–effectiveness = US$ 7250 / life–year saved**

From Brown and Fintor (1993)

effective when compared with no screening (see Chapter 4). On the basis of the early outcomes of three Swedish screening trials, a 16% reduction in breast cancer mortality, i.e. 600 fewer women dying from breast cancer annually, was estimated to be realistic for a nationwide programme of breast cancer screening every 2 years for women aged 50–69 in The Netherlands (de Koning *et al.*, 1991). Integration of more data from five Swedish screening trials published in 1993 (Nyström *et al.,* 1993) indicated a probable 17% reduction in total breast cancer mortality in The Netherlands, that is to say 800 fewer breast cancer deaths per year and 15 life–years gained per individual (de Koning *et al.*, 1995a). In the United Kingdom, it was estimated before implementation of the nationwide breast cancer screening programme that screening of women aged 50–64 every 3 years should reduce breast cancer mortality by 25%, assuming 70% participation.

If screening is effective, it also leads to a reduction in advanced stage disease. This is important not only from the point of view of reduced costs due to less radical treatment but especially from the perspective of improved quality of life, less morbidity and fewer out-patient clinic visits (de Haes *et al.,* 1991; de Koning *et al.*, 1992).

## Unfavourable effects

The impact of national programmes on quality of life has been the subject of much discussion. The potential negative effects of the screening examination itself (Ellman *et al.*, 1989), the referral of a significant number of women with benign lesions (Gram *et al.*, 1990) and the consequences of earlier and often more intensive treatment cannot be ignored.

Many factors determine the favourable and unfavourable effects of screening and, possibly, its cost–effectiveness. Important variables are improved prognosis of cases detected at screening, the predictive value of the screening test and the detection of DCIS that would have progressed to invasive carcinoma. Although mortality reduction is the fundamental effect, other desirable and undesirable consequences of screening may influence a woman's quality of life.

Figure 44 summarizes the most important favourable and unfavourable effects of a screening programme (per million screens), other than mortality reduction or gain in crude number of life–years. The scale represents the relative weights given to various types of morbidity at different phases, 100 representing perfect quality of life and 0 representing the worst possible state. The value 82 for adjuvant hormonal treatment implies an estimated 18% loss in effect during this phase as compared with the situation of perfect health (de Haes *et al.,* 1991; de Koning *et al.*, 1991). Screening 1 million women is expected to make adjuvant hormonal treatment unnecessary for 525 women, owing to the smaller number of women with lymph-node metastases. Therefore, this effect would lead to an increase of (525 × 0.18 × 2 years) = 189 quality-adjusted life–years.

The screening examination itself is estimated to have only a slight, short-term (1 week) negative impact, resulting in a decrease of (1 million × 0.006 × 1/52 year) = 115 quality-adjusted life–years. Even though it is estimated that 15.8 million women will have been screened during the period 1990–2017, only 7% of the total negative quality adjustment is incurred by these examinations. More importantly, breast cancer will be diagnosed in approximately 4500 women an average of 4 years earlier

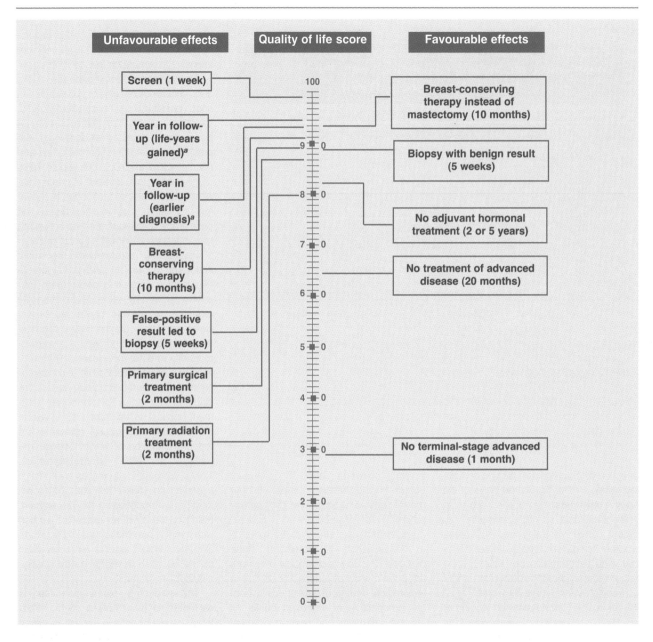

**Figure 44** Unfavourable and favourable effects, other than reduction in mortality, of 2-yearly screening of women aged 50–70

Differences are given per million screens (not discounted). Scale represents relative weights given to various types of morbidity, with decreases in quality of life due to unfavourable changes on the left and increases due to favourable changes on the right. Effects on morbidity are classified as short-term (treatment phase; 2 months), intermediate (first year after treatment; 10 months) and long-term (life–years). Durations (in parentheses) are assumed durations of impact on health-related quality of life for each episode.

From de Koning *et al.* (1991)

*a* Appear on negative side of the balance to correct the total gain in life-years for quality of life (lead time), and more than 1000 patients will experience a longer disease-free interval (16 500 life–years gained). In Figure 43, both types of additional years appear on the negative side of the balance, in order to correct the total gain in life–years for quality of life. The small loss in cost–effectiveness during follow-up is explained by the introduction of several medical follow-up procedures and by the negative impact on a woman's quality of life resulting from breast surgery and the knowledge that she has had breast cancer. The large increase in woman–years in follow-up is almost entirely responsible for the negative quality-of-life adjustment, whereas the decrease in the number of patients with advanced breast cancer as a result of screening is responsible for 70% of the positive quality-of-life adjustment. In the 27-year programme, a total of 252 000 quality-adjusted life–years are gained, which is a very small decrease from the 260 000 unadjusted life–years gained. As the more favourable effects are preceded by unfavourable effects, this difference becomes larger when effects and costs are discounted.

Differences in quality-adjusted life–years is a preferable measure to crude life–years gained. When associated morbidity in all possible phases is taken into account, favourable and unfavourable effects other than mortality reduction have only a limited impact and appear to cancel each other out. More extreme assumptions about expected cost–effectiveness in the various phases result in an adjustment of between – 20% (most unfavourable) and + 3% (most favourable) on life–years gained for 2-yearly screening of women aged 50–69 (de Haes et al., 1991).

It can be estimated that only one-quarter of the women in whom breast cancer is detected by screening benefit, in the sense that they do not die from breast cancer (de Koning, 1995). Even then, they have to live for longer with the knowledge of having cancer, which can

negatively affect their quality of life. Some women in whom breast cancer is diagnosed at a screening will die from it. Other women with screen-detected breast cancer might not have died from the disease, depending on the general diagnostic and therapeutic quality and survival rate. Screening generates a number of false-positive results, leading to temporary anxiety and additional assessment. False-negative, and also true-negative, results may falsely reassure women, so that they are less aware of symptoms and wait too long to see their general practitioner.

## Costs

The costs of systematic breast cancer screening can be divided roughly into those for organizing and implementing the programme, those for assessment, including that for false-positive results, those for additional primary treatment and savings in treatment costs due to a decreased number of cases of advanced disease. There has been debate about whether costs for health care not related to the treatment of breast cancer should be considered as well (Johnston, 2001).

The direct costs for screening include all those for inviting and screening women, e.g. for employing and training staff and for housing and material. These depend not only on the characteristics of a country but also on the organization of the screening programme. Separate screening units require high investment but guarantee high performance and better use of capacity. A centralized organization will keep overhead costs for coordination, quality assurance and monitoring low. Other determinants of the costs of screening are the type of invitation (personal letter or only general announcement), the number of views per screening examination, single or double reading of films and, especially, the total number and age range of the women invited and the frequency of screening examinations.

The costs of assessment depend initially on the number of recalled or referred screen-positive cases and secondly on the setting in which the further diagnostic assessment is carried out. In general, the higher the recall or referral rate, the higher will be the proportion of false-positive screen results. As diagnostic assessment of women with a true-positive result will almost always result in some kind of biopsy, the costs can be estimated precisely; however, this is not the case for false-positive results. In some cases, assessment will be limited to clinical investigation and a review of screening mammograms; in others, the assessment will be extended by magnification views and/or ultrasound examination, and a proportion of women with false-positive results will undergo a diagnostic biopsy. It is therefore difficult to estimate the costs related to false-positive screening results, and reliable data on the distribution of diagnostic procedures are often available only in an ongoing programme.

In the first few years after implementation of a screening programme, the treatment costs will rise owing to the increase in breast cancer detection. Thereafter, when most women have been invited for incidence screening rounds, the number of breast cancers detected in an advanced stage can be expected to decrease, and the costs of extensive breast cancer treatment can be saved (de Koning et al., 1992; Richards et al., 1993).

Implementation of a breast cancer screening programme can lead to a broad tendency to earlier detection of symptomatic breast cancers, as a consequence of publicity, increased awareness and improved early detection methods in clinical care. Although this generates additional costs, it will ultimately lead to a shift towards prognostically more favourable tumour stages and the possible saving of treatment costs for palliative care. A screening programme may also lead to less diagnostic assessment of breast symptoms among screened women. This assumption in the Dutch cost–effectiveness analysis was confirmed later by other studies in The Netherlands, showing that the demand for mammography outside the screening programme decreased among targeted women and remained stable in groups that were not targeted (Beemsterboer *et al.*, 1999; van Leiden *et al.*, 1999). Interestingly, during the first 2 years after the start of implementation of the screening programme, use of mammography outside the programme increased in all age groups but was significant only in the targeted age band. After 2 years, the frequency of spontaneous mammography returned to the previous level in the age groups that were not targeted but was significantly lower than before the start of the screening programme in the targeted population (Beemsterboer *et al.*, 1999).

## Discounting effects and costs

The costs and savings of a screening programme are not all seen at the same time. For example, the costs of the screening test(s) itself (seen at the start of the screening) represent the largest share, while much of the savings is due to avoidance of future treatment of disease. Furthermore, various target populations can be screened for the same disease, leading to different time profiles. It is generally accepted that earning an amount of money today is preferable to earning the same amount next year, because it can be put into a bank account where it will 'grow' by earning interest. This concept is called 'time preference' in economics. For example, if the 'real' interest rate (the interest without inflation) is 3%, a sum of 1000 will grow to 1000 + (1000 × 3%) = 1030 in 1 year. Conversely, the amount of 1030 of next year can be regarded as equivalent to an amount of 1000 in this year, provided the interest rate is 3%. The interest rate in this reverse reasoning is called the 'discount rate', and the amounts obtained by applying discount rates to future costs and savings are called 'present values'.

Table 59 gives an example of how cost–effectiveness indices should be presented, for the Dutch situation. First, the table presents the number of breast cancer deaths and the number of life–years lost as a result of breast cancer in the absence of mass screening and in the presence of mass screening, respectively. All effects are evaluated without discounting, but discount rates are applied to the costs. The effect of discounting is that the later certain costs arise, the less heavily they weigh in the cost–effectiveness analysis. The higher the discount rate, the more strongly this mechanism works. Various discount rates have been proposed (3%, 5%, 6%, 10%). In this table, a discount rate of 3% was used. The costs for screening, diagnosis and breast cancer therapy are

## Table 59. Effectiveness, cost and cost–effectiveness of mammographic breast cancer screening in The Netherlands

| | No screening | Screening (difference from no screening) |
|---|---|---|
| **No discounting** | | |
| *Effectiveness* | | |
| No. of deaths from breast cancer | 351 364 | – 31 195 |
| Life–years lost from breast cancer (× 1000) | 6 374 | – 514 |
| Quality-adjusted life–years lost (× 1000) | 7 168 | – 468 |
| **3% discounted** | | |
| *Effectiveness* | | |
| No. of deaths from breast cancer | 140 520 | – 16 180 |
| Life–years lost from breast cancer (× 1000) | 2 395 | – 203 |
| Quality-adjusted life–years lost (× 1000) | 2 715 | – 179 |
| **Costs (x $10^6$ euros)** | | |
| Screening | 0 | + 630 |
| Diagnosis | 2 921 | – 58 |
| Primary treatment | 4 159 | + 119 |
| Follow-up | 1 456 | + 43 |
| Palliative care | 5 481 | – 287 |
| Total | 14 017 | + 448 |
| **Cost–effectiveness (euros)** | | |
| Cost per life–year gained | | 2 209 |
| Cost per quality-of-life year gained | | 2 496 |

Adapted from de Koning *et al.* (1991)
Assuming women aged 50–69 screened every 2 years

distinguished to provide insight into the costs and savings at various stages of breast cancer. Finally, in the computation of cost–effectiveness ratios, a discount rate equal to that used for the cost should be applied to the effects. Although this principle has been debated, it is based on theoretical grounds. One is that not discounting effects will always lead to a situation in which postponing a programme (discounted less cost) is more cost–effective than starting the programme today. The cost–effectiveness is expressed as the cost per breast cancer death prevented or as the cost per life–year gained. If the effects have been adjusted for quality of life, the outcome is cost per quality-adjusted life–year gained.

## Modelling for policy decisions

The Netherlands was one of the first European countries to begin organized breast cancer screening. In 1974 and 1975, population-based, experimental, mammographic screening programmes were started in the cities of Utrecht and Nijmegen. The two programmes differed with respect to the targeted age groups, the screening interval and the re-invitation policy. In a case–control study, the two programmes were estimated to have resulted in a reduction in breast cancer mortality among screened women of 50–70% (Collette et al., 1984; Verbeek et al., 1984).

In the 1980s, the Department of Public Health at Erasmus University, Rotterdam, developed a computer-simulation package for analysing the effects of screening (MIcrosimulation SCreening ANalysis, MISCAN). The natural history and epidemiology of the disease, the design of the screening programme and the performance of screening are incorporated in this application. Roughly summarized, it simulates life histories in the absence of a screening programme and evaluates how these would be changed by various screening strategies

(van Oortmarssen et al., 1990; de Koning et al., 1995a). At the request of the Dutch Ministry of Health in 1986, a national research group was set up to determine the expected effects of a nationwide breast cancer screening programme based on model calculations with data from three randomized screening trials and from the two Dutch experimental programmes. With the inclusion of estimates of various cost aspects, this evaluation became an extensive cost–effectiveness analysis (de Koning et al., 1991). It takes into account various screening strategies with respect to the total number of screen examinations per woman, the length of the interval between successive screening rounds and referral modalities.

In general, the age at which a programme is started, the interval at which the test is applied and the age at which the programme is stopped are considered the major organizational aspects (Commission of the European Communities, 2000). Unfortunately, these aspects cannot be simply copied from experience elsewhere, because each country and trial is unique in terms of the underlying incidence and stage distribution of breast cancer and the screening design, which must be taken into account in interpreting 'efficacy' (de Koning et al., 1995a; de Koning, 2000b). Small differences in general circumstances or in design can have heavy consequences on both effects and costs. The same applies to modelling and its assumptions.

### Policy decisions on age categories to be screened

Whereas, in general, screening of postmenopausal women by mammography is considered to result in a reduction in breast cancer mortality, there remains uncertainty about its effect in women under 50.

#### Younger ages
It appears to be more cost–effective to increase the frequency of screening

examinations in a programme for women aged 50–69 than to screen women under 50 (de Koning et al., 1991). The same conclusion was drawn from a study on the screening programme for breast cancer in Catalonia, Spain, for women aged 50–64: on the basis of proven benefits and costs, extension of the programme to older women would be more effective than including younger women (Beemsterboer et al., 1998a). This conclusion was drawn in spite of the fact that in the Catalonian study extension to older and to younger ages appeared to be almost equally cost–effective and that, theoretically, younger women could gain more life–years. Extension to older women, however, would prevent more breast cancer deaths. Furthermore, screening has proved to be effective for women aged 50–69 years, whereas the effectiveness in younger women remains uncertain.

The lower cost–effectiveness of screening younger women is due to the lower breast cancer incidence and the poorer performance of the screening test due to denser breast tissue, resulting in a lower positive predictive value of an abnormal mammogram and higher rates of false-positive and false-negative results. These disadvantages could be partly outweighed by a higher frequency of screening examinations; that, however, would increase not only the costs but also the risk for radiation-induced breast cancers (Beemsterboer et al., 1998b).

Figure 45 shows the marginal costs per additional life–year gained and the corresponding changes in total costs with different screening policies, on the basis of inequal effectiveness by age group (de Koning et al., 1991). In comparison with increasing the invitation frequency of a 2-yearly screening programme for women aged 50–69, extension to women aged 40–49 would lead to a relatively high marginal cost–effectiveness ratio (additional cost

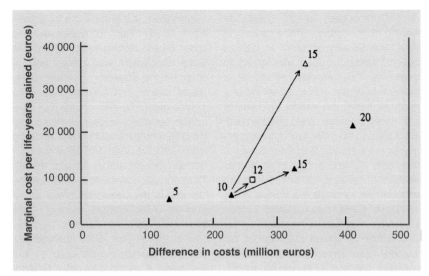

**Figure 45** Marginal cost–effectiveness (additional euros per additional life–year gained) of six breast cancer screening policies: 5, 10, 15 or 20 invitations to women aged 50–69 (filled triangles), 12 invitations to women aged 50–75 (square) and 5 invitations to women aged 40–49 followed by 10 invitations when they are 50–69 (open triangle). The corresponding differences in cost for each screening policy are shown on the horizontal axis; 5% discount rate.
From de Koning et al. (1991)

per additional life–year gained) of 35 500 euros. This finding is in line with the analyses of Salzmann et al. (1997), who showed that the cost–effectiveness was almost five times that in older women.

### Upper age limit
Another point that has not been completely resolved is the upper age limit for mass screening. The increasing breast cancer incidence with age favours better performance of a screening test among older women in contrast to younger women. Nevertheless, participation rates among older women may be lower, relatively more of the breast cancers detected may be of lesser clinical importance, and competing causes of death will play a greater role and limit the number of life–years gained. All these factors will affect the cost–effectiveness of screening older populations unfavourably (Commission of the European Communities, 2001). However, few empirical data are available from screening trials and pilot programmes on

women over 70; thus, the choice of an upper age limit of 69 or 70 would seem arbitrary. Some studies have suggested that mortality from breast cancer is also reduced among women aged ≥ 70 (Tabár et al., 1989; van Dijck et al., 1996), but no large-scale randomized controlled trials have been performed to settle this question.

Model simulations show that breast cancer screening is cost–effective for women aged > 69 years, on the assumption that the efficacy is the same as in women aged 50–69 (Boer et al., 1995; Kerlikowske et al., 1999). It is likely that, in organized programmes, reasonable attendance rates can be achieved for this age group. However, it is conceivable that, after a certain age, the balance between the benefits and harms of screening will become unfavourable. This depends theoretically on the 'behaviour' of the preclinical sojourn time of breast tumours, i.e. whether it increases continuously with age or whether it remains stable in women over

a certain age, for instance 65 years (Figure 46). In the first case—a continuous increase with age—unfavourable effects of screening, such as detection of clinically less important cancers and concomitant loss of quality of life, will outweigh the benefit of screening from a certain age (Boer et al., 1995).

### Policy decisions on screening interval
The choice of frequency of screening depends directly on the epidemiology and natural history of the disease and especially on the sojourn time. If this increases with age, as is generally assumed for breast cancer, a longer screening interval would be justified for older women. A study in which an increase in the sojourn time for preclinical breast cancer was observed showed a more favourable cost–effectiveness ratio in women aged ≥ 65 when they were screened less frequently than younger women (Boer et al., 1999a). However, the logistics of a population-based breast cancer screening programme with different invitation schedules for different subgroups, especially for a programme in which mobile units are used, may become complex and expensive. In the Swedish trials, the screening intervals varied from 18 to 33 months. Currently, most organized breast cancer screening programmes invite eligible women every 2 years (Shapiro et al., 1998).

Of the large-scale nationwide programmes, that in the United Kingdom represents the most important exception, as it provided mammographic screening only every 3 years. Despite this important difference in programme design from the Dutch programme, the cost–effectiveness ratios are similar, but the effectiveness is expected to be lower (de Koning, 2000b). A study in 1998 showed the cost–effectiveness of shortening the screening interval in the programme in the United Kingdom from 3 to 2 years, and estimated that 2-yearly

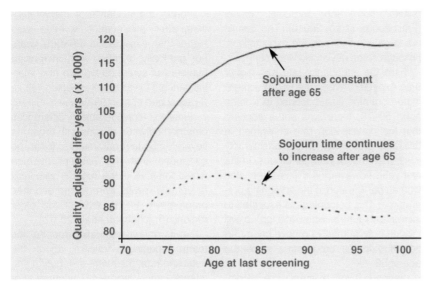

**Figure 46** Numbers of 5% discounted quality-adjusted life–years gained as a function of the upper age limit of invitation to screening in a programme with a 2-year screening interval, starting at age 51 From Boer *et al.* (1995)

screening would cost UK£ 2709 per life–year gained versus UK£ 2522 with the current policy (Boer *et al.*, 1998). In the same study, it was calculated that extending the upper age limit for invitation from 64 to 69 years would increase the cost per life–year gained from UK£ 2522 to UK£ 2990. The study, which concluded that either of the two alternatives, shortening the screening interval or extending the age range, would be effective, demonstrates that the policy choice of screening interval is related to the choice of age group to invite and vice versa (see also Figure 44).

### Policy decisions on high-risk groups

Instead of screening large populations at relatively low average risk of developing the disease in question, one alternative could be to limit screening to persons at high(er) risk, in order to reduce costs and unfavourable effects. This alternative approach would require accurate identification of 'high-risk' individuals. In the case of breast cancer, this is unrealistic,

as there are no clear markers of risk. To date, high-risk breast cancer screening is an option for women at high lifetime risk for familial breast cancer (see Chapter 4). This concerns predominantly young women, however, for whom mammography is probably not the most effective screening method. It is therefore still uncertain whether, from the public health point of view, screening high-risk groups would be cost–effective.

### Policy decisions on recall or referral

The method used for reading screening mammograms and the recall or referral policy affect the cost of screening and its effectiveness. A low recall threshold results in a high proportion of screened women with a false-positive result and thus lower specificity; a (too) high threshold leads to an inadequate rate of breast cancer detection and a high frequency of interval cancers. These aspects depend on the number of views used, the quality of the films and the training and experience of the readers. At the start of a

screening programme, a decision must be taken whether one, two or more readers, generally radiologists, are to read the screening mammograms. If there is to be double (or multiple) reading, various strategies are possible, such as independent double-reading of all films or pre-screening of all films by a first reader followed by double-reading of the initially selected mammograms. In the near future, computer-aided detection may play a role in supporting the reading process. All double or multiple readings will lead to discrepant findings, interpretation and referral recommendations in a proportion of cases, and clear guidelines should be drawn up to deal with the discrepancies and to decide which of them requires a recommendation for recall or referral, e.g. always referral, decision by one reader, decision by a third reader or after consensus of the two readers.

Several studies of the effect of single versus double reading on sensitivity and specificity generally agree that double reading leads to a higher detection rate and to lower specificity (Anderson *et al.*, 1994; Denton & Field, 1997; Blanks *et al.*, 1998). However, it is not clear whether the increased effect of double reading compared with single reading is also cost–effective (Haiart & Henderson, 1991; Brown *et al.*, 1996; Leivo *et al.*, 1999).

## Participation

Inadequate data are available to allow estimation of the cost–effectiveness of recruitment strategies or the effects of different attendance rates.

## Cost-effectiveness in practice

The continuing cost-effectiveness of a breast cancer screening programme in actual practice should be monitored carefully. Breast cancer screening should be offered only if there are concomitant efforts to maximize the ratio of benefits to harm. This requires effective routine monitoring of performance (Commission of the European Communities, 2001). Any unfavourable development with regard to effects or cost might adversely affect the cost–effectiveness and will require interventions.

In The Netherlands, a national team is responsible for evaluating and monitoring the effects of the Dutch breast cancer screening programme (Fracheboud et al., 2001a). In general, the results of subsequent screens are considered the most important indicator of the effectiveness of the programme. Subsequent examinations account for over 85% of all screening examinations now that the Dutch programme has been fully implemented.

As the decision to implement the Dutch nationwide breast cancer screening programme was based on the favourable outcomes of computer simulations with the validated MISCAN model, the observed effects have regularly been measured against those expectations. Now, more than 10 years after the start of screening, it is still not possible to answer the question of whether the programme has resulted in a reduction in breast cancer mortality. Although the mortality rate has been decreasing throughout the past decade in both The Netherlands and the United Kingdom, it is not clear to what extent the screening programmes contributed to this reduction. In anticipation of the answer to this question, the monitoring and evaluation of the programme concentrate on short-term results, such as participation rate, breast cancer detection rate, tumour stage distribution, false-positive and false-negative screening rates and sensitivity and specificity.

Although favourable short-term results do not guarantee a reduction in mortality, they are essential prerequisites. In Table 60, the short-term results of the Dutch screening programme for 1990–97 are compared with the expected

results from the MISCAN model (Fracheboud et al., 2001b). The results are largely in line with the expectations, although some deviations were seen.

First, the attendance rate was higher than expected. When the Dutch screening programme was extended to women aged 69–75, there was some concern that the participation rate of women in this age group would be considerably lower than that of younger groups. In the first year, however, 64.6% of the invited women participated in the screening programme. This percentage is expected to increase in future, when this group will include only women who have been participating in the programme since the age of 50.

Second, fewer women were recommended for further diagnostic testing than expected. In initial screens, the high predictive value of referral resulted in a breast cancer detection rate that conformed to expectation (taking into account the falling average age of the women attending initial screens over the course of the years). The breast cancer detection rate at subsequent screens, however, was lower than expected. The question is whether the relatively low referral rate—which is four to six times lower than that in the United Kingdom—is the cause. Efforts must be made to increase the referral rate, in order to increase the detection rate without a disproportionate increase in the number of false-positive screening results.

Third, the stage distribution of cancers detected at subsequent screens was similar to that at initial screens, although it had been expected that the distribution at subsequent screens would be more favourable. Possible explanations are that the natural history of breast cancer is different from that currently assumed, shortcomings in the quality and assessment of the mammograms or a difference in the interpretation or policy in national screening programmes from that in some of the trials (Boer et al., 1999b).

Fourth, the incidence of interval cancers after subsequent screens was higher than expected in the early years but gradually changed with increasing numbers of screened women and interval cancers towards the expected values (Fracheboud et al., 1999).

Finally, considerable differences emerged between regions with regard to several important parameters. It can be concluded that the national average would improve if the regions with less favourable results were to improve their programmes to the level of the other regions (Fracheboud et al., 2001b).

In its annual evaluation reports, the team expressed concern about the detection rate, the stage distribution and interval cancer incidence observed at or after subsequent screens. A study was initiated in 1999 to find ways of optimizing the effectiveness of the Dutch screening programme and to reduce the variation in regional results.

## Quality of life

In the early 1990s, there was little empirical evidence for the effects of screening on the short-term quality of life of women who participated or for the long-term quality of life resulting from the expected shift in the number of women experiencing early and advanced disease. The adjustment for quality of life in the MISCAN model was based on the results of a literature review and on the assignment of values to various disease and treatment phases by experts in breast cancer and public health (de Haes et al., 1991). The early computer simulations predicted that 2-yearly mammographic screening for women aged 50–70 would be 8% 'less effective' after adjustment for quality of life. The conclusion was that quality of life was not a major issue in the decision to undertake a large-scale breast cancer screening programme.

Since 1990, there has been increased interest in health-related quality of life, and this aspect has been assessed in

## Table 60. Observed and expected results of initial and subsequent screening examinations in The Netherlands, 1990–97

| Result | Initial screen | | Subsequent screens (< 2.5 years after previous screen) | |
|---|---|---|---|---|
| | Observed | Expected | Observed | Expected |
| Attendance (%) | 78.5 | 70.0 | 78.5 | 70.0 |
| Referrals/1000 | 13.1 | 16.0 | 6.9 | 7.5 |
| Biopsies/1000 | 9.2 | 12.0 | 4.5 | 6.0 |
| PPV of referral (%) | 47 | 41 | 51 | 57 |
| PPV of biopsy (%) | 66 | 54 | 78 | 72 |
| Screen-detected cancers/1000 | 6.1 | 6.5 | 3.5 | 4.3 |
| Tumour size distribution of screen-detected cancers (all carcinomas) | | | | |
| Ductal carcinoma *in situ* (%) | 14 | 13 | 14 | 14 |
| T1a–T1c (%) | 61 | 65 | 64 | 73 |
| ≥ T2 (%) | 20 | 18 | 17 | 9 |
| Unknown | 5 | 5 | 5 | 5 |
| Axillary lymph node status (% of invasive carcinomas) | | | | |
| Positive | 27 | 26 | 23 | 23 |
| Negative | 67 | 68 | 71 | 71 |
| Unknown | 6 | 6 | 6 | 6 |
| Interval cancers/1000 woman–years of follow-up | 0.96 | 1.00 | 0.93 | 0.96 |

PPV, positive predictive value
From Fracheboud et al. (2001b)

the various phases of breast cancer diagnosis and treatment. The Interdisciplinary Group for Cancer Care Evaluation (GIVIO, 1994) has undertaken programmes to assess the health-related quality of life of patients with early breast cancer since 1980 and in 1994 compared the quality of life in groups with intensive and conservative follow-up. Cockburn et al. (1994) and many others have reported on the psychological consequences of mammographic screening (see also Chapter 3).

The measurements of quality of life made about a decade ago are still largely valid; however, their influence on cost–effectiveness may have changed. For instance, with less invasive treatment such as breast-conserving therapy, quality of life will be better than with invasive treatment such as mastectomy. Any shift towards less invasive treatment, resulting not only from mass screening but also from improved medical techniques or new insights, will result in a more favourable cost–effectiveness ratio.

## Cost

In the late 1980s, much effort was made to obtain an overview of all the relevant costs of breast cancer screening, diagnosis and treatment. In order to adjust for time preference, the cost–effectiveness ratio was calculated with 3% and 5% discount rates. The development of costs that has been observed subsequently in The Netherlands is largely in line with the estimates. However, some changes warrant renewed cost–effectiveness analysis. For instance, the duration of hospital stay after surgical procedures has been reduced, which will lower the cost.

Developments in the costs of diagnosis and treatment were not monitored as continuously as the effects. Treatment for breast cancer in particular has become more expensive during the past decade, but that will be partly outweighed by the shortening of in-patient stays. Furthermore, the increased costs will be accompanied by increased savings.

## Cost–effectiveness

There is no sign that the cost–effectiveness of the Dutch breast cancer screening programme is less favourable than was expected. Many surrogate measures have been monitored and evaluated, and the results do not refute most of the assumptions made in earlier cost–effectiveness analyses. The participation rates, detection rates, size distribution, interval cancer rates and referral rates have been fairly stable or improved over time, suggesting possible effectiveness at the nationwide level. In The Netherlands, assumptions on effectiveness were based initially on three, and later five Swedish randomized controlled trials (de Koning et al., 1991, 1995a). Although recent reviews have given rise to discussion and the results can be used in sensitivity analyses for cost–effectiveness, they do not change the general picture that breast cancer screening can be very cost–effective.

Assumptions of 50% lower effectiveness lead to ratios in the order of those of the Dutch cervical cancer screening programme.

## Limitations of cost-effectiveness analysis

Evaluation of the cost–effectiveness of any screening programme is highly recommended. This requires adequate quantification of all the relevant effects and costs, which, in turn, requires continuous collection and registration of relevant data. The effort required to accomplish this is often enormous. In practice, a number of obstacles may limit a comprehensive cost–effectiveness analysis. These include practical limitations, gaps in knowledge, current and future developments in the diagnosis and treatment of breast cancer and alternative screening policies. Model-based cost–effectiveness analysis can provide relevant estimates of these long-term effects, but comparison with published analyses is often hampered by differences or lack of clarity in the assumptions made. Many so-called model-based cost–effectiveness analyses have been published which do not have the scientific rigour, clarity about assumptions and sensitivity analyses that should be provided. The box below provides an overview of the shortcomings of cost–effectiveness. Some of these shortcomings are discussed below in the context of the Dutch breast cancer screening programme.

### Practical limitations

All the information considered important for an optimal cost–effectiveness evaluation of the Dutch breast cancer

---

### Shortcomings in cost–effectiveness analysis

**Practical problems**

Limitations of obtaining data (privacy regulations, informed consent)

Limitations of registries (incompleteness, not national)

**Gaps in knowledge**

Natural history of breast cancer (duration of preclinical detectable phase with increasing age, biology of ductal carcinoma in situ)

False reassurance

**New developments**

Diagnosis and treatment of cancer (such as large-core needle biopsy)

Screening methods (digital mammography)

Alternative screening strategies (< 50 years)

**Quality of life evaluation**

Empirical data on episodes induced and prevented

screening programme is simply not available.

- Monitoring the effects of screening, particularly the effect on breast cancer mortality, is hindered by privacy regulations. All women participating in the Dutch screening programme are asked to give informed consent for use of their data in evaluating the screening programme. As such permission is not obtained from unscreened women, evaluation of breast cancer mortality at an individual level is impossible.
- The increasing amount of data registered by the screening organizations and regional cancer registries leads to a longer delay until delivery of the data.
- Some relevant data are not available nationally. For instance, in The Netherlands, there are no national data on the grade of malignancy of breast cancers.

## Gaps in knowledge

The model-based cost–effectiveness analysis of 1990 was based partly on a number of assumptions, because of lack of empirical data. Some of the assumptions and uncertainties are discussed below.

- The duration of the preclinical detectable phase with increasing age ($\geq 65$) is unknown. In order to estimate this duration, it is essential to have information about the detection rate in prevalence rounds and in subsequent rounds at an interval longer than 2.5 years and about the interval cancer rate. In The Netherlands, empirical evidence is expected to become available around 2003, 5 years after introduction of mass screening for women aged 70–75. At that time, the balance between favourable and unfavourable effects of breast

cancer screening for women aged $\geq$ 75 will be estimated more carefully;
- The 1990 cost–effectiveness analysis was based on the assumption that the number of requests by the target population for mammography outside the programme (opportunistic screening) would decrease. Opportunistic screening in a target population can negatively influence the effectiveness of screening and the costs of health care, and opportunistic screening of women in adjacent age groups would be another negative effect of screening from the public health perspective. In order to quantify these aspects, the effect of the start of the Dutch screening programme on the number of mammographies requested in general practice was examined (Beemsterboer *et al.*, 1999). The study showed an increased number of requests by general practitioners after the start of the screening programme, for women in all age groups. More than 2 years after the start of screening, however, the number of requests for mammography in all age groups had decreased to that before the start. In the age group 50–69, the number of mammographies was significantly lower than before screening started, probably due to the introduction of the national screening programme. Opportunistic screening was not clearly demonstrated in adjacent age groups.
- Negative results in a screening examination may falsely reassure screened women and lead to delayed diagnosis of symptomatic breast cancer, either during the interval or at the next screening examination. However, it is not known whether false reassurance indeed plays an important role and, if so, to what extent.

- At the time the decision was made to introduce breast cancer screening in The Netherlands, the radiation dose used in modern medicine was assumed to be negligible (Health Council, 1987). As a result of new techniques and continuous improvement of image quality, the radiation dose has probably increased from 0.5 mGy to about 2 mGy per examination. In order to study the risk of mammographic radiation and the implications for screening programmes for different age groups and intervals, model-based estimates were made of the number of breast cancer deaths induced by low-dose radiation (2 mGy per view) in breast cancer screening programmes and the numbers prevented (Beemsterboer *et al.*, 1998b). This study showed that the balance between the number of deaths induced and those prevented was favourable in the age group 50–69, assuming a screening programme with a 2-year interval. If screening is extended to the age group 40–49, the results are less favourable: one induced breast cancer death versus 66 prevented with a 1-year interval and one versus 97 with a 2-year interval.
- Little is known about how the effects of adjuvant systemic therapy interact with the proposed benefits of screening in trials performed in periods when such treatment was not available.

## New developments

New developments in breast cancer diagnosis and treatment may also necessitate a review of cost–effectiveness analysis, as they may have consequences for both the effectiveness and the costs of breast cancer screening and for quality of life. Important developments are:

- *New diagnostic procedures for impalpable breast lesions.* Less invasive diagnostic procedures, such as stereotactic core biopsy, have increasingly replaced needle-localized biopsy for the evaluation and treatment of impalpable breast lesions. In general, these procedures are cheaper and are assumed to have fewer negative effects on quality of life than open breast biopsy. Introduction of these procedures will lead to fewer unnecessary open surgical biopsies, thus lowering health care costs and, as a consequence, influencing cost–effectiveness.
- *Digital mammography.* Replacing conventional screen–film mammography by digital mammography will require heavy initial financial investment (purchase of expensive equipment) but in the long run may save costs (transport, files, archives). Another favourable aspect of digital mammography may be a reduction in risk from radiation and better performance of screening programmes due to high-quality imaging.

Computer-assisted pre-selection and enlargement of mammographic images are related techniques. The possible consequences are not yet clear.

Cost–effectiveness analysis is essential if an alternative screening policy is being considered, such as extension of the age limit of the target population, an increase or decrease in the screening interval or choice of another screening instrument. For instance, the results of current screening trials involving women under the age of 50, such as the trial in the United Kingdom for women aged ≥ 40 (Moss, 1999), may warrant reconsideration of the lower age limit in the Dutch breast cancer screening programme and an update of the cost–effectiveness analysis.

Because of the relatively unfavourable detection rate after subsequent screens, in combination with the relatively low referral rate, in the Dutch programme, an alternative referral strategy might be considered. Currently, all screening mammographies are read by two readers, and women are referred only if there is consensus between the two. An alternative strategy would be to refer women if at least one of the two readers recommends further assessment of the mammographic lesion. This would result in a higher referral rate and a larger number of false-positive results, but with an expected increase in the detection rate. A revision of the cost–effectiveness analyses would then be required.

The differences found between observed and expected outcomes in The Netherlands may have several implications. There may be some dysfunction in actual screening practice, which should be corrected. The regional differences in particular imply that some improvement is possible. Another explanation is that the expectations were too optimistic. It is not unlikely that the results of 10 years' screening in The Netherlands are more representative of reality than the model-based expectations. In that case, the model used to estimate cost–effectiveness should be reconsidered and revised. At least in The Netherlands, both explanations may be true.

# Chapter 7

# Summary

## Breast cancer and screening

### World-wide burden

Breast cancer is the commonest cancer among women in both high-income and low-income countries, accounting for 22% of the 4.7 million new cases of cancer occurring annually among females worldwide. Improvements in treatment and possibly breast screening by mammography have reduced mortality from breast cancer in high-income countries, but the risk continues to increase in eastern Europe and Latin America. Substantial improvements in survival have been reported in high-income countries such as the USA, where the prevalence of breast cancer is estimated to be 1.5% of the female population, whereas survival from this cancer in middle- and low-income countries remains poor, mainly because of late presentation of cases.

### Biology, pathology and natural history

Breast cancer appears to be a heterogeneous disease. The introduction of mammographic screening has altered the range of benign lesions and the patterns of neoplastic entities that are removed surgically. In general, there are three categories of breast abnormalities: benign conditions, in-situ conditions and invasive cancer. Benign conditions are associated with a risk for breast cancer ranging from one- to fivefold, depending on the degree of epithelial proliferation and atypia. In-situ lesions are lobular or ductal. Lobular carcinoma *in situ* is associated with an increased risk for invasive breast cancer but is usually an incidental finding and is not generally detected by mammography. Although data on the natural history of ductal carcinoma *in situ* are limited, it is likely that poorly differentiated cytonuclear lesions (high grade) are associated with a significantly higher risk for development of invasive carcinoma than well-differentiated cytonuclear lesions (low grade). High-grade lesions appear to be more biologically aggressive, with a higher rate of recurrence after breast-conserving surgery. Low-grade ductal carcinoma *in situ* is associated with low-grade invasive cancer, which is generally characterized by indolent behaviour and a good prognosis. Molecular markers may become available that will improve evaluation of prognosis.

Reliable classification of in-situ and invasive breast cancers provides important clinical information and can contribute to the evaluation and quality assurance of breast cancer screening programmes. The grading of in-situ cancers is evolving, and standardized staging of invasive cancers has become possible.

### Conceptual considerations

The main concept in cancer screening is that detection of early disease will make it possible to reduce mortality, because treatment at early stages is more effective than treatment at later stages. The purpose of modelling the screening process is to identify the characteristics of both a screening test and a screening programme that will determine the extent to which cancers are detected earlier, and thus the potential for reducing mortality. A model is presented, which is based on the assumption that the aim of screening for cancer is to detect lesions that, if left untreated, would progress to clinical cancers. The definitions of sensitivity, specificity and positive predictive value are therefore based on the proportion of cancers that would otherwise be diagnosed clinically during some specified period after screening but which are diagnosed at screening. The model allows for the considerable heterogeneity among cancers indicated by increasing knowledge of tumour biology. This heterogeneity is expressed partly as variation in the preclinical detectable phase, which results in variation in the potential lead time of lesions. The models can be used to identify intermediate outcomes of a screening programme that predict future reductions in mortality from the cancer in question and, as such, are valuable monitors.

## Screening techniques

### Screening mammography

Modern mammography machines are equipped with devices to reduce scatter, automatically control exposure and optimize the quality of the image in relation to the dose of radiation. The mean absorbed dose to the average-sized breast is in the order of 1.0–2.0 mGy. The sensitivity and specificity of mammography depend on several factors, including the density of the breast parenchyma, which in turn is related to age, parity, menopausal status and use of hormone replacement therapy, and technical variability. Sensitivity is also determined by the number of image projections used. Variability in interpretation by readers can be partly offset by training and by double reading of films. Continuing training and monitoring of the imaging process is a crucial part of a quality assessment programme for mammographic screening.

## Other and emerging imaging techniques

Many techniques have been suggested for breast cancer screening. Although several of them hold promise, a systematic review showed that few have been used to screen populations, and the studies were generally small and of poor quality, so that the evidence for the following statements is weak. A combination of ultrasound and mammography may increase sensitivity, especially in women with radiographically dense breasts, but with a concomitant reduction in specificity. Magnetic resonance imaging is more sensitive than mammography in women at high risk for breast cancer but has less specificity. Computer-aided diagnosis may improve sensitivity when used in combination with conventional mammography, although it is unclear whether the improvement is greater than with other techniques, such as double reading and special training of film readers. The role of computer-aided diagnosis in specificity is unclear. The sensitivity of full-field digital mammography may be similar to that of film mammography. Only one small study has been reported of use of positron emission tomography in screening, and none has been reported for computed tomography scanning, magnetic resonance spectroscopy, scintimammography, electrical impedance, infrared spectroscopy, light scanning or recent thermography.

## Clinical breast examination

No one technique for clinical breast examination has been shown to be better than any other for breast cancer screening. The technique generally recommended involves visual examination and systematic palpation of the entire breast and regional axillary nodes. The sensitivity of clinical breast examination alone in large studies ranged from 55% to 70% and the specificity from 85% to 95%.

## Breast self-examination

Women often find their own breast cancers. Detailed protocols for breast self-examination have been designed, and competence in the practice has been evaluated by use of silicone models of the breast. Training and reinforcement improve the quality and increase the frequency of use of breast self-examination. While many programmes have been designed to promote breast self-examination, a minority of women practise it and fewer do it well.

## Use of breast cancer screening

## Delivery and uptake of screening

Breast cancer screening is delivered in a variety of ways, including organized programmes and 'opportunistic' activities, which involve referral to mammography facilities by clinicians and self-referral by women themselves. Organized programmes include an administrative structure responsible for implementation, quality assurance and evaluation. Most programmes emphasize mammography. The characteristics of screening in various regions are summarized below.

### Europe

Organized breast cancer screening programmes were first established in northern Europe and the United Kingdom. Currently, screening is done through organized screening programmes in 19

countries, although opportunistic screening co-exists. Seven of the programmes are organized nationally, nine are organized regionally, and three are pilot programmes. The programmes target at least women aged 50–69, but some extend invitations to women aged up to 74 or under 50. In most of the programmes, women are invited to mammography about every 2 years; in the United Kingdom, women are invited every 3 years. Seven countries offer clinical breast examination in addition to mammography in their screening policies

The proportion of women with access to organized screening programmes varies markedly, from 2% in the German pilot programme to nearly 100% in six countries. Quality review is extensive, following European or national guidelines for addressing the technical quality of mammography, external and internal control, recall rates and cancer detection rates and a wide range of other relevant indicators.

### The Americas

In Canada, screening is done primarily through a nationally organized programme that is funded and administered at provincial level, targeting women aged 50–69. Although all women have access to screening, 79% of those aged 50–69 reported ever having had mammography, and 54% reported having had one within the previous 2 years. The technical quality of mammography is reviewed within programmes according to national standards.

In contrast, in the USA, screening is primarily opportunistic, and few organized programmes exist. The recommendations of the Preventive Services Task Force now include mammography for women aged 40–69. Assessment of mammography use in a state-based telephone survey showed that 85% of women over 40 had ever had a mammogram, and 71% had had one in the previous 2 years. Quality assurance is nationally based and focuses on certification of mammography facilities.

Mammography is available on demand in Latin America and the Caribbean; however, most countries report either no policy regarding breast cancer screening or policies that may not completely reflect the available scientific evidence. No population-based estimates of mammography use are available.

### Oceania and Asia

Australia and New Zealand have organized national mammographic screening programmes; a few other countries have initiated local screening, usually not based on mammography. Screening in the organized programmes is targeted at women aged 50–69 in Australia and 50–64 in New Zealand and involves invitation for a mammogram every 2 years. In Australia, women aged 40–49 and ≥ 70 years may also attend, but they are not systematically invited. In Australia in 1997–98 and in New Zealand in 1999–2000, 54% of all eligible women had had mammograms in the previous 2 years. The Australian and New Zealand programmes have management structures for quality assurance and national standards for participation, recall rates, technical radiological performance, cancer detection rates and data monitoring.

## Behavioural considerations in screening participation

Women should be fully informed about the potential benefits and harms of periodic screening so that they can decide whether to take part. Most women tend to overestimate both the likelihood of developing breast cancer and the sensitivity and specificity of screening; they vary in their preference for numerical and verbal information about risk, and this information is often not well understood.

Some women are anxious about mammographic screening, primarily because of fear of an abnormal result. Women experience a moderate increase in anxiety after a false-positive mammogram, although this is usually short.

Factors associated with participation in mammographic screening include: an invitation or reminder to attend within an organized programme, a recommendation from a doctor to attend, good understanding of the benefits of mammographic screening, a belief that breast cancer can be treated, a perception of personal risk, moderate anxiety about breast cancer and having had other preventive health interventions.

The effects of a number of intervention strategies on participation have been studies, including programmes targeting individual women, community strategies, health care provider programmes and strategies for special groups. Most of these strategies were found under trial conditions to be effective to some extent in increasing participation; however, the feasibility and cost–effectiveness of these strategies as part of routine programme implementation is unknown.

## Efficacy of screening

### Methodological and analytical issues in assessing efficacy

The efficacy of screening is best evaluated by means of randomized screening trials. Such trials, with mortality from the cancer of interest as the end-point, avoid selection bias and the biases associated with studying survival after diagnosis, including lead-time bias, length bias and overdiagnosis bias. Trials must be planned and conducted with attention to the necessary quality standards, particularly in the areas of randomization, confirmation that balance is achieved by randomization (especially if cluster randomization is used), delivery of the screening intervention, participation by the intervention group and little contamination from screening in the control group, comparison of cases in the two arms of the trial with regard to early indicators of an effect of the intervention such as tumour size and nodal status, treatment according to stage of detection applied equally in both groups and adequate documentation of the study end-point, preferably after an independent review of cause of death by persons unaware of the allocation of the woman to intervention or control. Observational studies of screening, such as cohort and case–control studies, may give biased measures of effect because of self-selection of women for screening. There are no certain ways of eliminating this bias.

### Conventional screening mammography

The screening modality use mainly as a public health intervention at present is mammography alone. The Working Group therefore focused its attention on trials in which the efficacy of mammography alone was compared with no screening.

Of the 10 randomized trials of breast cancer screening, the effect of invitations to mammography alone was compared with that of usual care in six studies, all conducted in Sweden. In two of these, women were randomized by cluster, while various forms of individual randomization were used in the others: two according to randomly ordered birth cohort and the other two by date of birth, either exclusively or in part. Various analytical approaches confirmed that these processes achieved balance. In addition, for a short period at the beginning of the Finnish national programme, women born in even-numbered years were invited to be screened. This is equivalent to randomization, and the results of this experience were incorporated into the evaluation of screening for women aged 50–69.

The findings from the latest follow-ups for women aged 50–69 in the five trials of mammography alone that included this age group and the Finnish programme gave a combined rate ratio of 0.75 (95% confidence interval, 0.67–0.85) and displayed no heterogeneity.

The findings for women aged 40–49 (43–49 in one trial and 45–49 in another) in the six trials of mammography alone that included this age group gave an overall rate ratio of 0.81 (95% confidence interval, 0.65–1.01). It is uncertain how much of this effect could have been due to screening after the age of 50.

The possibility of the introduction of bias into the results of the studies of screening with mammography alone by a range of methodological factors was considered. The available evidence suggested that none, if any, bias was present that could have had a sufficiently large effect to affect the overall rate ratios appreciably.

The other trials involved combined screening with mammography and clinical breast examination. In one, conducted in the 1960s in New York, USA, the results for both age groups were similar to those in the trials with mammography alone. One, conducted in Edinburgh, Scotland, as a randomized component of the Trial of Early Detection of Breast Cancer and involving combined mammography and clinical breast examination, was based on cluster randomization. There was evidence that the randomization had failed, as there were appreciable differences between the two groups in distribution by social class and mortality from causes other than breast cancer. The Working Group was not convinced that the adjustments undertaken in the analysis of the trial would satisfactorily have removed any bias due to differences between the two groups.

Of the two trials in Canada, both of which involved individual randomization of volunteers, one addressed combined screening with mammography and clinical breast examination of women aged 40–49 in comparison with usual care. The women were also taught breast self-examination. After an average of 13 years of follow-up, there was no evidence of a reduction in mortality from breast cancer, although the confidence interval was compatible with the overall estimate of effect in this age group in the trials of mammography alone.

The other trial in Canada, of women aged 50–59, was a comparison of screening with mammography plus clinical breast examination with clinical breast examination alone. Thus, its results do not allow a direct evaluation of the efficacy of screening for breast cancer with mammography alone.

In addition to the trials, there have been one quasi-experimental study, one cohort study and four case–control studies, conducted independently of the trials. In general, the observational studies showed greater reductions in the relative risk for death from breast cancer than the trials. This difference has often been attributed to the fact that observational studies address the effect of attendance for screening rather than that of invitation to screening, as is measured in trials. However, observational studies have an inherent potential for bias, due, for example, to self-selection of women for screening, which would make such interpretation inappropriate. Estimates of efficacy should rather be based on the results of trials, after adjustment for non-participation and contamination. By making such adjustments, the Working Group estimated that attendance for screening would reduce mortality from breast cancer by about 35%.

Various frequencies of screening were used in the trials, ranging from 12 to 33 months. In view of the small number of trials, which also had many other differences, it is impossible to assess the effect of screening frequency on the reduction in mortality. One subsequent randomized trial was designed to compare the effect of annual versus three-yearly screening on the size, stage and grade of tumours. Predictive models based on these data suggest that the effect of shortening the screening interval is modest.

The conclusions of the Working Group differ from those of the review published by the Cochrane Collaboration. In particular, the Group disagreed with the exclusion in that review of several of the randomized trials carried out in Sweden.

## Clinical breast examination

The efficacy of screening by clinical breast examination alone in reducing mortality from breast cancer has not been demonstrated in randomized controlled studies. A case–control study and an ecological study in Japan provided very weak evidence for a reduction in mortality in women screened by clinical breast examination as compared with no screening. One randomized controlled trial showed similar rates of mortality from breast cancer in women screened by clinical examination alone and by a combination of clinical examination and mammography.

## Breast self-examination

Among women who present clinically with breast cancers, the tumours detected in those who practise self-examination tend to be smaller and to be associated with longer survival than those in women who do not examine themselves. Cohort and case–control studies provide some evidence for a reduction in the risk for death from breast cancer among women who practise breast self-examination frequently and competently. Randomized trials in the Russian Federation (of which only one of two components has been reported) and in China showed that women who were taught breast self-examination were more likely than women in the control groups to detect benign breast lesions but not more likely to detect breast cancers at a less advanced stage of progression. Neither the trial in the

Russian Federation, where participation was relatively limited, nor the trial in China, where participation was high, showed a reduction in mortality from breast cancer among women taught this technique.

## Women at high risk

Women who carry mutations in either the *BRCA1* or the *BRCA2* gene have a very high lifetime risk for breast cancer, and many clinicians recommend annual mammographic screening of carriers of such mutations, beginning some time between the ages of 25 and 35. It has not yet been proven that screening of this predisposed group by mammography reduces their mortality from breast cancer, and no randomized trials with mortality as the end-point have been conducted in this group of women. Because of their high risk for cancer, both the prevalence of cancer at screening and the positive predictive value of the screening test are higher than in other women. Because the *BRCA1* and *BRCA2* genes participate in the repair of radiation-induced DNA breaks, it has been suggested that women who carry these mutations are at greater risk for radiation-induced breast cancer than are women in the general population; however, no relevant data are available. The sensitivity of magnetic resonance imaging has been reported to be greater than that of screening mammography for women at high risk because of a *BRCA* mutation or a family history. These studies, however, were based on small numbers of women.

## Effectiveness of population-based screening

### Implementation of population-based screening in accordance with results of screening trials

The results of randomized trials of mammographic screening compared with no intervention have been used as the basis for centrally organized screening programmes, to decide the age range of women to be screened and the screening interval. All national screening programmes cover at least women aged 50–64, and all programmes involve an interval of 3 years or fewer. Older and younger women are invited in some countries. Other components of a screening programme, such as the number of film readers and the number of mammographic views, are based largely on considerations other than the results of trials.

### Indicators of the effectiveness of population-based screening programmes

The basic indicator used for effectiveness is the standardized mortality ratio (SMR). From the point of view of public health, a relative measure such as the SMR may be an incomplete indicator; absolute measures will provide additional information on effectiveness. In none of the national mammographic screening programmes has a reduction in mortality from breast cancer of the order demonstrated in the randomized trials yet been observed. If such a reduction is achievable in practice, it will take many years to occur.

Indicators of performance can be used as a basis for corrective action to a screening programme in the early stages and can be used to predict whether a reduction in mortality is likely to be found in the long term. These indicators include measures of coverage, participation, age-specific or age-standardized rates of detection of cancer and rates of detection of advanced disease and interval cancers (by stage). Predictions of mortality reduction can be based on modelling, and several techniques with various assumptions can be used and validated by comparison with the results of randomized experiments. The microsimulation screening analysis (MISCAN) model has been used for several populations.

Intermediate indicators and surrogate measures are important in order to obtain an early estimate of effect. They are necessary but not sufficient for an effective screening programme. The interval cancer rate is a useful determinant of programme sensitivity and the rate of advanced disease of programme effectiveness. Both are predicated on the availability of cancer registration in the target population; the identification of interval cancers also requires linkage of data sources into a coherent information system, and measurement of the rate of advanced cancer also requires that the cancer registry records clinical stage.

In the few instances in which assessment of advanced cancer rates has been possible, screening appears to have been followed by a decline in the rates of advanced disease (albeit more than offset by the large numbers of early and in situ cancers detected). In all the programmes examined, the decreases in advanced disease rates have been smaller than predicted from the data of the Two-county study in Sweden.

Given the natural history of the disease and the long implementation period of national programmes, it is too early to expect a substantial reduction in breast cancer mortality. Evidence from the United Kingdom has shown that the recent substantial declines are probably due to multifactorial causes, and the precise roles of screening and other factors, including improved therapy, are hard to determine. This is even truer in areas that depend only on overall rates of breast cancer mortality for evaluating effectiveness, as the quality of screening and the extent of information are likely to be correlated.

Cases of breast cancer diagnosed before the start of screening contribute to the mortality rates, and removal of these cases results in a better estimate of effect. Such estimates of 'refined' mortality require the existence of a cancer registry and the possibility of linkage to data on screening. Refined mortality should be estimated for screened and unscreened populations to ensure comparability. Furthermore, cancer registration with data on treatment is likely to be the only means for differentiating the confounding effect of changes in treatment from the effect of screening.

Studies on effectiveness, including those based on modelling, have so far resulted in estimates of 5–10% reductions in mortality in the the target population due to screening. The estimates of refined mortality have been higher, around 20%, closer to the effect indicated by the screening trials. In terms of prolongation of life, the effect per screen remains small.

## Hazards of screening
### *False-positive mammograms*:
False-positive results are inevitable in screening. However, the rate varies dramatically from one area to another; it is particularly high in the USA. Depending on the setting and the frequency of examinations, the cumulative risk of a woman who receives a false-positive result after completing a screening programme can be extrapolated to be as low as 2% or as high as 50%. False-positive results increase health care use associated with screening. Women experience considerable anxiety after being told they have a positive result; this effect is largely transient and is an accepted part of screening for most women. The greatest opportunity for reducing false-positive results is in improving radiological interpretation.

### *Overdiagnosis*
"Overdiagnosis' is the term used to describe the detection of cancers that would never have been found without screening. Patients who have such indolent cancers experience only harm: the anxiety associated with a cancer diagnosis and the complications of therapy. Overdiagnosis increases the cost of screening and complicates evaluation of the programme.

There is evidence of some over-diagnosis of breast cancer in the randomized trials of mammography and from population-based incidence rates. From 5 to 25% of cancers detected by mammography may represent overdiagnosis. The finding of a substantial breast cancer reservoir suggests that perhaps the most pressing challenge for breast cancer screening is to determine which lesions should be treated.

### *Ductal carcinoma* in situ
Evidence from clinical studies suggests that a proportion of ductal carcinomas *in situ* will progress to invasive cancer. How small this proportion is for non-palpable lesions detected by mammography is, however, less clear. The results of the trials in Canada suggested that detection of ductal carcinoma *in situ* by mammography and its subsequent treatment did not lead to a reduction in the incidence of invasive cancer within 11 years. As current work suggests that the prognosis of ductal carcinoma *in situ* differs according to its nuclear grade, screening might offer greater benefit to women with some types of lesion than to others. It is an open question, therefore, whether the potential benefits of detecting and treating ductal carcinoma *in situ* outweigh the harmful effects of treatment (anxiety, operations, radiotherapy).

### *Radiation*
Exposure to radiation ia a known risk factor for breast cancer. The mean absorbed dose of radiation to the breast during mammography is now generally below 3 mGy per screen, and the dose of radiation to the thyroid and other organs is assumed to be negligible. The risk for radiation-induced breast cancer decreases with age and is particularly low for women after the menopause. In a model based on the assumption of a linear relationship between risk for breast cancer and dose of radiation, the number of deaths from radiation-induced breast cancer during the remaining life span when screening is begun at the age of 50 is estimated to be 10–50 per million in regularly screened women (10–20 screens, 2–5 mGy per screen), These numbers can be compared with the 30 000–40 000 deaths from breast cancer over a lifespan after 50 years of age per million women in the whole population, of which some 10 000–15 000 may be preventable by screening. If screening is begun at the age of 40, the number of radiation-induced breast cancers is estimated to be 100–200 per million regularly screened women.

In relation to the expected benefit, the risk is negligible when screening is started at the age of 50 but is higher when screening is begun between the ages of 40 and 50. The risk for radiation-induced breast cancer should be taken into account if screening is started at a younger age.

## Cost–effectiveness of population-based screening

In many countries, it has become routine policy to assess the costs of new, promising health care interventions in relation to their expected benefits, before implementation. The screening policy for breast cancer that is most cost–effective in a particular country depends on various factors, including the incidence of breast cancer, its stage distribution and mortality rate, the expected quality of the screening programme, the national health care setting and economics. Although the final ratio, cost per life–year gained, is considered most important by some, the hierarchy in cost–effectiveness analyses is, first, to assess the benefits (breast cancer mortality reduction and life–years gained), second, to assess the possible harm and benefits other than reduction in mortality (quality of life) and, finally, to weigh these against induced costs and possible savings.

Given the evidence about reduction of mortality from breast cancer in randomized trials of breast cancer screening, screening programmes for women aged 50–69 at a 2- or 3-year interval are expected to be cost–effective in high-incidence countries with well-organized programmes. National reductions in breast cancer mortality may be of the order of 10–20%; women who do not die from breast cancer may gain approximately 15 years of life, and the cost–effectiveness ratio is 3000–8000 euros per life–year gained. Very high referral rates of about 10% unfavourably influence cost–effectiveness ratios, as does the delicate balance between favourable and unfavourable effects. In general, the harm inflicted on a group of screened women is less than the benefits achieved by some part of the same screened group. Correction for all anticipated unfavourable effects in terms of quality-adjusted life–years gained may diminish the total number of life–years gained by 5–15%.

The most important cost elements to consider are the cost of screening and the cost of treating advanced disease. Savings in the cost of screening of up to 30% may be achieved by the reduction in the cost of treating advanced disease, but breast cancer screening will always lead to substantial additional cost for a country. It should be compared with other health care priorities, preferably by cost–effectiveness ratios too. Low-risk and low-income countries are likely to give higher priority to other activities.

The marginal cost–effectiveness of expanding a programme to younger women (40–49) greatly depends on its effect on reducing breast cancer mortality as estimated from randomized controlled trials. Under the assumption of less or relatively low benefits of screening younger women, it would be more cost–effective to increase the upper age limit to 74 or to narrow the screening interval from 3 to 2 years for the age group 50–69, rather than expand the programme to women aged 40–49.

# Chapter 8

# Evaluation

## Evaluation of the efficacy of breast cancer screening

There is *sufficient evidence* for the efficacy of screening women aged 50–69 years by mammography as the sole screening modality in reducing mortality from breast cancer.

There is *limited evidence* for the efficacy of screening women aged 40–49 years by mammography as the sole screening modality in reducing mortality from breast cancer.

There is *inadequate evidence* for the efficacy of screening women under 40 or over 69 years by mammography in reducing mortality from breast cancer.

There is *inadequate evidence* for the efficacy of screening women by clinical breast examination in reducing mortality from breast cancer.

There is *inadequate evidence* for the efficacy of screening women by breast self-examination in reducing mortality from breast cancer.

## Overall evaluation

### Effect of screening with mammography on mortality from breast cancer

There is *sufficient evidence* from randomized trials that inviting women 50–69 years of age to screening with mammography reduces their mortality from breast cancer; the best current estimate of the average reduction is 25%. There is only *limited evidence* for this effect in women 40–49 years of age, in whom the reduction, if real, is estimated at 19% but could be less, depending on the extent to which it is due to screening of the women after they reached the age of 50. No direct conclusions can be drawn about the efficacy of inviting women younger than 40 or older than 69 years of age to screening with mammography.

The reduction in mortality from breast cancer in women 50–69 years of age who accept an invitation to screening has been estimated to be about 35%, by adjustment of the results of the trials for the effect of non-acceptance of the invitation by some women.

Both apparent and real deficiencies of the randomized trials that were considered in making this evaluation of the efficacy of invitation to screening were carefully assessed for their impact on its validity. They were judged not to invalidate the trials' findings and therefore the evaluation.

### Influence of inter-screening interval on effect of screening by mammography

There is little evidence on which to base recommendations on the frequency with which women should be offered mammographic screening. In most of the randomized trials on which the evidence of efficacy of screening was based, women were invited to be screened at intervals of about 24 months. Modelling has suggested that about a further 5% reduction in mortality is gained for women 50–69 years of age for each reduction in the inter-screening interval of one year, between three years and one year. These estimates are compatible with the results of a randomized trial of the effects of annual compared with three-yearly screening, which predicted breast cancer mortality on the basis of the prognostic characteristics of breast cancers at the time of diagnosis.

## Effect of breast screening by clinical breast examination on mortality from breast cancer

There is *inadequate evidence* that breast screening with clinical breast examination, whether alone or in addition to screening mammography, can reduce mortality from breast cancer.

## Effect of breast screening by breast self-examination on mortality from breast cancer

There is *inadequate evidence* that breast self-examination can reduce mortality from breast cancer.

## Effectiveness in practice of breast cancer screening with mammography

There is some evidence for the effectiveness of programmes of screening with mammography, with or without clinical breast examination, in reducing mortality from breast cancer in targeted populations. Estimates made in some European countries with organized breast screening programmes suggest that reductions of some 20% can be expected in the long term in the target populations of screening. Estimates of the actual reduction achieved so far have ranged between 5% and 20%. The lower early figures are probably due to the length of time taken to achieve full implementation of national programmes, a substantial proportion of the breast cancer deaths in the first 5–10 years after implementation being due to cancers diagnosed before screening began or lower quality screening in the early years of implementation.

Changes in breast cancer mortality due to screening are difficult to distinguish from other trends in breast cancer mortality in many populations. An alternative would be to measure intermediate indicators of the effectiveness of screening programmes, such as participation rate, rate of detection of small cancers, rate of interval cancers and the incidence rate of later-stage cancers, to show whether the programme is adequate to achieve the desired long-term outcomes. These indicators will also be valuable for improving the quality of service.

## Adverse effects of breast screening

Between 50% and 90% of women who are referred for assessment after a positive screening mammogram will prove not to have breast cancer. These false-positive mammograms generate anxiety, additional physician visits and diagnostic tests, and some excision biopsies. If a false-positive result is not recognized as such during assessment, some such referrals may also lead to unnecessary treatment for breast cancer.

Some 20% of women in whom breast cancer is diagnosed have ductal carcinoma *in situ*, a cancerous change that has not extended beyond the tissue lining the breast ducts. Treatment of some forms of this lesion will prevent development of an invasive cancer in the affected tissue. In a currently unknown, but possibly high, proportion of women in whom ductal carcinoma *in situ* is diagnosed as a result of breast cancer screening, invasive cancer would not develop in the in-situ cancer within the lifetime of the woman. Some of these women, however, will be treated for breast cancer, with little prospect of long-term benefit from the therapy.

In some women in whom an abnormality is detected by breast cancer screening, an invasive cancer may be diagnosed that would never have progressed to produce symptoms and be diagnosed clinically in their lifetime. This possibility is suggested by the persistence of the increased incidence rates of breast cancer that occurs with the introduction of screening to a population and, initially at least, can be attributed to earlier detection of cancers that would otherwise be incident in a later period. No population into which breast screening has been introduced has yet been reported to show an unequivocal return of incidence rates to the baseline expected from pre-screening trends; but there have been no rigorous analyses.

As irradiation of the breasts with X-rays is known to increase a woman's risk for breast cancer, the exposure of women from mammography should be the lowest compatible with adequate image quality. In women 50–69 years of age, the increase in risk for breast cancer due to this exposure is extremely small and is substantially outweighed by the benefits of mammography. This balance is probably not as favourable, however, for women 40–49 years of age. In women under 40 years of age, the risk for radiation-induced breast cancer is higher, and there is no evidence of benefit for this age group.

## Cost–effectiveness of a programme of screening with mammography

A recent summary of analyses of the cost–effectiveness of breast cancer screening programmes in a number of countries, done with similar methods, has shown costs per year of life saved varying from 3000 to 8000 euros for two-yearly screening of women 50–69 years of age. If, in addition, the impact of screening on quality of life is considered and account is taken, on the negative side, of the longer period of life with a diagnosis of breast cancer and of the the consequences of false-positive diagnoses, the costs per quality-adjusted year of life saved may, depending on the assumptions, be up to 23% higher or 3% lower than those stated above.

## Implications for public health

Health policy-makers can make decisions about the screening services they offer women, and women themselves can take decisions about whether to seek or accept an offer of breast cancer screening, in the knowledge that quality screening mammography done every two years in women 50–69 years of age should reduce their risk for death from breast cancer by about 35%.

When such a programme is offered and there is a high participation rate, it would be reasonable for a health service to expect a fall in the mortality rate from breast cancer in the target population for screening of some 20% in the long term. This reduction may be less if there is a high level of opportunistic screening before an organized programme is introduced.

The cost–effectiveness of a programme of screening mammography is comparable to that of other cancer screening programmes. As in all screening programmes, there are adverse consequences. For breast cancer screening, these include costs to the quality and, to a very small extent, the quantity of a woman's life due to false-positive diagnoses, and the diagnosis of some in-situ and possibly invasive breast cancers that would not otherwise have been diagnosed. A few rare cases of breast cancer may be caused by mammographic radiation, but this adverse effect is substantially offset by the net reduction in mortality due to screening.

When mammographic screening cannot be offered, for practical or economic reasons, or women cannot afford to accept it, there is no other method of screening that is known to reduce the risk for death from breast cancer. Specifically, it is unlikely on present evidence that a programme to encourage breast self-examination alone would reduce mortality from breast cancer. Women should, however, be encouraged to seek medical advice immediately if they detect any change in a breast that suggests breast cancer.

# Chapter 9

# Recommendations

## Research recommendations

### Improving conventional mammography

The sensitivity and specificity of conventional mammography could be improved by conducting studies to explore:

- the relative sensitivity, specificity and cost–effectiveness of various approaches to double reading;
- the sensitivity, specificity and cost–effectiveness of computer-assisted reading and tactics to improve interpretation; and
- the effects of training film readers, of their experience and volume of practice and of peer evaluation.

### Implementing mammographic screening programmes

A better understanding of factors affecting the acceptability, cost and implementation of mammographic screening programmes is needed. Studies should be conducted:

- in a variety of cultural settings to understand women's preferences for information and how best to communicate the harms and benefits of participation in mammographic screening;
- into the costs and benefits of initiating screening at various ages, particularly to evaluate the cost–effectiveness of starting screening of women at 45 years and stopping screening at 70 years; and
- to determine why some women with a suspect mammogram do not present for further evaluation for the presence of breast cancer.

### Accuracy of mammographic screening

Research should be conducted on the effect of menopausal status, with or without hormone replacement therapy, on the accuracy of mammography.

### Clinical breast examination

The efficacy and effectiveness of clinical breast examination in reducing mortality from breast cancer are unknown, and the trials in which clinical breast examination was combined with mammography cannot answer the question. A beneficial effect of clinical breast examination was suggested, however, in the Canadian comparison of mammography plus clinical breast examination with clinical breast examination alone, in which there appeared to be no additional benefit from the addition of mammography.

Clinical breast examination may be of particular importance in countries where there are insufficient resources for mammography and where disease is usually at an advanced stage at the time of diagnosis.

Many of these countries cannot afford mammography at all; others need evidence to allow them to decide whether to introduce mamography or clinical breast examination. Multi-country studies would be feasible in some regions of the world. Therefore:

- a randomized trial of clinical breast examination versus no screening should be conducted in a country or countries where resources are unlikely to permit implementation of mammographic screening in the foreseeable future, and
- a randomized trial of clinical breast examination versus mammography should be conducted in a country or countries where resources may permit some mammographic screening but are insufficient to cover the entire population at risk.

## Breast self-examination

The efficacy of the practice of breast self-examination in reducing mortality from breast cancer is unproven. It is unlikely that teaching breast self-examination as the sole method for breast cancer screening would reduce mortality from this disease. It could, however, be a useful adjunct to screening by other means, by allowing detection of interval cancers earlier. Therefore:

- a randomized trial should be conducted of the efficacy of breast self-examination versus no breast self-examination in detecting interval cancers in women who receive periodic mammographic screening.

## Consequences of diagnosis of breast cancer

By leading to earlier diagnosis of breast cancer, screening lengthens the period during which a woman lives with the knowledge that she has or has had cancer, whether ot not her life is actually lengthened as a result of the earlier diagnosis. To better understand the consequences of longer life with breast cancer:

- studies should be conducted to evaluate the psychological and physical consequences of living with a diagnosis of breast cancer and the sequelae of treatment for breast cancer.

## Biology of breast tumours in relation to screening

The natural history of breast cancer and its relevance for screening programmes are not yet fully understood. Studies should therefore be conducted:

- to study the natural history of ductal carcinoma *in situ* of various grades;
- to evaluate the likely impact of detection and treatment of ductal carcinoma *in situ* on the incidence of invasive cancer;
- to improve differentiation of high-grade and low-grade ductal carcinoma *in situ* during reading of mammograms.

There is probably wide heterogeneity in the malignant potential of the many small invasive tumours detected by screening. Molecular and histological markers might be useful in classifying such small cancers according to their malignant potential and thus to allow treatment to be designed in accordance with the expected behaviour of the cancer. Therefore:

- rigorous studies should be done of the predictive value of combinations of histological and recent molecular markers for the behaviour and outcome of small invasive breast cancers; and
- measurement of promising markers should be included in clinical trials of treatment of small invasive breast cancers, to determine whether some categories of cancers defined by these markers could be treated less aggressively without loss of efficacy.

## New techniques

Mammographic screening has imperfect sensitivity and specificity. The sensitivity, specificity and cost–effectiveness of new screening modalities should be compared with those of mammographic screening. Studies with rigorous designs should be conducted to evaluate:

- the effectiveness of new techniques, including magnetic resonance imaging, full-field digital mammography and positron emission tomography;
- the use of ultrasound as a screening modality in conjunction with mammography for women with dense breasts; and
- the usefulness of computer-assisted diagnosis in combination with full-field digital mammography: its impact on sensitivity and specificity, possible use as a 'second reader' and interaction with the 'experience' of film readers.

## Women at high risk

The issues for high-risk women associated with participating in mammographic screening should be better understood. Mammographic screening has potentially adverse effects on women with a genetic predisposition to breast cancer. Studies should be conducted:

- to identify high-risk women, with a variety of methods for estimating risk, including family history, results of genetic tests, nipple aspirates and biological markers; and
- on the use of density and characteristics of calcifications and other initial mammographic images as sensitive markers for estimating future risk and adapting screening.

# Public health recommendations

## Information systems

Before establishing a new screening programme:

- Surveillance systems should be ideally available to provide estimates of incidence, morbidity, survival and mortality from breast cancer in the community and its impact on the health status of the population, and to allow follow-up to ensure that women are treated.
- Information systems should be in place to measure rates of participation, cancer detection, interval cancers and deaths from breast cancer. This can be done in the absence of a full cancer registry.
- Efforts should be made to establish standard approaches to reporting breast cancer by agreed protocols, including: stage of cancer, tumour size, histological grading and differentiation of both invasive and in-situ cancers.

## Implementation of mammographic screening programmes

- Women should be given information about the potential harms and benefits of mammographic screening to enable them to make an informed decision about whether to participate.
- Mammography equipment should be monitored regularly and the radiation emitted minimized, while preserving the sensitivity to detect cancer.
- Screening programmes should be implemented, where possible, in a step-wise fashion, for example by introducing mammography in selected geographical areas or inviting women by birth cohort. This approach will help to circumscibe the scope of the programme in its early stages, ensuring that the available resources are not overwhelmed. In addition, it would provide a temporary control group for determining the effectiveness of the programme.

# Chapter 10

# References

Abdel-Fattah, M., Zaki, A., Bassili, A., El-Shazly, M. & Tognoni, G. (2000) Breast self-examination practice and its impact on breast cancer diagnosis in Alexandria, Egypt. *East. Mediterr. Health J.*, **6**, 34–40

Abdullah, A. & Leung, T. (2001) Factors associated with the use of breast and cervical cancer screening services among Chinese women in Hong Kong. *Public Health*, **115**, 212–217

Abe, R., Sakuma, A., Yoshida, K., Hariu, T., Kanno, H., Takahashi, K., Kumagai, N. & Sato, T. (1983) Mass screening for breast cancer. *Tohoku J. Exp. Med.*, **141**, 125–131

Adair, F.E. (1933) Clinical manifestations of early cancer of the breast. *New Engl. J. Med.*, **208**, 1250–1255

Adami, H.O., Sparen, P., Bergstrom, R., Holmberg, L., Krusemo, U.B. & Ponten, J. (1989) Increasing survival trend after cancer diagnosis in Sweden: 1960–1984. *J. Natl Cancer Inst.*, **81**, 1640–1647

Agurto, I. (2001) *Preventive Practices among Women: Bridging the Gap*, Washington DC, PAHO, Program on Noncommunicable Diseases

van den Akker-van Marle, M.E., Reep-van den Bergh, C.M., Boer, R., del Moral Aldaz, A., Ascunce, N. & de Koning, H.J. (1997) Breast cancer screening in Navarra: Interpretation of a high detection rate at the first screening round and a low rate at the second round. *Int. J. Cancer*, **73**, 464–469

van den Akker-van Marle, M.E., de Koning, H., Boer, R. & van der Maas, M.P. (1999) Reduction in breast cancer mortality due to the introduction of mass screening in The Netherlands: Comparison with the United Kingdom. *J. Med. Screen.*, **6**, 30–34

van den Akker-van Marle, M.E., van Ballegooijen, M., van Oortmarssen, G.J., Boer, R. & Habbema, J.D. (2002) Cost–effectiveness of cervical cancer screening: Comparison of screening policies. *J. Natl Cancer Inst.*, **94**, 193–204

Alexander, F., Roberts, M.M., Lutz, W. & Hepburn, W. (1989) Randomisation by cluster and the problem of social class bias. *J. Epidemiol. Community Health*, **43**, 29–36

Alexander, F.E., Anderson, T.J., Brown, H.K., Forrest, A.P., Hepburn, W., Kirkpatrick, A.E., Muir, B.B., Prescott, R.J. & Smith, A. (1999) 14 years of follow-up from the Edinburgh randomized trial of breast-cancer screening. *Lancet*, **353**, 1903–1908

Ali-Abarghoui, F., Simoes, E.J., Newschaffer, C.J., Tao, X., Mack, N.E. & Brownson, R.C. (1998) Predictors of mammography utilization in Missouri, 1993–1994. *J. Public Health Manag. Pract.*, **4**, 29–42

Alizadeh, A.A., Ross, D.T., Perou, C.M. & van de Rijn, M. (2001) Towards a novel classification of human malignancies based on gene expression patterns. *J. Pathol.*, **195**, 41–52

Alpers, C.E. & Wellings, S.R. (1985) The prevalence of carcinoma in situ in normal and cancer-associated breasts. *Hum. Pathol.*, **16**, 796–807

Alveryd, A., Andersson, I., Aspegren, K., Balldin, G., Bjurstam, N., Edstrom, G., Fagerberg, G., Glas, U., Jarlman, O. & Larsson, S.A. (1990) Lightscanning versus mammography for the detection of breast cancer in screening and clinical practice. A Swedish multicenter study. *Cancer*, **65**, 1671–1677

American College of Radiology (1995) *Breast Imaging and Reporting Data System (BI-RADS)*, 2nd Ed., Reston, Virginia

American Joint Committee on Cancer (2002) *Cancer Staging Manual*, 6th Ed., New York. Springer

Amsel, Z., Prakash, L., Grover P.L. & Balshem A.M. (1984) The impact of physician reinforcement on breast self-examination practice. *J. Fam. Pract.*, **19**, 236–238

Ancelle-Park, R. & Nicolau, J. (1999) [Breast Cancer Screening, Report on Evaluation of Epidemiological Follow-up], Paris, Institut de la Veille Sanitaire (in French)

Ancelle-Park, R., Séradour, B., Schaffer, P., Allemand, H. & Tubiana, M. (1997) [National breast screening programme: Organization and results.] *Bull. Epidémiolo. Hebd.*, **10**, 39–40 (in French)

Anderson, T.J., Lamb, J., Donnan, P., Alexander, F.E., Huggins, A., Muir, B.B., Kirkpatrick, A.E., Chetty, U., Hepburn, W. & Smith, A. (1991) Comparative pathology of breast cancer in a randomised trial of screening. *Br. J. Cancer*, **64**, 108–113

Anderson, E.D., Muir, B.B., Walsh, J.S. & Kirkpatrick, A.E. (1994) The efficacy of double reading mammograms in breast screening. *Clin. Radiol.*, **49**, 248–251

Andersson, I. (1981) Radiographic screening for breast carcinoma. III. Appearance of carcinoma and number of projections to be used at screening. *Acta Radiol. Diagn.*, **22**, 407–420

Andersson, I. & Janzon, L. (1997) Reduced breast cancer mortality in women under age 50: Updated results from the Malmö mammographic screening program. *Natl Cancer Inst. Monogr.*, **22**, 63–67

Andersson, I., Janzon, L. & Pettersson, H. (1981) Radiographic patterns of the mammary parenchyma. Variation with age at examination and age at first birth. *Radiology*, **138**, 59–62

Andersson, I., Aspegren, K., Janzon, L., Landberg, T., Lindholm, K., Linell, F., Ljungberg, O., Ranstam, J. & Sigfusson, B. (1988) Mammographic screening and mortality from breast cancer: The Malmö mammographic screening trial. *Br. Med. J.*, **297**, 943–948

Angèle, S. & Hall, J. (2000) The *ATM* gene and breast cancer: Is it really a risk factor? *Mutat. Res.*, **462**, 167–178

Anh, P.T., Parkin, D.M., Hanh, N.T. & Duc, N.B. (1993) Cancer in the population of Hanoi, Vietnam, 1988–1990. *Br. J. Cancer*, **68**, 1236–1242

Anim, J.T. (1993) Breast cancer in sub-Saharan African women. *Afr. J. Med. Sci.*, **22**, 5–10

Anttinen, I., Pamilo, M., Soiva, M. & Roiha, M. (1993) Double reading of mammography screening films—One radiologist or two? *Clin. Radiol.*, **48**, 414–421

Argentina Ministry of Health (2001) Secretaria de Atención Sanitaria, Subsecretaría de Programas de Prevención y Promoción. Programa Nacional de Control de Cáncer; Subprograma de Prevención secundaria de Cáncer de Mama, Buenos Aires

Armes, J.E., Egan, A.J., Southey, M.C., Dite, G.S., McCredie, M.R., Giles, G.G., Hopper, J.L. & Venter, D.J. (1998) The histologic phenotypes of breast carcinoma occurring before age 40 years in women with and without BRCA1 or BRCA2 germline mutations: A population-based study. *Cancer*, **83**, 2335–2345

Aro, A.R., de Koning, H.J., Absetz, P. & Schreck, M. (1999) Psychosocial predictors of first attendance for organised mammography screening. *J. Med. Screen.*, **6**, 82–88

Aro, A.R., de Koning, H.J., Absetz, P. & Schreck, M. (2001) Two distinct groups of non-attenders in an organized mammography screening program. *Breast Cancer Res. Treat.*, **70**, 145–153

Arredondo, A., Lockett, L. & de Icaza, E. (1995) Cost of diseases in Brazil: Breast cancer, enteritis, cardiac valve disease and bronchopneumonia. *Rev. Saude Publ.*, **29**, 349–354

Assaf, A., Cummings, K.M. & Walsh, D. (1983) The relationship between breast self-examination frequency, technique, and breast lump detection. *Prog. Clin. Biol. Res.*, **130**, 323–329

Atkinson, C., Warren, R., Bingham, S.A. & Day, N.E. (1999) Mammographic patterns as a predictive biomarker of breast cancer risk: Effect of tamoxifen. *Cancer Epidemiol. Biomarkers Prev.*, **8**, 863–866

Atri, J., Falshaw, M., Gregg, R., Robson, J., Omar, R. & Dixon, S. (1997) Improving uptake of breast screening in multiethnic populations: A randomised controlled trial using practice reception staff to contact non-attenders. *Br. Med. J.*, **315**, 1356–1359

Austoker, J. (1999) Gaining informed consent for screening is difficult but many misconceptions need to be undone. *Br. Med. J.*, **18**, 722–723

Austoker, J. & Ong, G. (1994) Written information needs of women who are recalled for further investigation of breast screening: Results of a multicentre study. *J. Med. Screen.*, **1**, 238–244

Australia–New Zealand Breast Cancer Trials Group (1996) Recommendations from the Pathology and Multidisciplinary DCIS Workshops. In: *Diagnosis of DCIS*, Hunter Valley

Australian Institute of Health and Welfare (1998) *Breast and Cervical Cancer Screening in Australia 1996–1997*, Canberra, pp. 1–94

Australian Institute of Health and Welfare (2000) *BreastScreen Australia Achievement Report 1997 and 1998*, Canberra, pp. 1–86

Autier, P., Shannoun, F., Scharpantgen, A., Lux, C., Back, C., Severi, G., Steil, S. & Hansen-Koenig, D. (2002) A breast cancer screening programme operating in a liberal health care system: The Luxembourg mammography programme, 1992–1997. *Int. J. Cancer*, **97**, 828–832

Auvinen, A., Elovainio, L. & Hakama, M. (1996) Breast self-examination and survival from breast cancer: A prospective follow-up study. *Breast Cancer Res. Treat.*, **38**, 161–168.

Axelsson, C.K., Mouridsen, H.T. & Zedeler, K. (1992) Axillary dissection of level I and II lymph nodes is important in breast cancer classification. The Danish Breast Cancer Cooperative Group (DBCG). *Eur. J. Cancer,* **28A**, 1415–1418

Azzopardi, J.G., Ahmed, A. & Millis, R.R. (1979) Problems in breast pathology. *Major Probl. Pathol.*, **11**, 1–466

Badve, S., A'Hern, R.P., Ward, A.M., Millis, R.R., Pinder, S.E., Ellis, I.O., Gusterson, B.A. & Sloane, J.P. (1998) Prediction of local recurrence of ductal carcinoma in situ of the breast using five histological classifications: A comparative study with long follow-up. *Hum. Pathol.*, **29**, 915–923

Bailar, J.C., III & MacMahon, B. (1997) Randomization in the Canadian National Breast Screening Study: A review for evidence of subversion. *Can. Med. Assoc. J.*, **156**, 193–199

Baines, C.J. (1987) Breast palpation technique: What is the finger pad? *J. Chron. Dis.*, **40**, 361–362

Baines, C.J. (1988) Breast-self-examination: The known and the unknown. In: Day, N.E. & Miller, A.B., eds, *Screening for Breast Cancer,* Toronto, Huber, pp. 85–91

Baines, C.J. (1989) Breast self-examination. *Cancer*, **64**, 2661–2663

Baines, C.J. (1992a) Physical examination of the breasts in screening for breast cancer. *J. Gerontol.*, **47** (Special No.), 63–67

Baines, C.J. (1992b) Breast self-examination. *Cancer*, **69**, 1942–1946

Baines, C.J. (1994) The Canadian National Breast Screening Study: A perspective on criticisms. *Ann. Intern. Med.*, **120**, 326–334

Baines, C.J. & Miller, A.B. (1997) Mammography versus clinical examination of the breasts. *Natl Cancer Inst. Monogr.*, **22**, 125–129

Baines, C.J. & To, T. (1990) Changes in breast self-examination behavior achieved by 89,835 participants in the Canadian National Breast Screening Study. *Cancer*, **66**, 570–576

Baines, C.J., McFarlane, D.V. & Wall, C. (1986a) Audit procedures in the National Breast Screening Study: Mammography interpretation. *Can. Assoc. Radiol. J.*, **37**, 256–260

Baines, C.J., Miller, A.B., Wall, C., McFarlane, D.V., Simor, I.S., Jong, R., Shapiro, B.J., Audet, L., Petitclerc, M. & Ouimet-Oliva, D. (1986b) Sensitivity and specificity of first screen mammography in the Canadian National Breast Screening Study: A preliminary report from five centers. *Radiology*, **160**, 295–298

Baines, C.J., Wall, C., Risch, H.A., Kuin, J.K. & Fan, I.J. (1986c) Changes in breast self-examination behavior in a cohort of 8214 women in the Canadian National Breast Screening Study. *Cancer*, **57**, 1209–1216

Baines, C.J., McFarlane, D.V. & Miller, A.B. (1988a) Sensitivity and specificity of first screen mammography in 15 NBSS centres. *Can. Assoc. Radiol. J.*, **39**, 273–276

Baines, C.J., Krasowski, T.P. & Wall, C. (1988b) Incentives for breast self-examination: Role of the calendar. *Cancer Detect. Prev.*, **13**, 109–114

Baines, C.J., Miller, A.B. & Bassett, A.A. (1989) Physical examination. Its role as a single screening modality in the Canadian National Breast Screening Study. *Cancer*, **63**, 1816–1822

Baines, C.J., To, T. & Wall, C. (1990) Women's attitudes to screening after participation in the National Breast Screening Study. A questionnaire survey. *Cancer*, **65**, 1663–1669

Baines, C.J., Vidmar, M., McKeown-Eyssen, G. & Tibshirani, R. (1997) Impact of menstrual phase on false-negative mammograms in the Canadian National Breast Screening study. *Cancer*, **80**, 720–724.

Baker, L.H. (1982) Breast Cancer Detection Demonstration Project: Five-year summary report. *CA Cancer J. Clin.*, **32**, 194–225

Ballard-Barbash, R., Taplin, S.H., Yankaskas, B.C., Ernster, V.L., Rosenberg, R.D., Carney, P.A., Barlow, W.E., Geller, B.M., Kerlikowske, K., Edwards, B.K., Lynch, C.F., Urban, N., Chrvala, C.A., Key, C.R., Poplack, S.P., Worden, J.K. & Kessler, L.G. (1997) Breast Cancer Surveillance Consortium: A national mammography screening and outcomes database. *Am. J. Roentgenol.*, **169**, 1001–1008

Ballard-Barbash, R., Klabunde, C., Paci, E., Broeders, M., Coleman, E.A., Fracheboud, J., Bouchard, F., Rennert, G. & Shapiro, S. (1999) Breast cancer screening in 21 countries: Delivery of services, notification of results and outcomes ascertainment. *Eur. J. Cancer Prev.*, **8**, 417–426

Banks, E., Beral, V., Cameron, R., Hogg, A., Langley, N., Barnes, I., Bull, D., Reeves, G., English, R., Taylor, S., Elliman, J. & Lole, H.C. (2002a) Comparison of various characteristics of women who do and do not attend for breast cancer screening. *Breast Cancer Res.*, **4**, R1

Banks, E., Reeves, G., Beral, V., Bull, D., Crossley, B., Simmonds, M., Hilton, E., Bailey, S., Barrett, N., Briers, P., English, R., Jackson, A., Kutt, E., Lavelle, J., Rockall, L., Wallis, M.G. & Wilson, M. (2002b) Predictors of outcome of mammography in the National Health Service breast screening programme. *J. Med. Screen.*, (in press)

Barchielli, A. & Paci, E. (2001) Trends in breast cancer mortality, incidence, and survival, and mammographic screening in Tuscany, Italy. *Cancer Causes Control*, **12**, 249–255

Barnes, G.T. (1999) Mammography imaging physics: X-ray equipment considerations. In: Haus, A.G. & Yaffe, M.J., eds, *Categorial Course in Diagnostic Radiology Physics: Physical Aspects of Breast Imaging—Current and Future Considerations*. Oak Brook, Ilinois, Radiological Society of North America, pp. 41–57

Barnes, G.T. & Brezovich, I.A. (1978) The intensity of scattered radiation in mammography. *Radiology*, **126**, 243–247

Barnes, G.T., Wu, X., Chakraborty, D.P. & Wagner, A.J. (1989a) Scanning slit mammography: A practical design. *Radiology*, **173**, 164

Barnes, G.T., Wu, X., Wagner, A.J. & Rubin, E. (1989b) Scatter control in mammography: Past, present and future. *Radiology*, **173**, 472

Barnes, D.M., Bartkova, J., Camplejohn, R.S., Gullick, W.J., Smith, P.J. & Millis, R.R. (1992) Overexpression of the c-erbB-2 oncoprotein: Why does this occur more frequently in ductal carcinoma in situ than in invasive mammary carcinoma and is this of prognostic significance? *Eur. J. Cancer*, **28**, 644–648

Barr, L.C. & Baum, M. (1992) Time to abandon TNM staging of breast cancer? *Lancet*, **339**, 915–917

Barr, J., Franks, A., Lee, N., Antonucci, D., Rifkind, S. & Schachter, M. (2001) A randomized intervention to improve ongoing participation in mammography. *Am. J. Managed Care*, **7**, 887–894

Barratt, A.L., Cockburn, J., Redman, S., Paul, C. & Perkins, J. (1997a) Mammographic screening: Results from the 1996 National Breast Health Survey. *Med. J. Aust.*, **167**, 521–524

Barratt, A., Cockburn, J., Lowe, J., Paul, C., Perkins, J. & Redman, S. (1997b) *Report on the 1996 Breast Health Survey*, Woolloomooloo (NSW), National Breast Cancer Centre

Barratt, A., Cockburn, J., Furnival, C., McBride, A. & Mallon, L. (1999) Perceived sensitivity of mammographic screening: Women's views on test accuracy and financial compensation for missed cancers. *J. Epidemiol. Community Health*, **53**, 716–720

Barton, M.B., Harris, R.H. & Fletcher, S.W. (1999) Does this patient have breast cancer? The screening clinical breast examination: Should it be done? How? *J. Am. Med. Assoc.*, **282**, 1270–1280

Barton, M.B., Moore, S., Polk, S., Shtatland, E., Elmore, J.G. & Fletcher, S.W. (2001) Increased patient concern after false-positive mammograms: Clinician documentation and subsequent ambulatory visits. *J. Gen. Intern. Med.*, **16**, 150–156

Bartow, S.A., Pathak, D.R., Black, W.C., Key, C.R. & Teaf, S.R. (1987) Prevalence of benign, atypical, and malignant breast lesions in populations at different risk for breast cancer. *Cancer*, **60**, 2751–2760

Bassett, A.A. (1985) Physical examination of the breast and breast self-examination. In: Miller, A.B., ed., *Screening for Cancer*, Orlando, FL, Academic Press, pp. 271–291

Bassett, L.W. (1995) Clinical image evaluation. *Radiol. Clin. N. Am.*, **33**, 1027–1039

Bassett, L.W., Hendrick, R.E. & Bassford, T.L. (1994a) *Quality Determinants of Mammography* (95-0632), Rockville, MD, Agency for Health Care Policy and Research, Public Health Service, US Department of Health and Human Services

Bassett, L.W., Shayestehfar, B. & Hirbawi, I. (1994b) Obtaining previous mammogramas for comparison: Usefulness and costs. *Am. J. Roentgenol.*, 163, 1083–1086

Beahrs, O.H., Shapiro, S. & Smart, C. (1979) Report of the working group to review the National Cancer Institute American Cancer Society Breast Cancer Detection Demonstration Projects. *J. Natl Cancer Inst.*, **62**, 642–709

Beam, C.A., Layde, P.M. & Sullivan, D.C. (1996a) Variability in the interpretation of screening mammograms by US radiologists. Findings from a national sample. *Arch. Intern. Med.*, **156**, 209–213

Beam, C.A., Sullivan, D.C. & Layde, P.M. (1996b) Effect of human variability on independent double reading in screening mammography. *Acad. Radiol.*, **3**, 891–897

Bedwani, R., Vana, J., Rosner, D., Schmitz, R.L. & Murphy, G.P. (1981) Management and survival of female patients with 'minimal' breast cancer: As observed in the long-term and short-term surveys of the American College of Surgeons. *Cancer*, **47**, 2769–2778

Beemsterboer, P.M., de Koning, H.J., Warmerdam, P.G., Boer, R., Swart, E., Dierks, M.L. & Robra, B.P. (1994) Prediction of the effects and costs of breast-cancer screening in Germany. *Int. J. Cancer*, **58**, 623–628

Beemsterboer, P.M., Warmerdam, P.G., Boer, R. & de Koning, H.J. (1998a) Radiation risk of mammography related to benefit in screening programmes: A favourable balance? *J. Med. Screen.*, **5**, 81–87

Beemsterboer, P.M., Warmerdam, P.G., Boer, R. & de Koning, H.J. (1998b) Screening for breast cancer in Catalonia. Which policy is to be preferred? *Eur. J. Public Health*, **8**, 241–246

Beemsterboer, P.M., de Koning, H.J., Looman, C.W., Borsboom, G.J., Bartelds, A.I. & van der Maas, P.J. (1999) Mammography requests in general practice during the introduction of nation-wide breast cancer screening, 1988–1995. *Eur. J. Cancer*, **35**, 450–454

Bell, T.S., Branston, L.K., Newcombe, R.G. & Barton, G.R. (1999) Interventions to improve uptake of breast screening in inner city Cardiff general practices with ethnic minority lists. *Ethn. Health*, **4**, 277–284

Bennett, S.E., Lawrence, R.S., Fleischmann, K.H., Gifford, C.S. & Slack, W.V. (1983) Profile of women practicing breast self-examination. *J. Am. Med. Assoc.*, **249**, 488–491

Bennett, S.E., Lawrence, R.S., Angiolillo, D.F., Bennett, S.D., Budman, S., Schneider, G.M., Assaf, A.R. & Feldstein, M. (1990) Effectiveness of methods used to teach breast self-examination. *Am. J. Prev. Med.*, **6**, 208–217

Berkowitz, J.E., Gatewood, O.M., Goldblum, L.E. & Gayler, B.W. (1990) Hormonal replacement therapy: Mammographic manifestations. *Radiology*, **174**, 199–201

Bernay, T., Porrath, S., Golding-Mather, J.M. & Murray, J. (1982) The impact of breast cancer screening on feminine identity: Implications for patient education. *Breast*, **8**, 2–5

Bernstein, A.B., Thompson, G.B. & Harlan, L.C. (1991) Differences in rates of cancer screening by usual source of medical care. Data from the 1987 National Health Interview Survey. *Med. Care*, **29**, 196–209

Berrino, F., Sant, M., Verdecchia, A., Capocaccia, R., Hakulinen, T. & Estève, J., eds (1995) *Survival of Cancer Patients in Europe: The EUROCARE Study* (IARC Scientific Publications No. 132), Lyon, IARCPress

Berry, D.A. (1998) Benefits and risks of screening mammography for women in their forties: A statistical appraisal. *J. Natl Cancer Inst.*, **90**, 1431–1439

Berx, G., Cleton-Jansen, A.M., Nollet, F., de Leeuw, W.J., van de Vijver, M., Cornelisse, C. & van Roy, F. (1995) E-cad-herin is a tumour/invasion suppressor gene mutated in human lobular breast cancers. *EMBO J.*, **14**, 6107–6115

Bettelheim, R., Penman, H.G., Thornton-Jones, H. & Neville, A.M. (1984) Prognostic significance of perituminal vascular invasion in breast cancer. *Br. J. Cancer*, **50**, 771–777

Bhathal, P.S., Brown, R.W., Lesueur, G.C. & Russell, I.S. (1985) Frequency of benign and malignant breast lesions in 207 consecutive autopsies in Australian women. *Br. J. Cancer*, **51**, 271–278

Bhatia, S., Robison, L.L., Oberlin, O., Greenberg, M., Bunin, G., Fossati-Bellani, F. & Meadows, A.T. (1996) Breast cancer and other second neoplasms after child-hood Hodgkin's disease. *N. Engl. J. Med.*, **334**, 745–751

Bijker, N., Peterse, J.L., Duchateau, L., Julien, J.P., Fentiman, I.S., Duval, C., Di Palma, S., Simony-Lafontaine, J., de Mascarel, I. & van de Vijver, M.J. (2001a) Risk factors for recurrence and metastasis after breast-conserving therapy for ductal carcinoma-in-situ: Analysis of European Organization for Research and Treatment of Cancer Trial 10853. *J. Clin. Oncol.*, **19**, 2263–2271

Bijker, N., Peterse, J.L., Duchateau, L., Robanus-Maandag, E.C., Bosch, C.A., Duval, C., Pilotti, S. & van de Vijver, M.J. (2001b) Histological type and marker expression of the primary tumour compared with its local recurrence after breast-conserving therapy for ductal carcinoma in situ. *Br. J. Cancer*, **84**, 539–544

Bird, J.A., McPhee, S.J., Ha, N.T., Le, B., Davis, T. & Jenkins, C.N. (1998) Opening pathways to cancer screening for Vietnamese–American women: Lay health workers hold a key. *Prev. Med.*, **27**, 821–829

Birdwell, R.L., Ikeda, D.M., O'Shaugh-nessy, K.F. & Sickles, E.A. (2001) Mammographic characteristics of 115 missed cancers later detected with screening mammography and the potential utility of computer-aided detection. *Radiology*, **219**, 192–202

Bjurstam, N., Björneld, L., Duffy, S.W., Smith, T.C., Cahlin, E., Eriksson, O., Hafström, L.-O., Lingaas, H., Mattsson, J., Persson, S., Rudenstam, C.-M. & Säve-Söderbergh, J. (1997) The Gothenburg breast screening trial. First results on mortality, incidence, and mode of detection for women ages 39–49 years at randomization. *Cancer*, **80**, 2091–2099

Black, M.M., Barclay, T.H. & Hankey, B.F. (1975) Prognosis in breast cancer utilizing histologic characteristics of the primary tumor. *Cancer*, **36**, 2048–2055

Black, W.C., Nease, R.F., Jr & Tosteson, A.N. (1995) Perceptions of breast cancer risk and screening effectiveness in women younger than 50 years of age. *J. Natl Cancer Inst.*, **87**, 720–731

Black, W.C., Haggstrom, D.A. & Welch, H.G. (2002) All-cause mortality in random-ized trials of cancer screening. *J. Natl Cancer Inst.* **94**, 167–173

Blackman, D.K., Bennett, E.M. & Miller, D.S. (1999) Trends in self-reported use of mammograms (1989–1997) and Papani-colaou tests (1991–1997)—Behavioral risk factor surveillance system. *Morbid. Mortal. Weekly Rep.*, **48**, 1–22.

Blamey, R.W., Elston, C.W., Pinder, S.E. & Ellis, I.O. (2000) When is a patient cured of breast cancer? *J. Pathol.*, **190** (Suppl.), A44

Blanks, R.G. & Moss, S.M. (1996) Monitoring the performance of the breast screening programmes: Allowing for geographical variation in breast cancer incidence. *J. Med. Screen.*, **3**, 82–84

Blanks, R.G. & Moss, S.M. (1999) Breast cancer screening sensitivity in the NHSB-SP: Recent results and implications. *Breast*, **8**, 301–302

Blanks, R.G., Day, N.E. & Moss, S.M. (1996) Monitoring the performance of breast screening programmes: Use of indirect standardisation in evaluating the invasive cancer detection rate. *J. Med. Screen.*, **3**, 79–81

Blanks, R.G., Moss, S.M. & Wallis, M.G. (1997) Use of two view mammography compared with one view in the detection of small invasive cancers; Further results from the National Health Service breast screening programme. *J. Med. Screen.*, **4**, 98–101

Blanks, R.G., Wallis, M.G. & Moss, S.M. (1998) A comparison of cancer detection rates achieved by breast cancer screening programmes by number of readers, for one and two view mammography: Results from the UK National Health Service breast screening programme. *J. Med. Screen.*, **5**, 195–201

Blanks, R.G., Moss, S.M. & Patnick, J. (2000a) Results from the UK NHS breast screening programme 1994–1999. *J. Med. Screen.*, **7**, 195–198

Blanks, R.G., Moss, S.M., McGahan, C.E., Quinn, M.J. & Babb, P.J. (2000b) Effect of NHS breast screening programme on mortality from breast cancer in England and Wales, 1990–8: Comparison of observed with predicted mortality. *Br. Med. J.*, **321**, 665–669

Blanks, R.G., Moss, S.M. & Wallis, M.G. (2001) Monitoring and evaluating the UK National Health Service Breast Screening Programme: Evaluating the variation in radiological performance between individual programmes using PPV-referral diagrams. *J. Med. Screen.*, **8**, 24–28

Blanks, R.G., Bennett, R.L., Wallis, M.G. & Moss, S.M. (2002) Does individual programme size affect screening performance? Results from the United Kingdom NHS breast cancer screening programme. *J. Med. Screen.* 9, 11–14

Blichert-Toft, M., Rose, C., Andersen, J.A., Overgaard, M., Axelsson, C.K., Andersen, K.W. & Mouridsen, H.T. (1992) Danish randomized trial comparing breast conservation therapy with mastectomy: Six years of life-table analysis. Danish Breast Cancer Cooperative Group. *J. Natl Cancer Inst. Monogr*, 19–25

Bloom, H.J. (1950a) Prognosis in carcinoma of the breast. *Br. J. Cancer*, **4**, 259–288

Bloom, H.J. (1950b) Further studies on prognosis of breast carcinoma. *Br. J. Cancer*, **4**, 347–367

Bloom, H.J. & Richardson, W.W. (1957) Histological grading and prognosis in breast cancer. A study of 1409 cases of which 359 have been followed for 15 years. *Br. J. Cancer*, **11**, 359–377

Bloom, H.J., Richardson, W.W. & Field, J.R. (1970) Host resistance and survival in carcinoma of breast: A study of 104 cases of medullary carcinoma in a series of 1,411 cases of breast cancer followed for 20 years. *Br. Med. J.*, **3**, 181–188

Bluman, L.G., Borstelmann, N.A., Rimer, B.K., Iglehart, J.D. & Winer, E.P. (2001) Knowledge, satisfaction, and perceived cancer risk among women diagnosed with ductal carcinoma in situ. *J. Womens Health Gend. Based. Med.*, **10**, 589–598

Blustein, J. (1995) Medicare coverage, supplemental insurance, and the use of mammography by older women. *N. Engl. J. Med.*, **332**, 1138–1143

Bobo, J.K., Lee, N.C. & Thames, S.F. (2000) Findings from 752,081 clinical breast examinations reported to a national screening program from 1995 through 1998. *J. Natl Cancer Inst.*, **92**, 971–976

Bodiya, A., Vorias, D. & Dickson, H.A. (1999) Does telephone contact with a physician's office staff improve mammogram screening rates? *Fam. Med.*, **31**, 324–326

Boer, R., Warmerdam, P., de Koning, H. & van Oortmarssen, G. (1994) Extra incidence caused by mammographic screening. *Lancet*, **343**, 979

Boer, R., de Koning, H.J., van Oortmarssen, G.J. & van der Maas, P.J. (1995) In search of the best upper age limit for breast cancer screening. *Eur. J. Cancer*, **31A**, 2040–2043

Boer, R., de Koning, H., Threlfall, A., Warmerdam, P., Street, A., Friedman, E. & Woodman, C. (1998) Cost effectiveness of shortening screening interval or extending age range of NHS breast screening programme: Computer simulation study. *Br. Med. J.*, **317**, 376–379

Boer, R., de Koning, H.J. & van der Maas, P.J. (1999a) A longer breast carcinoma screening interval for women age older than 65 years? *Cancer*, **86**, 1506–1510

Boer, R., de Koning, H., van Oortmarssen, G., Warmerdam, P. & van der Maas, P. (1999b) Stage distribution at first and repeat examinations in breast cancer screening. *J. Med. Screen.*, **6**, 132–138

Boice, J.D., Jr (2001) Radiation and breast carcinogenesis. *Med. Pediatr. Oncol.*, **36**, 508–513

Bolen, J.C., Rhodes, L., Powell-Griner, E.E., Bland, S.D. & Holtzman, D. (2000) State-specific prevalence of selected

health behaviors, by race and ethnicity— Behavioral Risk Factor Surveillance System, 1997. *Morbid. Mortal. Wkly Rep. CDC Surveill. Summ.*, **49**, 1–60

Bonadonna, G., Rossi, A., Valagussa, P., Banfi, A. & Veronesi, U. (1977) The CMF program for operable breast cancer with positive axillary nodes. Updated analysis on the disease-free interval, site of relapse and drug tolerance. *Cancer*, **39**, 2904–2915

Bonadonna, G., Valagussa, P., Moliterni, A., Zambetti, M. & Brambilla, C. (1995) Adjuvant cyclophosphamide, methotrexate, and fluorouracil in node-positive breast cancer: The results of 20 years of follow-up. *New Engl. J. Med.*, **332**, 901–906

Bonfill, X., Marzo, M., Pladevall, M., Marti, J. & Emparanza, J.I. (2001) Strategies for increasing women participation in community breast cancer screening. *Cochrane Database Syst. Rev.*, **1** (CD002943)

Bonneterre, J., Buzdar, A., Nabholtz, J.M., Robertson, J.F., Thurlimann, B., von Euler, M., Sahmoud, T., Webster, A. & Steinberg, M. (2001) Anastrozole is superior to tamoxifen as first-line therapy in hormone receptor positive advanced breast carcinoma. *Cancer*, **92**, 2247–2258

Borràs, J.M., Guillen, M., Sánchez, V., Juncà, S. & Vicente, R. (1999) Educational level, voluntary private health insurance and opportunistic cancer screening among women in Catalonia (Spain). *Eur. J. Cancer Prev.*, **8**, 427–434

Boyd, N.F., Lockwood, G.A., Byng, J.W., Tritchler, D.L. & Yaffe, M.J. (1998) Mammographic densities and breast cancer risk. *Cancer Epidemiol. Biomarkers Prev.*, **7**, 1133–1144

Boyd, N.F., Lockwood, G.A., Martin, L.J., Byng, J.W., Yaffe, M.J. & Tritchler, D.L. (2001) Mammographic density as a marker of susceptibility to breast cancer: A hypothesis. In: Miller, A.B., Bartsch, H., Boffetta, P., Dragsted, L. & Vainio, H. eds, *Biomarkers in Cancer Chemoprevention* (IARC Scientific Publications No. 154), Lyon: IARCPress, pp. 163–169

Braddick, M.R. (1991) Audit of a breast cancer screening programme using clinical examination and lightscanning. *Health Bull.*, **49**, 299–303

Bragg Leight, S., Deiriggi, P., Hursh, D., Miller, D. & Leight, V. (2000) The effect of structured training on breast self-examination search behaviors as measured using biomedical instrumentation. *Nurs. Res.*, **49**, 283–289

Brain, K., Norman, P., Gray, J. & Mansel, R. (1999) Anxiety and adherence to breast self-examination in women with a family history of breast cancer. *Psychosom. Med.*, **61**, 181–187

te Brake, G.M., Karssemeijer, N. & Hendriks, J.H. (1998) Automated detection of breast carcinomas not detected in a screening program. *Radiology*, **207**, 465–471

Breast Cancer Linkage Consortium (1997) Pathology of familial breast cancer: Differences between breast cancers in carriers of BRCA1 or BRCA2 mutations and sporadic cases. *Lancet*, **349**, 1505–1510

BreastScreen Aotearoa (1998) *Background to Breast Screening*. Aotearoa, New Zealand Ministry of Health, pp. 1–10

BreastScreen Aotearoa Independent Monitoring Group (2001) *Monitoring Report No. 7*, Otago, University of Otago

Breast Screening Frequency Trial Group (2002) The frequency of breast cancer screening. Results from the UKCCCR Randomised Trial. *Eur. J. Cancer*, **38**, 1458–1464

Breast Screening Programme (1999) England 1997–98. Available at: www.doh.gov.uk/pub/docs/doh/bcscreen.pdf

BreastScreen NSW (2000) *Ten Year Statistical Report 1988–1998*, Sydney

BreastScreen Queensland (2000) *Annual Statistical Report 1998*, Queensland Health, Women's Cancer Screening Services, pp. 1–45

BreastScreen SA (1999) *BreastScreen SA at 10 Years (Incorporating the 1997 Statistical Report)*, South Australia, pp. 1–56

BreastScreen Victoria (2001) *Annual Statistical Report 1999*, Carlton South, Victoria, pp. 1–56

BreastScreen WA (2001) *Statistical Report 1997–1998*, West Australia, pp. 1–39

Breen, N., Wagener, D.K., Brown, M.L., Davis, W.W. & Ballard-Barbash, R. (2001) Progress in cancer screening over a decade: Results of cancer screening from the 1987, 1991, and 1998 National Health Interview Surveys. *J. Natl Cancer Inst.*, **93**, 1704–1713

Brekelmans, C.T., Seynaeve, C., Bartels, C.C., Tilanus-Linthorst, M.M., Meijers-Heijboer, E.J., Crepin, C.M., van Geel, A.A., Menke, M., Verhoog, L.C., van den, O.A., Obdeijn, I.M. & Klijn, J.G. (2001) Effectiveness of breast cancer surveillance in BRCA1/2 gene mutation carriers and women with high familial risk. *J. Clin. Oncol.*, **19**, 924–930

Brenner, R.J. & Pfaff, J.M. (1996) Mammographic changes after excisional breast biopsy for benign disease. *Am. J. Roentgenol.*, **167**, 1047–1052

Brett, J., Austoker, J. & Ong, G. (1998) Do women who undergo further investigation for breast screening suffer adverse psychological consequences? A multi-centre follow-up study comparing different breast screening result groups five months after their last breast screening appointment. *J. Public Health Med.*, **20**, 396–403

Brocca, P.P. (1866) *Traité des Tumeurs*, Paris, Asselin

Broeders, M.J.M., Peer, P.G.M., Straatman, H., Beex, L.V.A.M., Hendriks, J.H.C.L., Holland, R. & Verbeek, A.L.M. (2001) Diverging breast cancer mortality rates in relation to screening? A comparison of Nijmegen to Arnhem and the Netherlands, 1969–1997. *Int. J. Cancer*, **92**, 303–308

Brown, M.L. (1992) Sensitivity analysis in the cost-effectiveness of breast cancer screening. *Cancer*, **69**, 1963–1967

Brown, M.L. & Fintor, L. (1993) Cost–effectiveness of breast cancer screening: Preliminary results of a systematic review of the literature. *Breast Cancer Res. Treat.*, **25**, 113–118

Brown, M.L., Houn, F., Sickles, E.A. & Kessler, L.G. (1995) Screening mammography in community practice: Positive predictive value of abnormal findings and yield of follow-up diagnostic procedures. *Am. J. Roentgenol.*, **165**, 1373–1377

Brown, J., Bryan, S. & Warren, R. (1996) Mammography screening: An incremental cost effectiveness analysis of double versus single reading of mammograms. *Br. Med. J.*, **312**, 809–812

de Bruin, A., de Koning, H. & van Ballegooijen, M. (1993) Pap smears and mammography. HIS 1991. *Mnbar Gezondh.*, **5**, 4–21

Buchberger, W., Niehoff, A., Obrist, P., DeKoekkoek-Doll, P. & Dunser, M. (2000) Clinically and mammographically occult breast lesions: Detection and classification with high-resolution sonography. *Semin. Ultrasound CT MR*, **21**, 325–336

Buerger, H., Otterbach, F., Simon, R., Poremba, C., Diallo, R., Decker, T., Riethdorf, L., Brinkschmidt, C., Dockhorn-Dworniczak, B. & Boecker, W. (1999) Comparative genomic hybridization of ductal carcinoma in situ of the breast—Evidence of multiple genetic pathways. *J. Pathol.*, **187**, 396–402

Buerger, H., Mommers, E.C., Littmann, R., Simon, R., Diallo, R., Poremba, C., Dockhorn-Dworniczak, B., van Diest, P.J. & Boecker, W. (2001) Ductal invasive G2 and G3 carcinomas of the breast are the end stages of at least two different lines of genetic evolution. *J. Pathol.*, **194**, 165–170

Bull, A.R. & Campbell, M.J. (1991) Assessment of the psychological impact of a breast screening programme. *Br. J Radiol.*, **64**, 510–515

Bundred, N.J. (2001) Prognostic and predictive factors in breast cancer. *Cancer Treat. Rev.*, **27**, 137–142

Bundred, N.J., Morgam, D.A. & Dixon, J.M. (2000) *ABC of Breast Diseases*, London, BMJ Books, pp. 44–49

Burack, R.C., Gimotty, P.A., George, J., Stengle, W., Warbasse, L. & Moncrease, A. (1994) Promoting screening mammography in inner-city settings: A randomized controlled trial of computerized reminders as a component of a program to facilitate mammography. *Med. Care*, **32**, 609–624

Burman, M.L., Taplin, S.H., Herta, D.F. & Elmore, J.G. (1999) Effect of false-positive mammograms on interval breast cancer screening in a health maintenance organization. *Ann. Intern. Med.*, **131**, 1–6

Burns, R.B., Freund, K.M., Ash, A.S., Shwartz, M., Antab, L. & Hall, R. (1996) As mammography use increases, are some providers omitting clinical breast examination? *Arch. Intern. Med.*, **156**, 741–744

Burrell, H.C., Pinder, S.E., Wilson, A.R., Evans, A.J., Yeoman, L.J., Elston, C.W. & Ellis, I.O. (1996) The positive predictive value of mammographic signs: A review of 425 non-palpable breast lesions. *Clin. Radiol.*, **51**, 277–281

Butow, P.N., Kazemi, J.N., Beeney, L.J., Griffin, A.M., Dunn, S.M. & Tattersall, M.H. (1996) When the diagnosis is cancer: Patient communication experiences and preferences. *Cancer*, **77**, 2630–2637

Cadman, B.A., Ostrowski, J.L. & Quinn, C.M. (1997) Invasive ductal carcinoma accompanied by ductal carcinoma in situ (DCIS): Comparison of DCIS grade with grade of invasive component. *Breast*, **6**, 132–137

Calle, E., Flanders, W., Thun, M. & Martin, L. (1993) Demography predictors of mammography and Pap smear screening in US women. *Am. J. Public Health*, **83**, 53–60

Campbell, H.S., Fletcher, S.W., Pilgrim, C.A., Morgan, T.M. & Lin, S. (1991) Improving physicians' and nurses' clinical breast examination: A randomized controlled trial. *Am. J. Prev. Med.*, **7**, 1–8

Campbell, H.S., McBean, M., Mandin, H. & Bryant, H. (1994) Teaching medical students how to perform a clinical breast examination. *Acad. Med.*, **69**, 993–995

Carstens, P.H., Greenberg, R.A., Francis, D. & Lyon, H. (1985) Tubular carcinoma of the breast. A long term follow-up. *Histopathology*, **9**, 271–280

Carter, A.C., Feldman, J.G., Tiefer, L. & Hausdorff, J.K. (1985) Methods of motivating the practice of breast self-examination: A randomized trial. *Prev. Med.*, **14**, 555–572

Carter, C.L., Allen, C. & Henson, D.E. (1989) Relation of tumor size, lymph node status, and survival in 24,740 breast cancer cases. *Cancer*, **63**, 181–187

Celentano, D.D. & Holtzman, D. (1983) Breast self-examination competency: An analysis of self-reported practice and associated characteristics. *Am. J. Public Health*, **73**, 1321–1323

Chamberlain, J., Coleman, D., Ellman, R., Moss, S., Thomas, B., Price, J., Boulter, P.S., Gibbs, N., Forrest, A.P.M., Alexander, F.E., Anderson, T.J., Kirkpatrick, A.E., Hill, A., Vessey, M., Summerly, M., Bradfield, P. & Preece, M. (1991) Sensitivity and specificity of screening in the UK trial of Early Detection of Breast Cancer. In: Miller, A.B., Chamberlain, J., Day, N.E., Hakama, M. & Prorok, P.C., eds, *Cancer Screening*, Cambridge, Cambridge University Press, pp. 3–17

Champion, V.L. (1987) The relationship of breast self-examination to health belief model variables. *Res. Nurs. Health*, **10**, 375–382

Chan, S. (1999) Practice of breast self-examination amongst women attending a Malaysian well person's clinic. *Med. J. Malaysia*, **54**, 433–437

Chan, L.K., Lam, H.S., Chan, E.S., Lau, Y., Chan, M., Gwi, E. & Leung, T.Y. (1998) Mammogram screening of Chinese women in Kwong Wah Hospital, Hong Kong. *Australas. Radiol.*, **42**, 6–9

Chang, J., Yang, W.T. & Choo, H.F. (1999) Mammography in Asian patients with BRCA1 mutations. *Lancet*, **353**, 2070–2071

Chappelon, S. & Jestin, C. (1998) [Screening mechanism.] *Act. Dossier Santé Publique*, **25**, 36–39 (in French)

Chattopadhyay, S.K., Hall, H.I., Wolf, R.B. & Custer, W.S. (1999) Sources of health insurance in the US: Analysis of state-level data and implications for public health programs. *J. Public Health Manag. Pract.*, **5**, 35–46.

Chenevix-Trench, G., Spurdle, A.B., Gatei, M., Kelly, H., Marsh, A., Chen, X., Donn, K., Cummings, M., Nyholt, D., Jenkins, M.A., Scott, C., Pupo, G.M., Dork, T., Bendix, R., Kirk, J., Tucker, K., McCredie, M.R., Hopper, J.L., Sambrook, J., Mann, G.J. & Khanna, K.K. (2002) Dominant negative ATM mutations in breast cancer families. *J. Natl Cancer Inst.*, **94**, 205–215

Chie, W.C., Huang, C.S., Chen, J.H. & Chang, K.J. (2000) Utility assessment for different clinical phases of breast cancer in Taiwan. *J. Formosa Med. Assoc.*, **99**, 677–683

Chow, C.K., Venzon, D., Jones, E.L., Premkumar, A., O'Shaughnessy, J. & Zujewski, J.A. (2000) Effect of tamoxifen on mammographic density. *Cancer Epidemiol. Biomarkers Prev.*, **9**, 917–921

Christiansen, C.L., Wang, F., Barton, M.B., Kreuter, W., Elmore, J.G., Gelfand, A.E. & Fletcher, S.W. (2000) Predicting the cumulative risk of false-positive mammograms. *J. Natl Cancer Inst.*, **92**, 1657–1666

Chu, K.C., Tarone, R.E., Kessler, L.G., Ries, L.A., Hankey, B.F., Miller, B.A. & Edwards, B.K. (1996) Recent trends in US breast cancer incidence, survival, and mortality rates. *J. Natl Cancer Inst.*, **88**, 1571–1579

Chuaqui, R.F., Zhuang, Z., Emmert-Buck, M.R., Liotta, L.A. & Merino, M.J. (1997) Analysis of loss of heterozygosity on chromosome 11q13 in atypical ductal hyperplasia and in situ carcinoma of the breast. *Am. J. Pathol.*, **150**, 297–303

Ciatto, S., Cecchini, S., Isu, A., Maggi, A. & Cammelli, S. (1992) Determinants of non-attendance to mammographic screening. Analysis of a population sample of the screening program in the district of Florence. *Tumori*, **78**, 22–25

Ciatto, S., del Turco, M.R., Morrone, D., Catarzi, S., Ambrogetti, D., Cariddi, A. & Zappa, M. (1995) Independent double reading of screening mammograms. *J. Med. Screen.*, **2**, 99–101

Clark, R.M., McCulloch, P.B., Levine, M.N., Lipa, M., Wilkinson, R.H., Mahoney, L.J., Basrur, V.R., Nair, B.D., McDermot, R.S., Wong, C.S. & Corbett, P.J. (1992) Randomized clinical trial to assess the effectiveness of breast irradiation following lumpectomy and axillary dissection for node-negative breast cancer. *J. Natl Cancer Inst.*, **84**, 683–689

Clarke, V. & Savage, S. (1999) Breast self-examination training: A brief review. *Cancer Nurs.*, **22**, 320–326

Clayton, F. (1986) Pure mucinous carcinomas of breast: Morphologic features and prognostic correlates. *Hum. Pathol.*, **17**, 34–38

Clover, K.A., Redman, S., Forbes, J.F., Sanson-Fisher, R.W. & Dickinson, J.A. (1992) Promotion of attendance for mammographic screening through general practice: A randomised trial of two strategies. *Med. J. Aust.*, **156**, 91–94

Clover, K., Redman, S., Forbes, J., Sanson-Fisher, R. & Callaghan, T. (1996) Two sequential randomized trials of community participation to recruit women for mammographic screening. *Prev. Med.*, **25**, 126–134

Coates, M., Kricker, A., & Armstrong, B. (1999) Breast cancer in NSW in 1997. Cancer information update. NSW Cancer Registry. No 7. Available at: http://www.nswcc.org.au/cncrinfo/research/updates/updatef.htm

Cobleigh, M.A., Vogel, C.L., Tripathy, D., Robert, N.J., Scholl, S., Fehrenbacher, L., Wolter, J.M., Paton, V., Shak, S., Lieberman, G. & Slamon, D.J. (1999) Multinational study of the efficacy and safety of humanized anti-HER2 monoclonal antibody in women who have HER2-over-expressing metastatic breast cancer that has progressed after chemotherapy for metastatic disease. *J. Clin. Oncol.*, **17**, 2639–2648

Cockburn, J., De Luise, T., Hill, D., Hurley, S., Reading, D. & Russell, I. (1990) Boosting recruitment to breast screening programmes. *Medical J. Aust.*, **152**, 332

Cockburn, J., Staples, M., Hurley, S.F. & De Luise, T. (1994) Psychological consequences of screening mammography. *J. Med. Screen.*, **1**, 7–12

Cockburn, J., Sutherland, M., Cappiello, M. & Hevern, M. (1997) Predictors of attendance at a relocatable mammography service for rural women. *Aust. NZ J. Public Health*, **21**, 739–742

Codd, M.B., Laird, O.H., Dowling, M., Dervan, P.A., Gorey, T.F., Stack, J.P., O'Herlihy, B. & Ennis, J.T. (1994) Screening for breast cancer in Ireland: The Eccles breast screening programme. *Eur. J. Cancer Prev.*, **3** (Suppl.), 21–28

Coe, K., Harmon, M., Castro, F., Campbell, N., Mayer, J. & Elder, J. (1994) Breast self-examination: Knowledge and practices of Hispanic women in two southwestern metropolitan areas. *J. Community Health*, **19**, 433–448

Cole, C.F. & Coleman, C. (1999) Breast imaging today and tomorrow. *Nurse Pract. Forum*, **10**, 129–136

Coleman, E.A. & Pennypacker, H. (1991) Measuring breast self-examination proficiency. A scoring system developed from a paired comparison study. *Cancer Nurs.*, **14**, 211–217

Coleman, E.A., Riley, M.B., Fields, F. & Prior, B. (1991) Efficacy of breast self-examination teaching methods among older women. *Oncol. Nurs. Forum*, **18**, 561–566

Collaborative Group on Hormonal Factors in Breast Cancer (2001) Familial breast cancer: Collaborative reanalysis of individual data from 52 epidemiological studies including 58 209 women with breast cancer and 101 986 women without the disease. *Lancet*, **358**, 1389–1399

Collette, H.J., Day, N.E., Rombach, J.J. & de Waard, F. (1984) Evaluation of screening for breast cancer in a non-randomised study (the DOM project) by means of a case–control study. *Lancet*, **1**, 1224–1226

Collette, H.J., de Waard, F., Rombach, J.J., Collette, C. & Day, N.E. (1992) Further evidence of benefits of a (non-randomised) breast cancer screening programme: The DOM project. *J. Epidemiol. Community Health*, **46**, 382–386

Commission of the European Communities (1996) *European Guidelines for Quality Assurance in Mammography Screening*, Europe Against Cancer Programme, Luxembourg, Office for Official Publications of the European Communities

Commission of the European Communities (2000) *Evaluation and Monitoring of Screening Programmes*, Luxembourg, Office for Official Publications of the European Communities

Commission of the European Communities (2001) *European Guidelines for Quality Assurance in Mammography Screening*, 3rd Ed., Europe Against Cancer Programme, Luxembourg, Office for Official Publications of the European Communities

Committee on the Biological Effects of Ionizing Radiation (BEIR; 1990) *Health Effects of Exposure to Low Levels of Ionizing Radiation*, Washington DC, National Research Council

Connolly, J.L., Fechner, R.E., Kempson, R.L., LiVolsi, V.A., Page, D.L., Patchefsky, A.A. & Silverberg, S.G. (1996) Recommendations for the reporting of breast carcinoma. Association of Directors of Anatomic and Surgical Pathology. *Hum. Pathol.*, **27**, 220–224

Connor, R.J. & Prorok, P.C. (1994) Issues in the mortality analysis of randomized controlled trials of cancer screening. *Control. Clin. Trials*, **15**, 81–99

Conry, C., Main, D., Miller, R., Iverson, D. & Calonge, B. (1993) Factors influencing mammogram ordering at the time of the office visit. *J. Fam. Pract.*, **37**, 356–360

Consensus Conference Committee (1997) Consensus Conference on the Classification of Ductal Carcinoma In Situ. *Cancer*, **80**, 1798–1802

Contesso, G., Mouriesse, H., Friedman, S., Genin, J., Sarrazin, D. & Rouesse, J. (1987) The importance of histologic grade in long-term prognosis of breast cancer: A study of 1,010 patients, uniformly treated at the Institut Gustave-Roussy. *J. Clin. Oncol.*, **5**, 1378–1386

Cooper, H.S., Patchefsky, A.S. & Krall, R.A. (1978) Tubular carcinoma of the breast. *Cancer*, **42**, 2334–2342

Cornford, E.J., Wilson, A.R., Athanassiou, E., Galea, M., Ellis, I.O., Elston, C.W. & Blamey, R.W. (1995) Mammographic features of invasive lobular and invasive ductal carcinoma of the breast: A comparative analysis. *Br. J. Radiol.*, **68**, 450–453

Costa Rica Ministry of Health (2000) Decreto No. 28851-S, *La Gaceta: Diario oficial*, **CXXII** (No. 177), San José

Cowan, W.K., Angus, B., Henry, J., Corbett, I.P., Reid, W.A. & Horne, C.H. (1991) Immunohistochemical and other features of breast carcinomas presenting clinically compared with those detected by cancer screening. *Br. J. Cancer*, **64**, 780–784

Cox, B. (1997) Variation in the effectiveness of breast screening by year of follow-up. *Natl Cancer Inst. Monogr.*, **22**, 69–72

Crane, L., Leakey, T., Rimer, B., Wolfe, P., Woodworth, M. & Warnecke, R. (1998) Effectiveness of a telephone outcall intervention to promote screening mammography among low income women. *Prev. Med.*, **25**, S39–S49

Craun, A.M. & Deffenbacher, J.L. (1987) The effects of information, behavioral rehearsal, and prompting on breast self-exams. *J. Behav. Med.*, **10**, 351–365

de Cremoux, P., Salomon, A.V., Liva, S., Dendale, R., Bouchind'homme, B., Martin, E., Sastre-Garau, X., Magdelenat, H., Fourquet, A. & Soussi, T. (1999) p53 mutation as a genetic trait of typical medullary breast carcinoma. *J. Natl Cancer Inst.*, **91**, 641–643

Cutler, S.J., Black, M.M., Friedell, G.H., Vidone, R.A. & Goldenberg, I.S. (1966) Prognostic factors in cancer of the female breast. II. Reproducibility of histopathologic classification. *Cancer*, **19**, 75–82

Cutler, S.J., Black, M.M., Mork, T., Harvei, S. & Freeman, C. (1969) Further observations on prognostic factors in cancer of the female breast. *Cancer*, **24**, 653–667

Cuzick, J., Edwards, R. & Segnan, N. (1997) Adjusting for non-compliance and contamination in randomized clinical trials. *Stat. Med.*, **16**, 1017–1029

Cuzick, J., Holland, R., Barth, V., Davies, R., Faupel, M., Fentiman, I., Frischbier, H.J., Lamarque, J.L., Merson, M., Sacchini, V., Vanel, D. & Veronesi, U. (1998) Electropotential measurements as a new diagnostic modality for breast cancer. *Lancet*, **352**, 359–363

Dalton, L.W., Page, D.L. & Dupont, W.D. (1994) Histologic grading of breast carcinoma. A reproducibility study. *Cancer*, **73**, 2765–2770

Davis, B.W., Gelber, R., Goldhirsch, A., Hartmann, W.H., Hollaway, L., Russell, I. & Rudenstam, C.M. (1985) Prognostic significance of peritumoral vessel invasion in clinical trials of adjuvant therapy for breast cancer with axillary lymph node metastasis. *Hum. Pathol.*, **16**, 1212–1218

Davis, N., Nash, E., Bailey, C., Lewis, M., Rimer, B. & Koplan, J. (1997) Evaluation of three methods for improving mammography rates in a managed care plan. *Am. J. Prev. Med.*, **13**, 298–302

Dawson, P.J., Ferguson, D.J. & Karrison, T. (1982) The pathological findings of breast cancer in patients surviving 25 years after radical mastectomy. *Cancer*, **50**, 2131–2138

Day, N.E. (1985) Estimating the sensitivity of a screening test. *J. Epidemiol Community Health*, **39**, 364–366

Day, N.E. (1991) Screening for breast cancer. *Br. Med. Bull.*, **47**, 400–415

Day, N.E. & Duffy, S.W. (1996) Trial design based on surrogate endpoints—Application to comparison of different screening frequencies. *J. R. Stat. Soc.*, **159**, 49–60

Day, N.E. & Walter, S.D. (1984) Simplified models of screening for chronic disease: Estimation procedures from mass screening programmes. *Biometrics*, **40**, 1–14

Day, N.E., Walter, S.D., Tabar, L., Fagerberg, C.J.B. & Collette, H.J.A. (1988) The sensitivity and lead time of breast cancer screening: A comparison of the results of different studies. In: Day, N.E. & Miller, A.B., eds, *Screening for Breast Cancer*, Toronto, Hans Huber, pp. 105–110

Day, N.E., Williams, D.R.R. & Khaw, K.T. (1989) Breast cancer screening programmes: The development of a monitoring and evaluation system. *Br. J. Cancer*, **59**, 954–958

Day, N., McCann, J., Camilleri-Ferrante, C., Britton, P., Hurst, G., Cush, S. & Duffy, S. (1995) Monitoring interval cancers in breast screening programmes: The East Anglian experience. Quality assurance management group of the East Anglian breast screening programme. *J. Med. Screen.*, **2**, 180–185

Dean, L. & Geshchicter, C.F. (1938) Comedocarcinoma of the breast. *Arch. Surg.*, **36**, 225–234

Dean, P.B. & Pamilo, M. (1999) Screening mammography in Finland—1.5 million examinations with 97 percent specificity. Mammography Working Group, Radiological Society of Finland. *Acta Oncol.*, **38** (Suppl. 13), 47–54

Demissie, K., Mills, O.F. & Rhoads, G.G. (1998) Empirical comparison of the results of randomized controlled trials and case–control studies in evaluating the effectiveness of screening mammography. *J. Clin. Epidemiol.*, **51**, 81–91

Denton, E.R. & Field, S. (1997) Just how valuable is double reporting in screening mammography? *Clin. Radiol.*, **52**, 466–468

Desnick, L., Taplin, S., Taylor, V., Coole, D. & Urban, N. (1999) Clinical breast examination in primary care: Perceptions and predictors among three specialties. *J. Women's Health*, **8**, 389–397

Diab, S.G., Clark, G.M., Osborne, C.K., Libby, A., Allred, D.C. & Elledge, R.M. (1999) Tumor characteristics and clinical outcome of tubular and mucinous breast carcinomas. *J. Clin. Oncol.*, **17**, 1442–1448

Dietrich, A., O'Connor, G., Keller, A., Carney, P., Levy, D. & Whaley, F. (1992) Cancer: Improving early detection and prevention. A community practice randomised trial. *Br. Med. J.*, **304**, 687–691

van Dijck, J.A., Holland, R., Verbeek, A.L., Hendriks, J.H. & Mravunac, M. (1994) Efficacy of mammographic screening of the elderly: A case–referent study in the Nijmegen program in The Netherlands. *J. Natl Cancer Inst.*, **86**, 934–938

van Dijck, J.A., Verbeek, A.L., Beex, L.V., Hendriks, J.H., Holland, R., Mravunac, M., Straatman, H. & Werre, J.M. (1996) Mammographic screening after the age of 65 years: Evidence for a reduction in breast cancer mortality. *Int. J. Cancer*, **66**, 727–731

Dinnes, J., Moss, S., Melia, J., Blanks, R., Song, F. & Kleijnen, J. (2001) Effectiveness and cost–effectivenes of double reading of mammograms in breast cancer screening: Findings of a systematic review. *Breast*, **10**, 455–463

Dixon, J.M., Anderson, T.J., Page, D.L., Lee, D. & Duffy, S.W. (1982) Infiltrating lobular carcinoma of the breast. *Histopathology*, **6**, 149–161

Dixon, J.M., Page, D.L., Anderson, T.J., Lee, D., Elton, R.A., Stewart, H.J. & Forrest, A.P. (1985) Long-term survivors after breast cancer. *Br. J. Surg.*, **72**, 445–448

Dixon-Woods, M., Baum, M. & Kurinczuk, J. (2001) Letter to the Editor: Screening for breast cancer with mammography. *Lancet*, **358**, 2166–2167

Doll, R., Payne, P. & Waterhouse, J., eds (1966) *Cancer Incidence in Five Continents. A Technical Report*, Heidelberg, Springer Verlag

Doll, R., Muir, C. & Waterhouse, J., eds (1970) *Cancer Incidence in Five Continents, Volume II*, Heidelberg, Springer Verlag

Donabedian, A. (1980) *Explorations in Quality Assessment and Monitoring*, Vol. I, *The Definition of Quality and Approaches to Its Assessment,* Chicago, Health Administration Press

Donato, F., Bollani, A., Spiazzl, R., Soldo, M., Pasquale, L., Monarca, S., Lucini, L. & Nardi, G. (1991) Factors associated with non-participation of women in a breast cancer screening programme in a town in northern Italy. *J. Epidemiol. Community Health*, **45**, 59–64

van Dongen, J.A., Fentiman, I.S., Harris, J.R., Holland, R., Peterse, J.L., Salvadori, B. & Stewart, H.J. (1989) In-situ breast cancer: The EORTC consensus meeting. *Lancet*, **ii**, 25–27

van Dongen, J.A., Holland, R., Peterse, J.L., Fentiman, I.S., Lagios, M.D., Millis, R.R. & Recht, A. (1992a) Ductal carcinoma in-situ of the breast: Second EORTC consensus meeting. *Eur. J. Cancer*, **28**, 626–629

van Dongen, J.A., Bartelink, H., Fentiman, I.S., Lerut, T., Mignolet, F., Olthuis, G., van der Scheueren, E., Sylvester, R., Winter, J. & van Zijl, K. (1992b) Randomized clinical trial to assess the value of breast-conserving therapy in stage I and II breast cancer, EORTC 10801 trial. *Natl Cancer Inst. Monogr*, 15–18

van Dongen, J.A., Voogd, A.C., Fentiman, I.S., Legrand, C., Sylvester, R.J., Tong, D., van der Scheueren, E., Helle, P.A., van Zijl, K. & Bartelink, H. (2000) Long-term results of a randomized trial comparing breast-conserving therapy with mastectomy: European Organization for Research and Treatment of Cancer 10801 trial. *J. Natl Cancer Inst.*, **92**, 1143–1150

Dork, T., Bendix, R., Bremer, M., Rades, D., Klopper, K., Nicke, M., Skawran, B., Hector, A., Yamini, P., Steinmann, D., Weise, S., Stuhrmann, M. & Karstens, J.H. (2001) Spectrum of ATM gene mutations in a hospital-based series of unselected breast cancer patients. *Cancer Res.*, **61**, 7608–7615

Dorsay, R.H., Cuneo, W.D., Somkin, C.P. & Tekawa, I.S. (1988) Breast self-examination: Improving competence and frequency in a classroom setting. *Am. J. Public Health*, **78**, 520–522

Douglas-Jones, A.G., Gupta, S.K., Attanoos, R.L., Morgan, J.M. & Mansel, R.E. (1996) A critical appraisal of six modern classifications of ductal carcinoma in situ of the breast (DCIS): Correlation with grade of associated invasive carcinoma. *Histopathology*, **29**, 397–409

Duffy, S.W. & Tabár, L. (2000) Screening mammography re-evaluated. *Lancet*, **355**, 747–748

Duffy, S.W., Day, N.E., Tabár, L., Chen, H.H. & Smith, T.C. (1997) Markov models of breast tumor progression: Some age-specific results. *Natl Cancer Inst. Monogr.*, **22**, 93–97

Dupont, W.D. & Page, D.L. (1985) Risk factors for breast cancer in women with proliferative breast disease. *New Engl. J. Med.*, **312**, 146–151

Dupont, W.D., Parl, F.F., Hartmann, W.H., Brinton, L.A., Winfield, A.C., Worrell, J.A., Schuyler, P.A. & Plummer, W.D. (1993) Breast cancer risk associated with proliferative breast disease and atypical hyperplasia. *Cancer*, **71**, 1258–1265

Dupont, W.D., Page, D.L., Parl, F.F., Vnencak-Jones, C.L., Plummer, W.D., Jr, Rados, M.S. & Schuyler, P.A. (1994) Long-term risk of breast cancer in women with fibroadenoma. *New Engl. J. Med.*, **331**, 10–15

Eggertsen, S.C., Berg, A.O. & Moe, R.E. (1983) An evaluation of individual components of breast self-examination. *J. Fam. Pract.*, **17**, 921–922

Eisinger, F., Jacquemier, J., Charpin, C., Stoppa-Lyonnet, D., Bressac-de Paillerets, B., Peyrat, J.P., Longy, M., Guinebretiere, J.M., Sauvan, R., Noguchi, T., Birnbaum, D. & Sobol, H. (1998) Mutations at BRCA1: The medullary breast carcinoma revisited. *Cancer Res.*, **58**, 1588–1592

Ellis, L.M. & Fidler, I.J. (1995) Angiogenesis and breast cancer metastasis. *Lancet*, **346**, 388–390

Ellis, I.O., Galea, M., Broughton, N., Locker, A., Blamey, R.W. & Elston, C.W. (1992) Pathological prognostic factors in breast cancer. II. Histological type. Relationship with survival in a large study with long-term follow-up. *Histopathology*, **20**, 479–489

Ellis, I.O., Galea, M.H., Locker, A., Rocbuck, E.J., Elston, C.W., Blamey, R.W. & Wilson, A.R. (1993) Early experience in breast cancer screening: Emphasis on development of protocols for triple assessment. *Breast*, **2**, 148–153

Ellman, R., Angeli, N., Christians, A., Moss, S., Chamberlain, J. & Maguire, P. (1989) Psychiatric morbidity associated with screening for breast cancer. *Br. J. Cancer*, **60**, 781–784

Ellman, R., Moss, S.M., Coleman, D. & Chamberlain, J. (1993) Breast self-examination programmes in the trial of early detection of breast cancer: Ten year findings. *Br. J. Cancer*, **68**, 208–212

Elmore, J.G., Wells, C.K., Lee, C.H., Howard, D.H. & Feinstein, A.R. (1994) Variability in radiologists' interpretations of mammograms. *New Engl. J. Med.*, **331**, 1493–1499

Elmore, J.G., Barton, M.B., Moceri, V.M., Polk, S., Arena, P.J. & Fletcher, S.W. (1998) Ten-year risk of false positive screening mammograms and clinical breast examinations. *New Engl. J. Med.*, **338**, 1089–1096

Elson, B.C., Helvie, M.A., Frank, T.S., Wilson, T.E. & Adler, D.D. (1993) Tubular carcinoma of the breast: Mode of presentation, mammographic appearance, and frequency of nodal metastases. *Am. J. Roentgenol.*, **161**, 1173–1176

Elston, C.W. & Ellis, I.O. (1991) Pathological prognostic factors in breast cancer. I. The value of histological grade in breast cancer: Experience from a large study with long-term follow-up. *Histopathology*, **19**, 403–410

Elston, C.W. & Ellis, I.O. (1998) *Systemic Pathology*, London, Churchill Livingstone

Elston, C.W., Gresham, G.A., Rao, G.S., Zebro, T., Haybittle, J.L., Houghton, J. & Kearney, G. (1982) The Cancer Research Campaign (King's/Cambridge) trial for early breast cancer: Clinico-pathological aspects. *Br. J. Cancer*, **45**, 655–669

Ernster, V.L., Barclay, J., Kerlikowske, K., Grady, D. & Henderson, C. (1996) Incidence of and treatment for ductal carcinoma in situ of the breast. *J. Am. Med. Assoc.*, **275**, 913–918

Ernster, V.L., Barclay, J., Kerlikowske, K., Wilkie, H. & Ballard-Barbash, R. (2000) Mortality among women with ductal carcinoma in situ of the breast in the population-based Surveillance, Epidemiology and End Results program. *Arch. Intern. Med.*, **160**, 953–958

Esserman, L., Cowley, H., Eberle, C., Kirkpatrick, A., Chang, S., Berbaum, K. & Gale, A. (2002) Improving the accuracy of mammography: Volume and outcome relationships. *J. Natl Cancer Inst.*, **94**, 369–375

European Network of Cancer Registries (2001) *Eurocim Version 4.0*, Lyon, IARC

Eusebi, V., Foschini, M.P., Cook, M.G., Berrino, F. & Azzopardi, J.G. (1989) Long-term follow-up of in situ carcinoma of the breast with special emphasis on clinging carcinoma. *Semin. Diagn. Pathol.*, **6**, 165–173.

Evans, A., Pinder, S., Wilson, R., Sibbering, M., Poller, D., Elston, C. & Ellis, I. (1994a) Ductal carcinoma in situ of the breast: Correlation between mammographic and pathologic findings. *Am. J. Roentgenol.*, **162**, 1307–1311

Evans, A.J., Pinder, S., Ellis, I.O., Sibbering, M., Elston, C.W., Poller, D.N. & Wilson, R. (1994b) Screening-detected and symptomatic ductal carcinoma in situ: Mammographic features with pathologic correlation. *Radiology*, **191**, 237–240

Evans, A.J., Pinder, S.E., Snead, D.R., Wilson, A.R., Ellis, I.O. & Elston, C.W. (1997) The detection of ductal carcinoma in situ at mammographic screening enables the diagnosis of small, grade 3 invasive tumours. *Br. J. Cancer*, **75**, 542–544

Evans, A.J., Pinder, S.E., Burrell, H.C., Ellis, I.O. & Wilson, A.R. (2001a) Detecting which invasive cancers at mammographic screening saves lives? *J. Med. Screen.*, **8**, 86–90

Evans, A.J., Pinder, S.E., Ellis, I.O., Wilson, A.R. (2001b) Screen detected ductal carcinoma in situ (DCIS): Overdiagnosis or an obligate precursor of invasive disease? *J. Med. Screen.*, **8**, 149–151

Fajardo, L.L., Hillman, B.J. & Frey, C. (1988) Correlation between breast parenchymal patterns and mammographers' certainty of diagnosis. *Invest. Radiol.*, **23**, 505–508

Feig, S.A. (1984) Radiation risk from mammography: Is it clinically significant? *Am. J. Roentgenol.*, **143**, 469–475

Feig, S.A. & Hendrick, R.E. (1997) Radiation risk from screening mammography of women aged 40–49 years. *Natl Cancer Inst. Monogr.*, **22**, 119–124

Feldman, J.G., Carter, A.C., Nicastri, A.D. & Hosat, S.T. (1981) Breast self-examination, relationship to stage of breast cancer at diagnosis. *Cancer*, **47**, 2740–2745

Ferguson, D.J., Meier, P., Karrison, T., Dawson, P.J., Straus, F.H. & Lowenstein, F.E. (1982) Staging of breast cancer and survival rates. An assessment based on 50 years of experience with radical mastectomy. *J. Am. Med. Assoc.*, **248**, 1337–1341

Ferlay, J., Pisani, P. & Parkin, D.M., eds (2001) Globocan 2000 (IARC Cancer Base No 5), Lyon, IARCPress

Ferro, S., Caroli, A., Nanni, O., Biggeri, A. & Gambi, A. (1996) A randomized trial on breast self-examination in Faenza (northern Italy). *Tumori*, **82**, 329–334

Fine, M., Rimer, B. & Watts, P. (1993) Women's responses to the mammography experience. *J. Am. Board Fam. Pract.*, **6**, 546–555

Fisher, B. & Saffer, E. (1989) Presence of a growth-stimulating factor in serum following primary tumour removal in mice. *Cancer Res.*, **49**, 1996–2001

Fisher, B., Carbone, P.C., Economou, S.G., Frelick, R., Glass, A., Lerner, H., Redmond, C., Zelen, M., Band, P., Katrych, D.L., Wolmark, N. & Fisher, E.R. (1975) L-Phenylalanine mustard (L-PAM) in the management of primary breast cancer. A report of early findings. *New Engl. J. Med.*, **292**, 117–122

Fisher, E.R., Gregorio, R.M., Fisher, B., Redmond, C., Vellios, F. & Sommers, S.C. (1975) The pathology of invasive breast cancer. A syllabus derived from findings of the National Surgical Adjuvant Breast Project (Protocol No. 4). *Cancer*, **36**, 1–85

Fisher, E.R., Gregorio, R.M., Redmond, C. & Fisher, B. (1977) Tubulolobular invasive breast cancer: A variant of lobular invasive cancer. *Hum. Pathol.*, **8**, 679–683

Fisher, E.R., Sass, R. & Fisher, B. (1984) Pathologic findings from the National Surgical Adjuvant Project for Breast Cancers (Protocol No. 4). X. Discriminants for tenth year treatment failure. *Cancer*, **53**, 712–723

Fisher, B., Redmond, C., Poisson, R., Margolese, R., Wolmark, N., Wickerham, L., Fisher, E., Deutsch, M., Caplan, R., Pilch, Y., Glass, A., Shibata, H., Lerner, H., Terz, J. & Sidorovich, L. (1989) Eight-year results of a randomized clinical trial comparing total mastectomy and lumpectomy with or without irradiation in the treatment of breast cancer. *New Engl. J. Med.*, **320**, 822–828

Fisher, E.R., Kenny, J.P., Sass, R., Dimitrov, N.V., Siderits, R.H. & Fisher, B. (1990) Medullary cancer of the breast revisited. *Breast Cancer Res. Treat.*, **16**, 215–229

Fisher, B., Wickerham, D.L. &, Redmont, C. (1992) Recent developments in the use of systemic adjuvant therapy for the treatment of breast cancer. *Semin. Oncol.*, **19**, 263–277

Fisher, B., Anderson, S., Redmond, C.K., Wolmark, N., Wickerham, D.L. & Cronin, W.M., (1995) Reanalysis and results after 12 years of follow-up in a randomized clinical trial comparing total mastectomy with lumpectomy with or without irradiation in the treatment of breast cancer. *New Engl. J. Med.*, **333**, 1456–1461

Fisher, E.R., Costantino, J., Fisher, B., Palekar, A.S., Paik, S.M., Suarez, C.M. & Wolmark, N. (1996) Pathologic findings from the National Surgical Adjuvant Breast Project (NSABP) Protocol B-17. Five-year observations concerning lobular carcinoma in situ. *Cancer*, **78**, 1403–1416

Fisher, B., Dignam, J., Wolmark, N., DeCillis, A., Emir, B., Wickerham, D.L., Bryant, J., Dimitrov, N.V., Abramson, N., Atkins, J.N., Shibata, H., Deschenes, L. & Margolese, R.G. (1997) Tamoxifen and chemotherapy for lymph node-negative, estrogen receptor-positive breast cancer. *J. Natl Cancer Inst.*, **89**, 1673–1682

Fisher, E.R., Dignam, J., Tan-Chiu, E., Costantino, J., Fisher, B., Paik, S. & Wolmark, N. (1999) Pathologic findings from the National Surgical Adjuvant Breast Project (NSABP) eight-year update of Protocol B-17: Intraductal carcinoma. *Cancer*, **86**, 429–438

Fishman, P., Taplin, S., Meyer, D. & Barlow, W. (2000) Cost-effectiveness of strategies to enhance mammography use. *Effective Clin. Pract.*, **3**, 213–220

Fitzgibbons, P.L., Page, D.L., Weaver, D., Thor, A.D., Allred, D.C., Clark, G.M., Ruby, S.G., O'Malley, F., Simpson, J.F., Connolly, J.L., Hayes, D.F., Edge, S.B., Lichter, A. & Schnitt, S.J. (2000) Prognostic factors in breast cancer. College of American Pathologists Consensus Statement 1999. *Arch. Pathol. Lab. Med.*, **124**, 966–978

Flagiello, D., Gerbault-Seureau, M., Sastre-Garau, X., Padoy, E., Vielh, P., Dutrillaux, B. (1998) Highly recurrent der(1;16)(q10;p10) and other 16q arm alterations in lobular breast cancer. *Genes Chromosomes Cancer,* **23**, 300–306

Fletcher, S.W. (1997) Whither scientific deliberation in health policy recommendations?—Alice in the wonderland of breast-cancer screening. *New Engl. J. Med.*, **336**, 1180–1183

Fletcher, S.W., O'Malley, M.S. & Bunce, L.A. (1985) Physicians' abilities to detect lumps in silicone breast models. *J. Am. Med. Assoc.*, **253**, 2224–2228

Fletcher, S.W., Morgan, T.M., O'Malley, M.S., Earp, J.A. & Degnan, D. (1989) Is breast self-examination predicted by knowledge, attitudes, beliefs, or sociodemographic characteristics? *Am. J. Prev. Med.*, **5**, 207–215

Fletcher, S.W., O'Malley, M.S., Earp, J.L., Morgan, T.M., Lin, S. & Degnan, D. (1990) How best to teach women breast self-examination. A randomized controlled trial. *Ann. Intern. Med.*, **112**, 772–779

Fletcher, S.W., Black, W., Harris, R., Rimer, B.K. & Shapiro, S. (1993) Report of the International Workshop on Screening for Breast Cancer. *J. Natl Cancer Inst.*, **85**, 1644–1656

Flynn, B., Gavin, P., Worden, J., Ashikaga, T., Gautam, S. & Carpenter, J. (1997) Community education programs to promote mammography participation in rural New York State. *Prev. Med.*, **26**, 102–108

Food & Drug Administration (1997) *Quality Mammography Standards. Final Rule.* 21 CFR Parts 16 and 900 [Docket No. 95N-0192], (RIN 0910-AA24), Washington DC, Department of Health and Human Services, pp. 55852–55873

Ford, D., Easton, D.F., Stratton, M., Narod, S., Goldgar, D., Devilee, P., Bishop, D.T.,

Weber, B., Lenoir, G., Chang-Claude, J., Sobol, H., Teare, M.D., Struewing, J., Arason, A., Scherneck, S., Peto, J., Rebbeck, T.R., Tonin, P., Neuhausen, S., Barkardottir, R., Eyfjord, J., Lynch, H., Ponder, B.A., Gayther, S.A. & Zelada-Hedman, M. (1998) Genetic heterogeneity and penetrance analysis of the BRCA1 and BRCA2 genes in breast cancer families. The Breast Cancer Linkage Consortium. *Am. J. Hum. Genet.*, **62**, 676–689

Forrest, A.P. (1986) *Breast Cancer Screening: Report to the Health Ministers of England, Wales, Scotland and Nothern Ireland*, London, Her Majesty's Stationery Office

Foster, R.S., Jr & Costanza, M.C. (1984) Breast self-examination practices and breast cancer survival. *Cancer*, **53**, 999–1005.

Foucar, E. (1996) Carcinoma-in-situ of the breast: Have pathologists run amok? *Lancet*, **347**, 707–708

Fowler, B.A. (2000) Variability in mammography screening legislation across the states. *J. Women's Health Gender-based Med.*, **9**, 175–184

Fox, S. & Roetzheim, R. (1994) Screening mammography and older Hispanic women: Current status and issues. *Cancer*, **74**, 2028–2033

Fox, S., Siu, A. & Stein, J. (1994) The importance of physician communication on breast cancer screening of older women. *Arch. Intern. Med.*, **154**, 2058–2068

Fox, S.A., Pitkin, K., Paul, C., Carson, S. & Duan, N. (1998) Breast cancer screening adherence: Does church attendance matter? *Health Educ. Behav.*, **25**, 742–758

Fracheboud, J., de Koning, H.J., Beemsterboer, P.M., Boer, R., Hendriks, J.H., Verbeek, A.L., van Ineveld, B.M., de Bruyn, A.E. & van der Maas, P.J. (1998) Nation-wide breast cancer screening in The Netherlands: Results of initial and subsequent screening 1990–1995. National evaluation team for breast cancer screening. *Int. J. Cancer*, **75**, 694–698

Fracheboud, J., de Koning, H.J., Beemsterboer, P.M., Boer, R., Verbeek, A.L., Hendriks, J.H., van Ineveld, B.M., Broeders, M.J., de Bruyn, A.E. & van der Maas, P.J. (1999) Interval cancers in the Dutch breast cancer screening programme. *Br. J. Cancer*, **81**, 912–917

Fracheboud, J., Otto, S.J., Groenewoud, J.H., van Ineveld, B.M., Broeders, M.J.M., Verbeek, A.L.M., Hendriks, J.H.C.L., de Bruyn, A.E., van der Maas, P.J. & de Koning, H.J. (2001a) *Nationwide Evaluation of Breast Cancer Screening among the Dutch Population*, Rotterdam, Department of Public Health, Erasmus University

Fracheboud, J., de Koning, H.J., Boer, R., Groenewoud, J.H., Verbeek, A.L., Broeders, M.J., van Ineveld, B.M., Hendriks, J.H., de Bruyn, A.E., Holland, R. & van der Maas, P.J. (2001b) Nationwide breast cancer screening programme fully implemented in the Netherlands. *Breast*, **10**, 6–11

Frank, J.W. & Mai, V. (1985) Breast self-examination in young women: More harm than good? *Lancet*, **ii**, 654–657

Frank, E., Rimer, B., Brogan, D. & Elon, L. (2000) US women physicians' personal and clinical breast cancer screening practices. *J. Women's Health Gender-based Med.*, **9**, 791–801

Frankel, S.D., Sickles, E.A., Curpen, B.N., Sollitto, R.A., Ominsky, S.H. & Galvin, H.B. (1995) Initial versus subsequent screening mammography: Comparison of findings and their prognostic significance. *Am. J. Roentgenol.*, **164**, 1107–1109

Frazier, E.L., Jiles, R.B. & Mayberry, R. (1996a) Use of screening mammography and clinical breast examinations among black, Hispanic and white women. *Prev. Med.*, **25**, 118–125

Frazier, E.L., Okoro, C.A., Smith, C. & McQueen, D.V. (1996b) State- and sex-specific prevalence of selected characteristics—Behavioral Risk Factor Surveillance System, 1992 and 1993. *Morbid. Mortal. Weekly Rep.*, **45**, 1–36

Freer, T.W. & Ulissey, M.J. (2001) Screening mammography with computer-aided detection: Prospective study of 12,860 patients in a community breast center. *Radiology*, **220**, 781–786

Friedman, D.R. & Dubin, N. (1991) Case–control evaluation of breast cancer screening efficacy. *Am. J. Epidemiol.*, **133**, 974–984

Friedman, L., Moore, A., Webb, J. & Puryear, L. (1999) Breast cancer screening among ethnically diverse low-income women in a general hospital psychiatry clinic. *Gen. Hosp. Psychiatry*, **21**, 374–381

Friedrich, M. (1975) The effect of scatter on film quality in mammography. *RöFo Fortschr. Geb. Röntgenstr. Nuklearmed.*, **123**, 556–566

Frierson, H.F., Jr, Wolber, R.A., Berean, K.W., Franquemont, D.W., Gaffey, M.J., Boyd, J.C. & Wilbur, D.C. (1995) Interobserver reproducibility of the Nottingham modification of the Bloom and Richardson histologic grading scheme for infiltrating ductal carcinoma. *Am. J. Clin. Pathol.*, **103**, 195–198

Frisell, J., Glas, U., Hellstrom, L. & Somell, A. (1986) Randomized mammographic screening for breast cancer in Stockholm. Design, first round results and comparisons. *Breast Cancer Res. Treat.*, **8**, 45–54

Frixen, U.H., Behrens, J., Sachs, M., Eberle, G., Voss, B., Warda, A., Lochner, D., Birchmeier, W. (1991) E-Cadherin-mediated cell–cell adhesion prevents invasiveness of human carcinoma cells. *J. Cell. Biol.*, **113**, 173–185.

Fujii, H., Szumel, R., Marsh, C., Zhou, W.B. & Gabrielson, E. (1996) Genetic progression, histological grade, and allelic loss in ductal carcinoma in situ of the breast. *Cancer Res.*, **56**, 5260–5265

Fukuda, M., Shimizu, K., Okamoto, N., Arimura, T., Ohta, T., Yamaguchi, S. & Faupel, M.L. (1996) Prospective evaluation of skin surface electropotentials in Japanese patients with suspicious breast lesions. *Jpn. J. Cancer Res.*, **87**, 1092–1096

Fung, S. (1998) Factors associated with breast self-examination behaviour among Chinese women in Hong Kong. *Patient Educ. Couns.*, **33**, 233–243

Galea, M.H., Blamey, R.W., Elston, C.E. & Ellis, I.O. (1992) The Nottingham Prognostic Index in primary breast cancer. *Breast Cancer Res. Treat.*, **22**, 207–219

Gallager, H.S. & Martin, J.E. (1971) An orientation to the concept of minimal carcinoma. *Cancer*, **28**, 1505–1507

Gamallo, C., Palacios, J., Suarez, A., Pizarro, A., Navarro, P., Quintanilla, M. & Cano, A. (1993) Correlation of E-cadherin expression with differentiation grade and histological type in breast carcinoma. *Am. J. Pathol.*, **142**, 987–993

Gao, Y.T., Shu, X.O., Dai, Q., Potter, J.D., Brinton, L.A., Wen, W., Sellers, T.A., Kushi, L.H., Ruan, Z., Bostick, R.M., Jin, F. & Zheng, W. (2000) Association of menstrual and reproductive factors with breast cancer risk: Results from the Shanghai breast cancer study. *Int. J. Cancer*, **87**, 295–300

Garas, I., Pateras, H., Triandafilou, D., Georgountzos, V., Mihas, A., Abatzoglou, M. & Tricholopoulos, D. (1994) Breast cancer screening in southern Greece. *Eur. J. Cancer Prev.*, **3** (Suppl.), 35–39

Gästrin, G. (1981) *Breast Cancer Control*, Stockholm, Almquist & Wilsell International

Garne, J.P., Aspegren, K. & Balldin, G. (1996) Breast cancer as cause of death — A study over the validity of the officially registered cause of death in 2631 breast cancer patients dying in Malmo, Sweden 1964–1992. *Acta Oncol.*, **35**, 671–675

Gästrin, G., Miller, A.B., To, T., Aronson, K.J., Wall, C., Hakama, M., Louhivuori, K. & Pukkala, E. (1994) Incidence and mortality from breast cancer in the Mama Program for Breast Screening in Finland, 1973–1986. *Cancer*, **73**, 2168–2174

Gaudette, L.A., Altmayer, C.A., Nobrega, M.P. & Lee, J. (1996) Trends in mammography utilization, 1981 to 1994. *Health Rep.*, **8**, 17–27

Geddes, M., Parkin, D.M., Khlat, M., Balzi, D. & Buiatti, E., eds (1993) *Cancer in Italy: Incidence and Mortality* (IARC Scientific Publications No. 123), Lyon, IARCPress

Geoffroy-Perez, B., Janin, N., Ossian, K., Lauge, A., Croquette, M.F., Griscelli, C., Debre, M., Bressac-de-Paillerets, B., Aurias, A., Stoppa-Lyonnet, D. & Andrieu, N. (2001) Cancer risk in heterozygotes for ataxia-telangiectasia. *Int. J. Cancer*, **93**, 288–293

van Gessel-Dauekaussen, A. & de Koning, H. (1995) Participating in population survey programme for breast cancer. *Mndbar Gezondh.*, **4**, 1–12

Gilbert, F.J., Cordiner, C.M., Affleck, I.R., Hood, D.B., Mathieson, D. & Walker, L.G. (1998) Breast screening: The psychological sequelae of false-positive recall in women with and without a family history of breast cancer. *Eur. J. Cancer*, **34**, 2010–2014

Giles, J., Kennedy, D., Dunn, E., Wallace, W., Meadows, S. & Cafiero, A. (2001) Results of a community pharmacy-based breast cancer risk-assessment and education program. *Pharmacotherapy*, **21**, 243–253

van Gils, C.H., Otten, J.D., Verbeek, A.L., Hendriks, J.H. & Holland, R. (1998) Effect of mammographic breast density on breast cancer screening performance: A study in Nijmegen, The Netherlands. *J. Epidemiol. Community Health*, **52**, 267–271

Giordano, L., Giorgi, D., Fasolo, G., Segnan, N. & Rosselli del Turco, M. (1996) Breast cancer screening: Characteristics and results of the Italian programmes in the Italian group for planning and evaluating breast cancer screening programmes (GISMA). *Tumori*, **82**, 31–37

Giorgi, D., Paci, E., Zappa, M. & Rosselli del Turco, M. (1994) Breast cancer early diagnosis experience in Florence: Can a self referral policy achieve the results of service screening? *J. Epidemiol. Community Health*, **48**, 471–475

Giorgi, D., Giordano, L., Senore, C., Merlino, G., Negri, R., Cancian, M., Lerda, M., Segnan, N. & Rosselli del Turco, M. (2000) General practitioners and mammographic screening uptake: influence of different modalities of general practitioner participation. Working Group. *Tumori*, **86**, 124–129

Given-Wilson, R.M. & Blanks, R.G. (1999) Incident screening cancers detected with a second mammographic view: Pathological and radiological features. *Clin. Radiol.*, **54**, 724–735

Given-Wilson, R., Blanks, R., Moss, S.M., Ansell, J., Carter, R., Cooke, J., Dabon, L., Given-Wilson, R., Horton, P., Kissin, M., Rockall, L., Rust, A., Smee, S., Toon, E. & Vecchi, P. (1999) An evaluation of breast cancer screening in the South West (West) Region of the UK NHS Breast Screening Programme: The first 10 years. *Breast*, **8**, 66–71

GIVIO (1991) Practice of breast self-examination: Disease extent at diagnosis and patterns of surgical care. A report from an Italian study. *J. Epidemiol. Community Health*, **45**, 112–116

GIVIO (1994) Impact of follow-up testing on survival and health-related quality of life in breast cancer patients. A multicenter randomized controlled trial. The GIVIO Investigators. *J. Am. Med. Assoc.*, **271**, 1587–1592

Glanz, K., Resch, N., Lerman, C., Blake, A., Gorchov, P. & Rimer, B. (1992) Factors associated with adherence to breast cancer screening among working women. *J. Occup. Med.*, **34**, 1071–1078

Glasziou, P.P. (1992) Meta-analysis adjusting for compliance: The example of screening for breast cancer. *J. Clin. Epidemiol.*, **45**, 1251–1256

Glasziou, P., Irwig, L., Bain, C. & Colditz, G. (1999) How to review the evidence: Systematic identification and review of the scientific literature. In: *Handbook Series on Preparing Clinical Practice Guidelines*, Cambridge, Cambridge University Press, pp. 1–115

Glockner, S., Holden, M., Hilton, S. & Norcross, W. (1992) Women's attitudes toward screening mammography. *Am. J. Prev. Med.*, **8**, 69–77

Goffin, J., Chappuis, P., Wong, N. & Foulkes, W.D. (2001) Magnetic resonance imaging and mammography in women with a high hereditary risk of breast cancer. *J. Natl Cancer Inst.*, **93**, 1754–1755

Gohagan, J.K., Darby, W.P., Spitznagel, E.L., Monsees, B.S. & Tome, A.E. (1986) Radiogenic breast cancer effects of mammographic screening. *J. Natl Cancer Inst.*, **77**, 71–76

Goldschmidt, R.A. & Victor, T.A. (1996) Lobular carcinoma in situ of the breast. *Semin. Surg. Oncol*, **12**, 314–320

Gornick, M.E., Eggers, P.W., Reilly, T.W., Mentnech, R.M., Fitterman, L.K. & Kucken, L.E. (1996) Effects of race and income on mortality and use of services among Medicare beneficiaries. *New Engl. J. Med.*, **335**, 791–799

Gotzsche, P.C. & Olsen, O. (2000) Is screening for breast cancer with mammography justifiable? *Lancet*, **355**, 129–134

Gould-Martin, K, Paganini-Hill, A., Casagrande, C., Mack, T. & Ross, R.K. (1982) Behavioral and biological determinants of surgical stage of breast cancer. *Prev. Med.*, **11**, 429–440

Goyder, E., Barratt, A. & Irwig, L. (2000) Telling people about screening programmes and screening test results: How can we do it better? *J. Med. Screen.*, **7**, 123–126

Grabau, D.A., Jensen, M.B., Blichert-Toft, M., Andersen, J.A., Dyreborg, U., Carstensen, B., Al-Suliman, N.N., Graversen, H.P. & Rose, C. (1998) The importance of surgery and accurate axillary staging for survival in breast cancer. *Eur. J. Surg. Oncol.*, **24**, 499–507

Grady, K.E. (1984) Cue enhancement and the long-term practice of breast self-examination. *J. Behav. Med.*, **7**, 191–204

Grady, K., Lemkau, J., McVay, J. & Reisine, S. (1992) The importance of physician encouragement in breast cancer screening of older women. *Prev. Med.*, **21**, 766–780

Gram, I.T., Lund, E. & Slenker, S.E. (1990) Quality of life following a false positive mammogram. *Br. J Cancer*, **62**, 1018–1022

Greendale, G.A., Reboussin, B.A., Sie, A., Singh, H.R., Olson, L.K., Gatewood, O., Bassett, L.W., Wasilauskas, C., Bush, T. & Barrett-Connor, E. (1999) Effects of estrogen and estrogen–progestin on mammographic parenchymal density. Postmenopausal estrogen/progestin interventions (PEPI) investigators. *Ann. Intern. Med.*, **130**, 262–269

Greenhough, R.B. (1925) Varying degrees of malignancy in cancer of the breast. *J. Cancer Res.*, **9**, 452–463

Greenwald, P., Nasca, P.C., Lawrence, C.E., Horton, J., Mcgarrah, R.P., Gabriele, T. & Carlton, K. (1978) Estimated effect of breast self-examination and routine physician examinations on breast-cancer mortality. *New Engl. J. Med.*, **299**, 271–273

Gruvberger, S., Ringner, M., Chen, Y., Panavally, S., Saal, L.H., Borg, A., Ferno, M., Peterson, C. & Meltzer, P.S. (2001) Estrogen receptor status in breast cancer is associated with remarkably distinct gene expression patterns. *Cancer Res.*, **61**, 5979–5984

Güllberg, B., Andersson, I., Janzon, L. & Ranstam, J. (1991) Screening mammography. *Lancet*, **337**, 244

Gump, F.E. (1993) Lobular carcinoma in situ (LCIS): Pathology and treatment. *J. Cell. Biochem. Suppl.*, **17G**, 53–58

Gump, F.E., Kinne, D. & Schwartz, G.F. (1998) Current treatment for lobular carcinoma in situ. *Ann. Surg. Oncol.*, **5**, 33–36

Gunther, K., Merkelbach-Bruse, S., Amo-Takyi, B.K., Handt, S., Schroder, W. & Tietze, L. (2001) Differences in genetic alterations between primary lobular and ductal breast cancers detected by comparative genomic hybridization. *J. Pathol.*, **193**, 40–47

Haagensen, C.D. (1986) *Diseases of the Breast,* Philadelphia, Saunders

Haagensen, C.D., Lane, N., Lattes, R. & Bodian, C. (1978) Lobular neoplasia (so-called lobular carcinoma in situ) of the breast. *Cancer*, **42**, 737–769

Haagensen, C.D., Bodian, C. & Haagensen, D.E. (1981) Physicians' clinical role in the detection and diagnosis of breast carcinoma. In: *Breast Carcinoma : Risk and Detection,* Philadelphia, W.B. Saunders, pp. 395–474

de Haes, J.C., de Koning, H.J., van Oortmarssen, G.J., van Agt, H.M., de Bruyn, A.E. & van der Maas, P.J. (1991) The impact of a breast cancer screening programme on quality-adjusted life-years. *Int. J. Cancer*, **49**, 538–544

Hafslund, B. (2000) Mammography and the experience of pain and anxiety. *Radiography*, **6**, 269–272

Haiart, D.C. & Henderson, J. (1991) A comparison of interpretation of screening mammograms by a radiographer, a doctor and a radiologist: Results and implications. *Br. J. Clin. Pract.*, **45**, 43–45

Haiart, D.C., McKenzie, L., Henderson, J., Pollock, W., McQueen, D.V., Roberts, M.M. & Forrest, A.P. (1990) Mobile breast screening: Factors affecting uptake, efforts to increase response and acceptability. *Public Health*, **104**, 239–247

Hakama, M., Elovainio, L., Kajantie, R. & Louhivuori, K. (1991) Breast cancer screening as public health policy in Finland. *Br. J. Cancer*, **64**, 962–964

Hakama, M., Holli, K., Isola, J., Kallioniemi, O.P., Karkkainen, A., Visakorpi, T., Pukkala, E., Saarenmaa, I., Geiger, U. & Ikkala, J. (1995) Aggressiveness of screen-detected breast cancers. *Lancet*, **345**, 221–224

Hakama, M., Pukkala, E., Heikkilä, M. & Kallio, M. (1997) Effectiveness of the public health policy for breast cancer screening in Finland: Population based cohort study. *Br. Med. J.*, **314**, 864–867

Hakama, M., Pukkala, E., Söderman, B. & Day, N. (1999) Implementation of screening as a public health policy: Issues in design and evaluation. *J. Med. Screen.*, **6**, 209–216

Hall, D.C., Adams, C.K., Stein, G.H., Stephenson, H.S., Goldstein, M.K. & Pennypacker, H.S. (1980) Improved detection of human breast lesions following experimental training. *Cancer*, **46**, 408–414

Hammerstein, G.R., Miller, D.W., White, D.R., Masterson, M.E., Woodard, H.Q. & Laughlin, J.S. (1979) Absorbed radiation dose in mammography. *Radiology*, **130**, 485–491

Handley, R.S. (1972) Observations and thoughts on cancer of the breast. *Proc. R. Soc. Med.*, **65**, 437–444

Hankinson, S.E., Willett, W.C., Colditz, G.A., Hunter, D.J., Michaud, D.S., Deroo, B., Rosner, B., Speizer, F.E. & Pollak, M. (1998a) Circulating concentrations of insulin-like growth factor-I and risk of breast cancer. *Lancet*, **351**, 1393–1396

Hankinson, S.E., Willett, W.C., Manson, J.E., Colditz, G.A., Hunter, D.J., Spiegelman, D., Barbieri, R.L. & Speizer, F.E. (1998b) Plasma sex steroid hormone levels and risk of breast cancer in postmenopausal women. *J. Natl Cancer Inst.*, **90**, 1292–1299

Hartmann, W.H. (1984) Minimal breast cancer. An update. *Cancer*, **53**, 681–684

Hartveit, F. (1971) Prognostic typing in breast cancer. *Br. Med. J.*, **4**, 253–257

Harvey, B.J., Miller, A.B., Baines, C.J. & Corey, P.N. (1997) Effect of breast self-examination techniques on the risk of death from breast cancer. *Can. Med. Assoc. J.*, **157**, 1205–1212

Harvey, J.A., Pinkerton, J.V. & Herman, C.R. (1997) Short-term cessation of hormone replacement therapy and improvement of mammographic specificity. *J. Natl. Cancer Inst.*, **89**, 1623–1625

Hasert, V. (1988) [Radiation exposure and radiation risk of the patient in mammography]. *Radiol. Diagn. (Berl)*, **29**, 605–609 (in German)

Hatziioannou, K.A., Psarrakos, K., Molyvda-Athanasopoulou, E., Kitis, G., Papanastassiou, E., Sofroniadis, I. & Kimoundri, O. (2000) Dosimetric considerations in mammography. *Eur. Radiol.*, **10**, 1193–1196

Haughey, B.P., Marshall, J.R., Mettlin, C., Nemoto, T., Kroldart, K. & Swanson, M. (1984) Nurses' ability to detect nodules in silicone breast models. *Oncol. Nurs. Forum*, **11**, 37–42

Haus, A.G. (1999) Mammography imaging physics: Screen-film processing and viewing condition considerations. In: Haus, A.G. & Yaffe, M.J., eds, *Categorial Course in Diagnostic Radiology Physics: Physical Aspects of Breast Imaging—Current and Future Considerations*, Oak Brook, Illinois, Radiological Society of North America, pp. 59–77

Haus, A.G. & Yaffe, M.J. (2000) Screen–film and digital mammography.

Image quality and radiation dose considerations. *Radiol. Clin. North Am.*, **38**, 871–898

Haybittle, J.L. (1991) Curability of breast cancer. *Br. Med. Bull.*, **47**, 319–323

Haybittle, J.L., Blamey, R.W., Elston, C.W., Johnson, J., Doyle, P.J., Campbell, F.C., Nicholson, R.I. & Griffiths, K. (1982) A prognostic index in primary breast cancer. *Br. J. Cancer*, **45**, 361–366

Haybittle, J.L., Brinkley, D., Houghton, J., A'Hern, R.P., Baum, M. (1989) Postoperative radiotherapy and late mortality: Evidence from the Cancer Research Campaign trial for early breast cancer. *Br. Med. J.*, **298**, 1611–1614

Health Council (1987) [The early detection of breast cancer], The Hague (in Dutch)

Hedenfalk, I., Duggan, D., Chen, Y., Radmacher, M., Bittner, M., Simon, R., Meltzer, P., Gusterson, B., Esteller, M., Kallioniemi, O.P., Wilfond, B., Borg, A. & Trent, J. (2001) Gene-expression profiles in hereditary breast cancer. *New Engl. J. Med.*, **344**, 539–548

Hellman, S. (1994) Natural history of small breast cancers. Karnofsky memorial lecture. *J. Clin. Oncol.*, **12**, 2229–2234

Hendrick, R.E. & Berns, E.A. (1999) Optimizing mammographic techniques. In: Haus, A.G. & Yaffe, M.J., eds, *Categorical Course in Diagnostic Radiology Physics: Physical Aspects of Breast Imaging— Current and Future Considerations*, Oak Brook, Illinois, Radiological Society of North America, pp. 79–89

Hendrick, R.E., Botsco, M. & Plott, C.M. (1995) Quality control in mammography. *Radiol. Clin. N. Am.*, **33**, 1041–1057

Hendrick, R.E., Chrvala, C.A., Plott, C.M., Cutter, G.R., Jessop, N.W. & Wilcox-Buchall, P. (1998) Improvement in mammography quality control: 1987–1995. *Radiology*, **207**, 663–668

Hendrick, E., Klabunde, C., Grivegnee, A., Pou, G. & Ballard-Barbash, R. (2002) Quality control practices in mammography screening programs in 22 countries. *Int. J. Qual. Health Care* (in press)

Henry-Lee, A. & Yearwood, A. (1999) *Protecting the Poor and the Medically Indigent under Health Insurance: A Case Study of Jamaica* (Small Applied Research, No. 6), Bethesda, Maryland, Partnerships for Health Reform

Henson, D.E., Ries, L., Freedman, L.S. & Carriaga, M. (1991) Relationship among outcome, stage of disease, and histologic grade for 22,616 cases of breast cancer. The basis for a prognostic index. *Cancer*, **68**, 2142–2149

Hermon, C. & Beral, V. (1996) Breast cancer mortality rates are leveling off or beginning to decline in many western countries: Analysis of time trends, age–cohort and age–period models of breast cancer mortality in 20 countries. *Br. J. Cancer*, **73**, 955–960.

Hewitt, M., Breen, N. & Devesa, S.S. (1999) Cancer prevalence and survivorship issues: Analysis of the 1992 national health interview survey. *J. Natl Cancer Inst.*, **91**, 1480–1486

Heywang-Köbrunner, S.H., Hilbertz, T., Pruss, E., Wolf, A., Permanetter, W., Eiermann, W. & Lissner, J. (1988) [Dynamic contrast medium examination with FLASH during magnetic resonance imaging of the breast]. *Digitale Biddiagn*, **8**, 7–13 (in German)

Hildreth, N.G., Shore, R.E. & Dvoretsky, P.M. (1989) The risk of breast cancer after irradiation of the thymus in infancy. *New Engl. J. Med.*, **321**, 1281–1284

Hill, D., Rassaby, J. & Gray, N. (1982) Health education about breast cancer using television and doctor involvement. *Prev. Med.*, **11**, 43–55

Hislop, T.G., Coldman, A.J. & Skippen, D.H. (1984) Breast self-examination: Importance of technique in early diagnosis. *Can. Med. Assoc. J.*, **131**, 1349–1352

Hoare, T., Thomas, C., Biggs, A., Booth, M., Bradley, S. & Friedman, E. (1994) Can the uptake of breast screening by Asian women be increased? A randomized controlled trial of a linkworker intervention. *J. Public Health Med.*, **16**, 179–185

Hoeijmakers, J.H. (2001) Genomic maintenance mechanisms for preventing cancer. *Nature*, **441**, 366–367

Hoffman-Goetz, L., Breen, N. & Meissner, H. (1998) The impact of social class on the use of cancer screening within three racial/ethnic groups in the United States. *Ethnicity Dis.*, **8**, 43–51

Holland, R., Hendriks, J.H., Vebeek, A.L., Mravunac, M. & Schuurmans Stekhoven, J.H. (1990) Extent, distribution, and mammographic/histological correlations of breast ductal carcinoma in situ. *Lancet*, **335**, 519–522

Holland, R., Peterse, J.L., Millis, R.R., Eusebi, V., Faverly, D., van de Vijver, M.J. & Zafrani, B. (1994) Ductal carcinoma in situ: A proposal for a new classification. *Semin. Diagn. Pathol.*, **11**, 167–180

Holmberg, L., Ekbom, A., Calle, E., Mokdad, A. & Byers, T. (1997) Breast cancer mortality in relation to self-reported use of breast self-examination. A cohort study of 450,000 women. *Breast Cancer Res. Treat.*, **43**, 137–140

Hopkins, R. & Hensley, K. (1993) Breast cancer screening in Florida. Opportunities for prevention. *J. Florida Med. Assoc.*, **80**, 178–180

Horton Taylor, D., McPherson, K., Parbhoo, S. & Perry, N. (1996) Response of women aged 65–74 to invitation for screening for breast cancer by mammography: A pilot study in London, UK. *J. Epidemiol. Community Health*, **50**, 77–80

Howe, H.L. (1980) Proficiency in performing breast self-examination. *Patient Couns. Health Educ.*, **2**, 151–153

Howe, G.R., Sherman, G.J., Semenciw, R.M. & Miller, A.B. (1981) Estimated benefits and risks of screening for breast cancer. *Can. Med. Assoc. J.*, **124**, 399–403

Howe, H.L., Wingo, P.A., Thun, M.J., Ries, L.A., Rosenberg, H.M., Feigal, E.G. & Edwards, B.K. (2001) Annual report to the nation on the status of cancer (1973 through 1998), featuring cancers with recent increasing trends. *J. Natl Cancer Inst.*, **93**, 824–842

Huguley, C.M., Jr, Brown, R.L., Greenberg, R.S. & Clark, W.S. (1988) Breast self-examination and survival from breast cancer. *Cancer*, **62**, 1389–1396

Hurley, S.F., Huggins, R.M., Jolley, D.J. & Reading, D. (1994) Recruitment activities and sociodemographic factors that predict attendance at a mammographic screening program. *Am. J. Public Health*, **84**, 1655–1658

IARC (1997) *Biennal Report 1996–1997*, Lyon, IARC Press, p.131

IARC (2000) *IARC Monographs on the Evaluation of Carcinogenic Risks to Humans*, Vol. 75, *Ionizing Radiation, Part I, X- and Gamma-radiation and Neutrons*, Lyon, IARCPress

ICRP (1982) *Protection of the Patient in Diagnostic Radiology* (ICRP Publication No. 34), Oxford

ICRP (1987) *Statement from the 1987 Como Meeting of the ICRP* (ICRP Publication No. 52), Oxford

ICRP (1991) *Recommendations of the International Commission on Radiological Protection 1990* (ICRP Publication No. 60), Oxford

Ikeda, D.M., Andersson, I., Wattsgård, C., Janzon, L. & Linell, F. (1992) Interval carcinomas in the Malmö mammographic screening trial; radiographic appearance and prognostic considerations. *Am. J. Roentgenol.*, **159**, 287–294

Irwig, L., Turnbull, D. & McMurchie, M. (1990) A randomised trial of general practitioner-written invitations to encourage attendance at screening mammography. *Community Health Stud.*, **14**, 357–364

Isaacs, C., Stearns, V., Hayes, D.F. (2001) New prognostic factors for breast cancer recurrence. *Semin. Oncol.*, **28**, 53–67

Jacob, T.C., Penn, N.E., Giebink, J. & Bastien, R. (1994) A comparison of breast self-examination and clinical examination. *J. Natl Med. Assoc.*, **86**, 40–45

Jacobson, J.A., Danforth, D.N., Cowan, K.H., d'Angelo, T., Steinberg, S.M., Pierce, L., Lippman, M.E., Lichter, A.S., Glatstein, E. & Okunieff, P. (1995) Ten-year results of a comparison of conservation with mastectomy in the treatment of stage I and II breast cancer. *New Engl. J. Med.*, **332**, 907–911

Janz, N.K., Becker, M.H., Anderson, L.A. & Marcoux, B.C. (1989) Interventions to enhance breast self-examination practice: A review. *Public Health Rev.*, **17**, 89–163

Janz, N.K., Schottenfeld, D., Doerr, K.M., Selig, S.M., Dunn, R.L., Strawderman, M. & Levine, P.A. (1997) A two-step intervention of increase mammography among women aged 65 and older. *Am. J. Public Health*, **87**, 1683–1686

Janzon, L. & Andersson, I. (1990) *Cancer Screening*, New York, Cambridge University Press, pp. 37–44

Jenkins, C.N., McPhee, S.J., Bird, J.A., Pham, G.Q., Nguyen, B.H., Nguyen, T., Lai, K.Q., Wong, C. & Davis, T.B. (1999) Effect of a media-led education campaign on breast and cervical cancer screening among Vietnamese–American women. *Prev. Med.*, **28**, 395–406

Jensen, R.A., Page, D.L., Dupont, W.D. & Rogers, L.W. (1989) Invasive breast cancer risk in women with sclerosing adenosis. *Cancer*, **64**, 1977–1983

Joensuu, H. & Toikkanen, S. (1995) Cured of breast cancer? *J. Clin. Oncol.*, **13**, 62–69

Joensuu, H., Klemi, P.J., Tuominen, J., Räsänen, O. & Parvinen, I. (1992) Breast cancer found at screening and previous detection by women themselves. *Lancet*, **339**, 315

Johnston, K. (2001) Modelling the future costs of breast screening. *Eur. J. Cancer*, **37**, 1752–1758

Johnston, M. & Voegele, C. (1993) Benefits of psychological preparation for surgery: A meta-analysis. *Ann. Behav. Med.*, **15**, 205–246

Jonsson, H., Nystrom, L., Tornberg, S. & Lenner, P. (2001) Service screening with mammography of women aged 50–69 years in Sweden: Effects on mortality from breast cancer. *J. Med. Screen.*, **8**, 152–160

Julien, J.P., Bijker, N., Fontiman, I.S., Peterse, J.L., Delledonne, V., Rouanet, P., Avril, A., Sylvester, R., Mignolet, F., Bartelink, H. & van Dongen, J.A. (2000) Radiotherapy in breast-conserving treatment for ductal carcinoma in situ: first results of the EORTC randomised phase III trial 10853. EORTC Breast Cancer Cooperative Group and EORTC Radiotherapy Group. *Lancet*, **355**, 528–533

Jung, H. (2001) [Assessment of usefulness and risk of mammography screening with exclusive attention to radiation risk.] *Radiologe*, **41**, 385–395 (in German)

Kahn, K.L. & Goldberg, R.J. (1984) Screening for breast cancer in the ambulatory setting. *Clin. Res.*, **32**, A649

Kaiser, W.A. (1989) [Results of magnetic resonance imaging of the breast on 253 cases] *Dtsch. Med. Wochenschrift*, **114**, 1351–1357 (in German)

Kanemura, S., Tsuji, I., Ohuchi, N., Takei, H., Yokoe, T., Koibuchi, Y., Ohnuki, K., Fukao, A., Satomi, S. & Hisamichi, S. (1999) A case control study on the effectiveness of breast cancer screening by clinical breast examination in Japan. *Jpn. J. Cancer Res.*, **90**, 607–613

Kaufman, Z., Garstin, W.I., Hayes, R., Michell, M.J. & Baum, M. (1991) The mammographic parenchymal patterns of women on hormonal replacement therapy. *Clin. Radiol.*, **43**, 389–392

Kavanagh, A.M., Mitchell, H. & Giles, G.G. (2000) Hormone replacement therapy and accuracy of mammographic screening. *Lancet*, **355**, 270–274

Kee, F., Telford, A., Donaghy, P. & O'Doherty, A. (1992) Attitude or access: Reasons for not attending mammography in Northern Ireland. *Eur. J. Cancer Prev.*, **1**, 311–315

Keemers-Gels, M., Groenendijk, R., van den Heuvel, J., Boetes, C., Peer, P. & Wobbes, T. (2000) Pain experienced by women attending breast cancer screening. *Breast Cancer Res. Treat.*, **60**, 235–240

Kerlikowske, K., Grady, D., Barclay, J., Sickles, E.A., Eaton, A. & Ernster, V. (1993) Positive predictive value of screening mammography by age and family history of breast cancer. *J. Am. Med. Assoc.*, **270**, 2444–2450

Kerlikowske, K., Grady, D., Rubin, S.M., Sandrock, C. & Ernster, V.L. (1995) Efficacy of screening mammography. A meta-analysis. *J. Am. Med. Assoc.*, **273**, 149–154

Kerlikowske, K., Salzmann, P., Phillips, K.A., Cauley, J.A. & Cummings, S.R. (1999) Continuing screening mammography in women aged 70 to 79 years: Impact on life expectancy and cost–effectiveness. *J. Am. Med. Assoc.*, **282**, 2156–2163

Kerlikowske, K., Carney, P.A., Geller, B., Mandelson, M.T., Taplin, S.H., Malvin, K., Ernster, V., Urban, N., Cutter, G., Rosenberg, R. & Ballard-Barbash, R. (2000) Performance of screening mammography among women with and without a first-degree relative with breast cancer. *Ann. Intern. Med.*, **133**, 855–863

Kimme-Smith, C., Rothschild, P.A., Bassett, L.W., Gold, R.H. & Moler, C. (1989) Mammographic film processor and temperature, development time, and chemistry: Effect on dose, contrast, and noise. *Am. J. Roentgenol.*, **152**, 35–40

Kirkpatrick, A., Tornberg, S. & Thijssen, M.A. (1993) European Guidelines for Quality Assurance in Mammography Screening (EUR 14821 EN), Brussels, Commission of the European Communities

Kitahara, O., Furukawa, Y., Tanaka, T., Kihara, C., Ono, K., Yanagawa, R., Nita, M.E., Takagi, T., Nakamura, Y. & Tsunoda, T. (2001) Alterations of gene expression during colorectal carcinogenesis revealed by cDNA microarrays after laser-capture microdissection of tumor tissues and normal epithelia. *Cancer Res.*, **61**, 3544–3549

Klabunde, C., Bouchard, F., Taplin, S., Scharpantgen, A. & Ballard-Barbash, R. (2001a) Quality assurance for screening mammography: An international comparison. *J. Epidemiol. Community Health*, **55**, 204–212

Klabunde, C.N., Sancho-Garnier, H., Broeders, M., Thoresen, S., Rodrigues, V.J.L. & Ballard-Barbash, R. (2001b) Quality assurance for screening mammography: Data collection systems in 22 countries. *Int. J. Technol. Assess. Health Care*, **17**, 528–541

Klein, R., Aichinger, H., Dierker, J., Jansen, J.T., Joite-Barfuss, S., Sabel, M., Schulz-Wendtland, R. & Zoetelief, J. (1997) Determination of average glandular dose with modern mammography units for two large groups of patients. *Phys. Med. Biol.*, **42**, 651–671

Klemi, P.J., Joensuu, H., Toikkanen, S., Tuominen, J., Rasanen, O., Tyrkko, J. & Parvinen, I. (1992) Aggressiveness of breast cancers found with and without screening. *Br. Med. J.*, **304**, 467–469

Kliewer, E.V. & Smith, K.R. (1995) Breast cancer mortality among immigrants in Australia and Canada. *J. Natl Cancer Inst.*, **87**, 1154–1161

Kohatsu, N., Cramer, E. & Bohnstedt, M. (1994) Use of a clinician reminder system for screening mammography in a public health clinic. *Am. J. Prev. Med.*, **10**, 348–352

Koibuchi, Y., Iino, Y., Takei, H., Maemura, M., Horiguchi, J., Yokoe, T. & Morishita, Y. (1998) The effect of mass screening by physical examination combined with regular breast self-examination on clinical stage and course of Japanese women with breast cancer. *Oncol. Rep.*, **5**, 151–155

Kolb, T.M., Lichy, J. & Newhouse, J.H. (1998) Occult cancer in women with dense breasts: Detection with screening ultrasound–diagnostic yield and tumor characteristics. *Radiology*, **207**, 191–199

Kollias, J., Sibbering, D.M., Blamey, R.W., Holland, P.A., Obuszko, Z., Wilson, A.R., Evans, A.J., Ellis, I.O. & Elston, C.W. (1998) Screening women aged less than 50 years with a family history of breast cancer. *Eur. J. Cancer*, **34**, 878–883

de Koning, H.J. (1995) Screening for breast cancer, time to think—and stop? National Evaluation Team for Breast Cancer Screening (NETB). *Lancet*, **346**, 438–439

de Koning, H.J. (2000a) Assessment of nationwide cancer-screening programmes. *Lancet*, **355**, 80–81

de Koning, H.J. (2000b) Breast cancer screening: Cost–effective in practice? *Eur. J. Radiol.*, **33**, 32–37

de Koning, H.J., van Ineveld, B.M., van Oortmarssen, G.J., de Haes, J.C., Collette, H.J., Hendriks, J.H. & van der Maas, P.J. (1991) Breast cancer screening and cost–effectiveness: Policy alternatives, quality of life considerations and the possible impact of uncertain factors. *Int. J. Cancer*, **49**, 531–537

de Koning, H.J., van Ineveld, B.M., de Haes, J.C., van Oortmarssen, G.J., Klijn, J.G. & van der Maas, P.J. (1992) Advanced breast cancer and its prevention by screening. *Br. J. Cancer*, **65**, 950–955

de Koning, H.J., Boer, R., Warmerdam, P.G., Beemsterboer, P.M. & van der Maas, P.J. (1995a) Quantitative interpretation of age-specific mortality reductions from the Swedish breast cancer-screening trials. *J. Natl Cancer Inst.*, **87**, 1217–1223

de Koning, H.J., Fracheboud, J., Boer, R., Verbeek, A.L.M., Collette, H.J.A., Hendriks, J.H.C.L., van Ineveld, B.M., de Bruyn, A.E. & van der Maas, P.J. (1995b) Nation-wide breast cancer screening in The Netherlands: Support for breast-cancer mortality reduction. *Int. J. Cancer*, **60**, 777–780

Kopans, D.B. (1992) The positive predictive value of mammography. *Am. J. Roentgenol.*, **158**, 521–526

Kopans, D.B. (1993) Mammography [Letter]. *Lancet*, **341**, 957

Kopans, D.B. & Feig, S.A. (1993) The Canadian National Breast Cancer Screening Study: A critical review. *Am. J. Roentgenol.*, **161**, 755–760

Kopans, D.B., Moore, R.H., McCarthy, K.A., Hall, D.A., Hulka, C.A., Whitman, G.J., Slanetz, P.J. & Halpern, E.F. (1996) Positive predictive value of breast biopsy performed as a result of mammography: There is no abrupt change at age 50 years. *Radiology*, **200**, 357–360

Kotwall, C.A., Covington, D.L., Rutledge, R., Churchill, M.P. & Meyer. A.A. (1996) Patient, hospital and surgeon factors associated with breast conserving surgery. A statewide analysis in North Carolina. *Ann. Surg.*, **224**, 419–429

Krag, D., Weaver, D., Ashikaga, T., Moffat, F., Klimberg, V.S., Shriver, C., Feldman, S., Kusminsky, R., Gadd, M., Kuhn, J., Harlow, S. & Beitsch, P. (1998) The sentinel node in breast cancer—A multicenter validation study. *New Engl.J. Med.*, **339**, 941–946

Kramer, W.M. & Rush, B.F. (1973) Mammary duct proliferation in the elderly. A histopathologic study. *Cancer*, **31**, 130–137

Kricker, A., Farac, K., Smith, D., Sweeny, A., McCredie, M. & Armstrong, B.K. (1999) Breast cancer in New South Wales in 1972–1995: Tumor size and the impact of mammographic screening. *Int. J. Cancer*, **81**, 877–880

Kroman, N., Jensen, M.B., Wohlfahrt, J., Mouridsen, H.T., Andersen, P.K. & Melbye, M. (2000) Factors influencing the effect of age on prognosis in breast cancer: Population based study. *Br. Med. J.*, **320**, 474–479

Kuhl, C.K., Schmutzler, R.K., Leutner, C.C., Kempe, A., Wardelmann, E., Hocke, A., Maringa, M., Pfeifer, U., Krebs, D. & Schild, H.H. (2000) Breast MR imaging screening in 192 women proved or suspected to be carriers of a breast cancer susceptibility gene: Preliminary results. *Radiology*, **215**, 267–279

Kuroishi, T., Tominaga, S., Ota, J., Horino, T., Taguchi, T., Ishida, T., Yokoe, T., Izuo, M., Ogita, M., Itoh, S., Abe, R., Yoshida, K., Morimoto, T., Enomoto, K., Tashiro, H., Kashiki, Y., Yamamoto, S., Kido, C., Honda, K., Saskawa, M., Fukuda, M. & Watanabe, H. (1992) The effect of breast self-examination on early detection and survival. *Jpn. J. Cancer Res.*, **83**, 344–350

Kuroishi, T., Hirose, K., Suzuki, T. & Tominaga, S. (2000) Effectiveness of mass screening for breast cancer in Japan. *Breast Cancer*, **7**, 1–8

Läärä, E., Day, N. & Hakama, M. (1987) Trends in mortality from cervical cancer in the Nordic countries: Association with organized screening programmes. *Lancet*, **i**, 1247–1249

Lagerlund, M., Hedin, A., Sparen, P., Thurfjell, E. & Lambe, M. (2000a) Attitudes, beliefs, and knowledge as predictors of nonattendance in a Swedish population-based mammography screening program. *Prev. Med.*, **31**, 417–428

Lagerlund, M., Sparen, P., Thurfjell, E., Ekbom, A. & Lambe, M. (2000b) Predictors of non-attendance in a population-based mammography screening programme; socio-demographic factors and aspects of health behaviour. *Eur. J. Cancer Prev.*, **9**, 25–33

Lagerlund, M., Widmark, C., Lambe, M. & Tishleman, C. (2001) Rationales for attending or not attending mammography screening: A focus group study among women in Sweden. *Eur. J. Cancer Prev.*, **10**, 429–442

Lakhani, S.R., Collins, N., Stratton, M.R. & Sloane, J.P. (1995) Atypical ductal hyperplasia of the breast: Clonal proliferation with loss of heterozygosity on chromosomes 16q and 17p. *J. Clin. Pathol.*, **48**, 611–615

Lakhani, S.R., Jacquemier, J., Sloane, J.P., Gusterson, B.A., Anderson, T.J., van de Vijver, M.J., Farid, L.M., Venter, D., Antoniou, A., Storfer-Isser, A., Smyth, E., Steel, C.M., Haites, N., Scott, R.J., Goldgar, D., Neuhausen, S., Daly, P.A., Ormiston, W., McManus, R., Scherneck, S., Ponder, B.A., Ford, D., Peto, J., Stoppa-Lyonnet, D. & Easton, D.F. (1998) Multifactorial analysis of differences between sporadic breast cancers and cancers involving BRCA1 and BRCA2 mutations. *J. Natl Cancer Inst.*, **90**, 1138–1145

Lalloo, F., Boggis, C.R., Evans, D.G., Shenton, A., Threlfall, A.G. & Howell, A. (1998) Screening by mammography, women with a family history of breast cancer. *Eur. J. Cancer*, **34**, 937–940

Lampejo, O.T., Barnes, D.M., Smith, P. & Millis, R.R. (1994) Evaluation of infiltrating ductal carcinomas with a DCIS component: Correlation of the histologic type of the in situ component with grade of the infiltrating component. *Semin. Diagn. Pathol.*, **11**, 215–222

de Landtsheer, J.P., Delanoy-Ortega, O.B. & Jemelin, C. (2000) [Breast cancer screening: Comparative analysis of three Swiss programmes.] *Med. Hyg.*, **2306**, 1407–1410 (in French)

Lane, D. & Messina, C. (1999) Methodology for targeting physicians for interventions to improve breast cancer screening. *Am. J. Prev. Med.*, **16**, 289–297

Lane, D.S., Messina, C.R. & Grimson, R. (2001) An educational approach to improving physician breast cancer screening practices and counseling skills. *Patient Educ. Couns.*, **43**, 287–299

Lantz, P., Stencil, D., Lippert, M., Beversdorf, S., Jaros, L. & Remington, P. (1995) Breast and cervical cancer screening in a low-income managed care sample: The efficacy of physician letters and phone calls. *Am. J. Public Health*, **85**, 834–836

Larsson, L.G., Andersson, I., Bjurstam, N., Fagerberg, G., Frisell, J., Tabár, L. & Nyström, L. (1997) Updated overview of the Swedish randomized trials on breast cancer screening with mammography: Age group 40–49 at randomization. *Natl Cancer Inst. Monogr.*, **22**, 57–61

Last, J.M. (1995) *A Dictionary of Epidemiology*, New York, Oxford University Press, p. 52

Lau, Y., Lau, P.Y., Chan, C.M. & Yip, A. (1998) The potential impact of breast cancer screening in Hong Kong. *Aust. N.Z. J. Surg.*, **68**, 707–711

La Vecchia, C., Negri, E., Levi, F., Decarli, A. & Boyle, P. (1998) Cancer mortality in Europe: Effects of age, cohort of birth and period of death. *Eur. J. Cancer*, **34**, 118–141

Law, J. (1987) Cancers induced and cancers detected in a mammography screening programme. *Br. J. Radiol.*, **60**, 231–234

Lawson, H.W., Henson, R., Bobo, J.K. & Kaeser, M.K. (2000) Implementing recommendations for the early detection of breast and cervical cancer among low-income women. *Morbid. Mortal. Weekly Rep.*, **49**, 35–55

Laya, M.B., Gallagher, J.C., Schreiman, J.S., Larson, E.B., Watson, P. & Weinstein, L. (1995) Effect of postmenopausal hormonal replacement therapy on mammographic density and parenchymal pattern. *Radiology*, **196**, 433–437

Laya, M.B., Larson, E.B., Taplin, S.H. & White, E. (1996) Effect of oestrogen replacement therapy on the specificity and sensitivity of screening mammography. *J. Natl Cancer Inst.*, **88**, 643–649

Le Doussal, V., Tubiana-Hulin, M., Friedman, S., Hacene, K., Spyratos, F. & Brunet, M. (1989) Prognostic value of histologic grade nuclear components of Scarff-Bloom-Richardson (SBR). An improved score modification based on a multivariate analysis of 1262 invasive ductal breast carcinomas. *Cancer*, **64**, 1914–1921

Lee, B.J., Hauser, H. & Pack, G.T. (1934) Gelatinous carcinoma of the breast. *Surg. Gynecol. Obstet.*, **59**, 841–850

Le Geyte, M., Mant, D., Vessey, M.P., Jones, L. & Yudkin, P. (1992) Breast self-examination and survival from breast cancer. *Br. J. Cancer*, **66**, 917–918

van Leiden, H.A., Gessel-Dabekaussen, A.A., van der Maas, P.J. & de Koning, H.J. (1999) Trends in mammography 1991–96 and the impact of nationwide screening in The Netherlands. *J. Med. Screen.*, **6**, 94–98

Leivo, T., Salminen, T., Sintonen, H., Tuominen, R., Auerma, K., Partanen, K., Saari, U., Hakama, M. & Heinonen, O.P. (1999) Incremental cost-effectiveness of double-reading mammograms. *Breast Cancer Res. Treat.*, **54**, 261–267

Lenner, P. (1990) The excess mortality rate. A useful concept in cancer epidemiology. *Acta Oncol.*, **29**, 573–576

Lenner, P. & Jonsson, H. (1997) Excess mortality from breast cancer in relation to mammography screening in northern Sweden. *J. Med. Screen.*, **4**, 6–9

Lerman, C., Trock, B., Rimer, B.K., Boyce, A., Jepson, C. & Engstrom, P.F. (1991) Psychological and behavioral implications of abnormal mammograms. *Ann. Intern. Med.*, **114**, 657–661

Lewin, J.M., Hendrick, R.E., D'Orsi, C.J., Isaacs, P.K., Moss, L.J., Karellas, A., Sisney, G.A., Kuni, C.C. & Cutter, G.R. (2001) Comparison of full-field digital mammography with screen–film mammography for cancer detection: Results of 4,945 paired examinations. *Radiology*, **218**, 873–880

Liberman, L., LaTrenta, L.R., van Zee, K.J., Morris, E.A., Abramson, A.F. & Dershaw, D.D. (1997) Stereotactic core biopsy of calcifications highly suggestive of malignancy. *Radiology*, **203**, 673–677

Libstug, A.R., Moravan, V. & Aitken, S.E. (1998) Results from the Ontario breast screening program, 1990–1995. *J. Med. Screen.*, **5**, 73–80

Lidbrink, E., Elfving, J., Frisell, J. & Jonsson, E. (1996) Neglected aspects of false positive findings of mammography in breast cancer screening: Analysis of false positive cases from the Stockholm trial. *Br. Med. J.*, **312**, 273–276

Lilford, R.J.B.D., Greenhalgh, R. & Edwards, S.J.L. (2000) Trials and fast changing technologies: The case for tracker studies. *Br. Med. J.*, **320**, 43–46

Lindfors, K.K., O'Connor, J. & Parker, R.A. (2001) False-positive screening mammograms: Effect of immediate versus later work-up on patient stress. *Radiology*, **218**, 247–253

Lindstrom, P., Janzon, L. & Sternby, N.H. (1997) Declining autopsy rate in Sweden: A study of causes and consequences in Malmo, Sweden. *J. Intern. Med.*, **242**, 157–165

Linver, M.N., Paster, S.B., Rosenberg, R.D., Key, C.R., Stidley, C.A. & King, W.V. (1992) Improvement in mammography interpretation skills in a community radiology practice after dedicated teaching courses: 2-year medical audit of 38,633 cases. *Radiology*, **184**, 39–43

Little, M.P. (2001) Comparison of the risks of cancer incidence and mortality following radiation therapy for benign and malignant disease with the cancer risks observed in the Japanese A-bomb survivors. *Int. J. Radiat. Biol.*, **77**, 431–464

Locker, A.P., Ellis, I.O., Morgan, D.A., Elston, C.W., Mitchell, A. & Blamey, R.W. (1989a) Factors influencing local recurrence after excision and radiotherapy for primary breast cancer. *Br. J. Surg.*, **76**, 890–894

Locker, A.P., Caseldine, J., Mitchell, A.K., Blamey, R.W., Roebuck, E.J. & Elston, C.W. (1989b) Results from a seven-year programme of breast self-examination in 89,010 women. *Br. J. Cancer*, **60**, 401–405

Lopez-Carrillo, L., Bravo-Alvarado, J., Poblano-Verastegui, O. & Ortega Altamirano, D. (1997) Reproductive determinants of breast cancer in Mexican women. *Ann. N.Y. Acad. Sci.*, **837**, 537–550

Lopez-Carrillo, L., Torres-Sanchez, L., Lopez-Cervantes, M. & Rueda-Neria, C. (2001) [Identification of malignant breast lesions in Health Mexico.]. *Publica Mexico*, **43**, 199–202 (in Spanish)

Lostao, L. & Joiner, T. (2001) Health-oriented behaviors: Their implication in attending for breast cancer screening. *Am. J. Health Behav.*, **25**, 21–32

Lostao, L., Joiner, T., Pettit, J., Chorot, P. & Sandin, B. (2001) Health beliefs and illness attitudes as predictors of breast cancer screening attendance. *Eur. J. Public Health*, **11**, 274–279

Lu, Z. (1995) Variables associated with breast self–examination among Chinese women. *Cancer Nurs.*, **18**, 29–34

Lu, Y.J., Osin, P., Lakhani, S.R., di Palma, S., Gusterson, B.A. & Shipley, J.M. (1998)

Comparative genomic hybridization analysis of lobular carcinoma in situ and atypical lobular hyperplasia and potential roles for gains and losses of genetic material in breast neoplasia. *Cancer Res.*, **58**, 4721–4727

Lungdren, B. (1977) The oblique view at mammography. *Br. J. Radiol.*, **50**, 626–628

Ma, L., Fishell, E., Wright, B., Hanna, W., Allan, S. & Boyd, N.F. (1992) Case–control study of factors associated with failure to detect breast cancer by mammography. *J. Natl Cancer Inst.*, **84**, 781–785

Maddox, W.A., Carpenter, J.T., Jr, Laws, H.L., Soong, S.J., Cloud, G., Urist, M.M. & Balch, C.M. (1983) A randomized prospective trial of radical (Halsted) mastectomy versus modified radical mastectomy in 311 breast cancer patients. *Ann. Surg.*, **198**, 207–212

Mainiero, M., Schepps, B., Clements, N. & Bird, C. (2001) Mammography-related anxiety: Effect of preprocedural patient education. *Women's Health Issues*, **11**, 110–115

Malich, A., Boehm, T., Facius, M., Freesmeyer, M.G., Fleck, M., Anderson, R. & Kaiser, W.A. (2001) Differentiation of mammographically suspicious lesions: Evaluation of breast ultrasound, MRI mammography and electrical impedance scanning as adjunctive technologies in breast cancer detection. *Clin Radiol.*, **56**, 278–283

Mammography Screening Evaluation Group (1998) Mammography screening for breast cancer in Copenhagen 1991–1997. *APMIS*, **83** (Suppl. 106), 1–44

Mamon, J. & Zapka, J. (1983) Determining the quality of breast self-examination and its relationship to other breast self-examination measures. *Prog. Clin. Biol. Res.*, **130**, 313–322

Man, S., Ellis, I.O., Sibbering, M., Blamey, R.W. & Brook, J.D. (1996) High levels of allele loss at the FHIT and ATM genes in non-comedo ductal carcinoma in situ and grade I tubular invasive breast cancers. *Cancer Res.*, **56**, 5484–5489

Mandelblatt, J. & Yabroff, K. (1999) Effectiveness of interventions designed to increase mammography use: A meta-analysis of provider-targeted strategies. *Cancer Epidemiol. Biomarkers Prev.*, **8**, 759–767

Mandelblatt, J., Traxler, M., Lakin, P., Kanetsky, P. & Kao, R. (1993a) Targeting

breast and cervical cancer screening to elderly poor black women: Who will participate? *Prev. Med.*, **22**, 20–33

Mandelblatt, J., Traxler, M., Lakin, P., Thomas, L., Chauhan, P., Matseoane, S. & Kanetsky, P. (1993b) A nurse practitioner intervention to increase breast and cervical cancer screening for poor, elderly black women. The Harlem study team. *J. Gen. Intern. Med.*, **8**, 173–178

Mandelblatt, J.S., Gold, K., O'Malley, A.S., Taylor, K., Cagney, K., Hopkins, J.S. & Kerner, J. (1999) Breast and cervix cancer screening among multiethnic women: Role of age, health, and source of care. *Prev. Med.*, **28**, 418–425

Mandelson, M.T., Oestreicher, N., Porter, P.L., White, D., Finder, C.A., Taplin, S.H. & White, E. (2000) Breast density as a predictor of mammographic detection: Comparison of interval- and screen-detected cancers. *J. Natl Cancer Inst.*, **92**, 1081–1087

Manfredi, C., Czaja, R., Freels, S., Trubitt, M., Warnecke, R. & Lacey, L. (1998) Prescribe for health. Improving cancer screening in physician practices serving low-income and minority populations. *Arch. Fam. Med.*, **7**, 329–337

Mant, D., Vessey, M.P., Neil, A., Mcpherson, K. & Jones, L. (1987) Breast self examination and breast cancer stage at diagnosis. *Br. J. Cancer*, **55**, 207–211

Maraste, R., Brandt, L., Olsson, H. & Ryde-Brandt, B. (1992) Anxiety and depression in breast cancer patients at start of adjuvant radiotherapy. Relations to age and type of surgery. *Acta Oncol.*, **31**, 641–643

Marcus, J.N., Watson, P., Page, D.L., Narod, S.A., Lenoir, G.M., Tonin, P., Linder-Stephenson, L., Salerno, G., Conway, T.A. & Lynch, H.T. (1996) Hereditary breast cancer: Pathobiology, prognosis, and BRCA1 and BRCA2 gene linkage. *Cancer*, **77**, 697–709

Margolese, R. (1999) Surgical considerations for invasive breast cancer. *Surg. Clin. North Am.*, **79**, 1031–1046

Margolis, K.L., Lurie, N., McGovern, P. & Slater, J.S. (1993) Predictors of failure to attend scheduled mammography appointments at a public teaching hospital. *J. Gen. Intern. Med.*, **8**, 602–605

Marshall, L.M., Hunter, D.J., Connolly, J.L., Schnitt, S.J., Byrne, C., London, S.J. & Colditz, G.A. (1997) Risk of breast cancer associated with atypical hyperplasia of lobular and ductal types. *Cancer Epidemiol. Biomarkers Prev.*, **6**, 297–301

Mattsson, A., Leitz, W. & Rutqvist, L.E. (2000) Radiation risk and mammographic screening of women from 40 to 49 years of age: Effect on breast cancer rates and years of life. *Br. J. Cancer*, **82**, 220–226

Maxwell, C.J., Bancej, C.M. & Snider, J. (2001) Predictors of mammography use among Canadian women aged 50–69: Findings from the 1996/97 National Population Health Survey. *Can. Med. Assoc. J.*, **164**, 329–334

May, D.S., Lee, N.C., Nadel, M.R., Henson, R.M. & Miller, D.S. (1998) The National Breast and Cervical Cancer Early Detection Program: Report on the first 4 years of mammography provided to medically underserved women. *Am. J. Roentgenol.*, **170**, 97–104

Mayer, J., Clapp, E., Bartholomew, S. & Offer, J. (1994) Facility-based inreach strategies to promote annual mammograms. *Am. J. Prev. Med.*, **10**, 353–356

McCann, J., Wait, S., Seradour, B. & Day, N. (1997) A comparison of the performance and impact of breast cancer screening programmes in East Anglia, UK, and Bouches du Rhone, France. *Eur. J. Cancer*, **33**, 429–435

McCann, J., Stockton, D. & Day, N.E. (1998) Breast cancer in East Anglia: The impact of the breast screening programme on stage at diagnosis. *J. Med. Screen.*, **5**, 42–48

McCann, J., Duffy, S., Day, N. & Warren, R. (2001) Predicted long-term breast cancer mortality reduction associated with the second round of breast screening in East Anglia. *Br. J. Cancer*, **84**, 423–428

McDermott, M.M., Dolan, N.C., Huang, J., Reifler, D. & Rademaker, A.W. (1996) Lump detection is enhanced in silicone breast models simulating postmenopausal breast tissue. *J. Gen. Intern. Med.*, **11**, 112–114

McDivitt, R.W., Boyce, W. & Gersell, D. (1982) Tubular carcinoma of the breast. Clinical and pathological observations concerning 135 cases. *Am. J. Surg. Pathol.*, **6**, 401–411

McFarlane, M.J., Feinstein, A.R., Wells, C.K. & Chan, C.K. (1987) The 'epidemiologic necropsy': Unexpected detections, demographic selections, and changing rates of lung cancer. *J. Am. Med. Assoc.*, **258**, 331–338

McNicholas, M.M., Heneghan, J.P., Milner, M.H., Tunney, T., Hourihane, J.B. & MacErlaine, D.P. (1994) Pain and increased mammographic density in women receiving hormone replacement therapy: A prospective study. *Am. J. Roentgenol.*, **163**, 311–315

McNoe, B., Richardson, A.K. & Elwood, J.M. (1996) Factors affecting participation in mammography screening. *N.Z. Med. J.*, **109**, 359–361

McPhee, S.J., Bird, J.A., Davis, T., Ha, N.T., Jenkins, C.N. & Le, B. (1997) Barriers to breast and cervical cancer screening among Vietnamese–American women. *Am. J. Prev. Med.*, **13**, 205–213

McPherson, C.P., Swenson, K.K., Jolitz, G. & Murray, C.L. (1997) Survival of women ages 40–49 with breast carcinoma according to method of detection. *Cancer*, **79**, 1923–1932

Meijers-Heijboer, H., van Geel, B., van Putten, W.L., Henzen-Logmans, S.C., Seynaeve, C., Menke-Pluymers, M.B., Bartels, C.C., Verhoog, L.C., van den Ouweland, A.M., Niermeijer, M.F., Brekelmans, C.T. & Klijn, J.G. (2001) Breast cancer after prophylactic bilateral mastectomy in women with a BRCA1 or BRCA2 mutation. *New Engl. J. Med.*, **345**, 159–164

Mejia, R.M., Recondo, M.M., Ross, A. & Casal, E. (1999) [Prevention of cancer of the breast with follow-up of patients.] *Medicina*, **59**, 314–315 (in Spanish)

Metsch, L., McCoy, C., McCoy, H., Pereyra, M., Trapido, E. & Miles, C. (1998) The role of the physician as an information source on mammography. *Cancer Pract.*, **6**, 229–236

Mettler, F.A., Upton, A.C., Kelsey, C.A., Ashby, R.N., Rosenberg, R.D. & Linver, M.N. (1996) Benefits versus risks from mammography: A critical reassessment. *Cancer*, **77**, 903–909

Michielutte, R., Dignan, M.B. & Smith, B.L. (1999) Psychosocial factors associated with the use of breast cancer screening by women age 60 years or over. *Health Educ. Behav.*, **26**, 625–647

Miettinen, O.S., Henschke, C.I., Pasmantier, M.W., Smith, J.P., Libby, D.M. & Yankelevitz, D.F. (2002) Mammographic screening: No reliable supporting evidence? *Lancet*, **359**, 404–405

Miller, A.B. (1992) Canadian national breast screening study: 1. Breast cancer detection and death rates among women age 40–49 years. [published erratum in *Can. Med. Assoc. J.* 1993, **148**, 718]. *Can. Med. Assoc. J.*, **147**, 1459–1476

Miller, A.B. (1994) Re: May we agree to disagree, or how do we develop guidelines for breast cancer screening in women? *J. Natl Cancer Inst.*, **86**, 1729–1731

Miller, A.B. (2001) Screening for breast cancer with mammography. *Lancet*, **358**, 2164

Miller, A.B. & Borges, A.M. (2001) Intermediate histologic effect markers for breast cancer. In: Miller, A.B., Bartsch, H., Boffetta, P., Dragsted, L. & Vainio, H., eds, *Biomarkers in Chemoprevention of Cancer* (IARC Scientific Publications No. 154), Lyon, IARCPress, pp. 171–175

Miller, A.B., Howe, G.R. & Wall, C. (1981) The national study of breast cancer screening. Protocol for a Canadian randomized controlled trial of screening for breast cancer in women. *Clin. Invest. Med.*, **4**, 227–258

Miller, A.B., Howe, G.R., Sherman, G.J., Lindsay, J.P., Yaffe, M.J., Dinner, P.J., Risch, H.A. & Preston, D.L. (1989) Mortality from breast cancer after irradiation during fluoroscopic examinations in patients being treated for tuberculosis. *New Engl. J. Med.*, **321**, 1285–1289

Miller, A.B., Baines, C.J. & Sickles, E.A. (1990) Canadian national breast screening study [Letter]. *Am. J. Roentgenol.*, **155**, 1133–1134

Miller, A.B., Baines, C.J. & Turnbull, C. (1991a) The role of the nurse–examiner in the national breast screening study. *Can. J. Public Health*, **82**, 162–167

Miller, A.B., Baines, C.J., To, T. & Wall, C. (1991b) The Canadian national breast screening study. In: Miller, A.B., Chamberlain, J., Day, N.E., Hakama, M. & Prorok, P.C., eds, *Cancer Screening*, Cambridge, Cambridge University Press, pp. 45–55

Miller, A.B., Baines, C.J., To, T. & Wall, C. (1992a) Canadian national breast screening study: 1. Breast cancer detection and death rates among women aged 40 to 49 years. *Can. Med. Assoc. J.*, **147**, 1459–1476

Miller, A.B., Baines, C.J., To, T. & Wall, C. (1992b) Canadian national breast screening study: 2. Breast cancer detection and death rates among women aged 50 to 59 years. *Can. Med. Assoc. J.*, **147**, 1477–1488

Miller, A.B., To, T., Baines, C.J. & Wall, C. (2000) Canadian national breast screening study-2: 13-year results of a randomized trial in women age 50–59 years. *J. Natl Cancer Inst.*, **92**, 1490–1499

Miller, A.B., Baines, C.J. & Wall, C. (2002) The Canadian National Breast Screening Study-1. A randomized screening trial of mammography in women age 40–49: Breast cancer mortality after 11–16 years of follow-up. *Ann. Intern. Med.*, **136** (in press)

Minister of Public Works and Government Services Canada (1999) *Organized Breast Cancer Screening Programs in Canada: 1996 Report* (Cat. No.:H1–9/13–1999), Ottawa, Health Canada

Ministerio de Salud (1998) Orientaciones para la pesquisa y control del cáncer de mama. *División de Salud de las Personas*, Santiago de Chile

Ministerio de Salud, Uruguay (2000) Evaluación del impacto del PRONACAM Junio 1999–Mayo 2000, Montevideo

Mishra, S.I., Luce, P.H. & Hubbell, F.A. (2001) Breast cancer screening among American Samoan women. *Prev. Med.*, **33**, 9–17

Mitnick, J.S., Vazquez, M.F., Kronovet, S.Z. & Roses, D.F. (1995) Malpractice litigation involving patients with carcinoma of the breast. *J. Am. Coll. Surg.*, **181**, 315–321

Mittra, I., Baum, M., Thornton, H. & Houghton, J. (2000) Is clinical breast examination an acceptable alternative to mammographic screening? *Br. Med. J.*, **321**, 1071–1073

Modeste, N.N., Cleb-Drayton, V.L. & Montgomery, S. (1999) Barriers to early detection of breast cancer among women in a Caribbean population. *Rev. Panam. Salud Publica*, **5**, 152–156

Mohler, P. (1995) Enhancing compliance with screening mammography recommendations: A clinical trial in a primary care office. *Fam. Med.*, **27**, 117–121

Moore, F.D. (1978) Breast self-examination. *New Engl. J. Med.*, **299**, 304–305

Moore, J.O.S. & Foote, J.F.W. (1949) The relatively favourable prognosis of medullary carcinoma of the breast. *Cancer*, **2**, 635–642

Moore, D.F. & Tsiatis, A.A. (1990) Robust examination of the variance in moment methods for extra-binomial and extra-Poisson variation. *Biometrics*, **47**, 383–401

del Moral Aldaz, A., Aupee, M., Batal-Steil, S., Cecchini, S., Chamberlain, J., Ciatto, S., Elizaga, N.A., Gairard, B., Grazzini, G. & Guldenfels, C. (1994) Cancer screening in the European Union. *Eur. J. Cancer*, **30A**, 860–872

Morimoto, T., Sasa, M., Yamaguchi, T., Kondo, H., Sagara, Y., Kuwamura, Y., Yamamoto, S. & Tada, T. (1997) Effectiveness of mammographic screening for breast cancer in women aged over 50 years in Japan. *Jpn. J Cancer Res*, **88**, 778–784

Morimoto, T., Sasa, M., Yamaguchi, T., Kondo, H., Akaiwa, H. & Sagara, Y. (2000) Breast cancer screening by mammography in women aged under 50 years in Japan. *Anticancer Res.*, **20**, 3689–3694

Morrison, A.S. (1992) *Screening in Chronic Disease*, 2nd Ed., New York: Oxford University Press, pp. 24, 33–35

Morrison, A.S., Brisson, J. & Khalid, N. (1988) Breast cancer incidence and mortality in the Breast Cancer Detection Demonstration Project [published erratum appears in *J. Natl Cancer Inst.*, 1989, **81**, 1513]. *J. Natl Cancer Inst.*, **80**, 1540–1547

Moskowitz, M. (1992) Guidelines for screening for breast cancer. Is a revision in order? *Radiol. Clin. North Am.*, **30**, 221–233

Moskowitz, M., Pemmaraju, S., Fidler, J.A., Sutorius, D.J., Russell, P., Scheinok, P. & Holle, J. (1976) On the diagnosis of minimal breast cancer in a screenee population. *Cancer*, **37**, 2543–2552

Moss, S. (1999) A trial to study the effect on breast cancer mortality of annual mammographic screening in women starting at age 40. Trial steering group. *J. Med. Screen.*, **6**, 144–148

Moss, S., Blanks, R., for the Interval Cancer Working Group (1998) Calculating appropriate target cancer detection rates and expected interval cancer rates for the UK NHS breast screening programme. *J. Epidemiol. Community Health*, **52**, 111–115

Moss, S.M., Summerley, M.E., Thomas, B.T., Ellman, R. & Chamberlain, J.O. (1992) A case_control evaluation of the effect of breast cancer screening in the United Kingdom trial of early detection of

breast cancer. *J. Epidemiol. Community Health*, **46**, 362–364

Moss, S.M., Coleman, D.A., Ellman, R., Chamberlain, J., Forrest, A.P., Kirkpatrick, A.E., Thomas, B.A. & Price, J.L. (1993) Interval cancers and sensitivity in the screening centres of the UK trial of early detection of breast cancer. *Eur. J. Cancer*, **29A**, 255–258

Moss, S.M., Michel, M., Patnick, J., Johns, L., Blanks, R. & Chamberlain, J. (1995) Results from the NHS breast screening programme 1990–1993. *J. Med. Screen.*, **2**, 186–190

Moss, S.M., Brown, J., Garvican, L., Coleman, D.A., Johns, L.E., Blanks, R.G., Rubin, G., Oswald, J., Page, A., Evans, A., Wilson, R., Lee, L., Liston, J., Sturdy, L., Sutton, G., Wardman, G., Patnick, J. & Winder, R. (2001) Routine breast screening for women aged 65–69: Results from evaluation of the demonstration sites. *Br. J. Cancer*, **85**, 1289–1294

Munn, E. (1993) Nonparticipation in mammography screening: Apathy, anxiety or cost? *N.Z. Med. J.*, **106**, 284–286

Murali, M.E. & Crabtree, K. (1992) Comparison of two breast self-examination palpation techniques. *Cancer Nurs.*, **15**, 276–282

Murray, M. & McMillan, C. (1993) Social behavioural predictors of women's cancer screening practices in Northern Ireland. *J. Public Health Med.*, **15**, 147–153

Muscat, J.E. & Huncharek, M.S. (1991) Breast self-examination and extent of disease: A population-based study. *Cancer Detect. Prev.*, **15**, 155–159

Narod, S.A. (2002) Modifiers of risk in hereditary breast cancer. *Nature Rev. Cancer*, **2**, 113–123

Narod, S.A. & Dubé, M.P. (2001) Re: Biologic characteristics of interval and screen-detected breast cancers. *J. Natl Cancer Inst.*, **93**, 151–152

Nass, S.J., Henderson, I.C. & Lashof, J.C. (2001) *Mammography and Beyond: Breast Imaging and Related Technologies*, Washington DC, National Academy Press

National Alliance of Breast Cancer Organizations (2001) *NABCO News*, January 2001. Update: Digital Mammography, pp. 1–2. Available at: http://www.nabco.org/resources/nabco_news/0101/digitalmammography.html

National Breast Cancer Centre (2001) *Breast Self-examination and the Early Detection of Breast Cancer: A Summary of the Evidence for Health Professionals*, Sydney

National Cancer Institute (2001a) *2003 Bypass Budget. Scientific Priorities for Cancer Research: NCI's Extraordinary Opportunities. Cancer Imaging.* Available at: http://plan.cancer.gov/scipri/imaging.htm

National Cancer Institute (2001b) *Surveillance, Epidemiology and End Results, November 2001 Submission (1973–1999)*, Bethesda, Maryland

National Coordinating Group for Breast Screening Pathology (1995) *Pathology Reporting in Breast Screening Pathology* (NHSBSP Publications No. 3), 2nd Ed., Sheffield, National Health Service Breast Screening Programme

National Council on Radiation Protection and Measurements (1986) *Mammography, A User Guide* (NCRP Report No. 85), Bethesda, MD

National Health Service Breast Screening Programme (1993) *Guidelines for Cytology Procedures and Reporting in Breast Cancer Screening* (NHSBSP Publication No. 22), Sheffield

National Health Service Breast Screening Programme (1997) *Guidelines for Breast Pathology Services* (NHSBSP Publication No. 2), Sheffield

National Health Service Breast Screening Programme (1998) *Guidelines on Quality Assurance Visits* (NHSBSP Publication No. 40), Sheffield

National Health Service Breast Screening Programme (2000) *Cancer Screening Programmes: Guidelines on Quality Assurance Visits* (NHSBSP Publications No. 40), 2nd Ed., Sheffield

National Institutes of Health (1997) Consensus Development Conference Statement: Breast Cancer Screening for Women Ages 40–49, January 21–23, 1997. National Institutes of Health Consensus Developmental Panel. *J. Natl Cancer Inst.*, **89**, 818–822

National Quality Management Committee of BreastScreen Australia (2001) *National Accreditation Standards BreastScreen Australia Quality Improvement Program*, Canberra, BreastScreen Australia, pp. 1–207

Nemoto, T., Vana, J., Bedwani, R.N., Baker, H.W., McGregor, F.H. & Murphy, G.P. (1980) Management and survival of female breast cancer: Results of a national survey by the American College of Surgeons. *Cancer*, **45**, 2917–2924

Neville, A.M., Bettelheim, R., Gelber, R.D., Save-Soderbergh, J., Davis, B.W., Reed, R., Torhorst, J., Golouh, R., Peterson, H.F., Price, K.N., *et al.* (1992) Factors predicting treatment responsiveness and prognosis in node-negative breast cancer. The International (Ludwig) Breast Cancer Study Group. *J. Clin. Oncol.*, **10**, 696–705

Newcomb, P.A., Weiss, N.S. Storer, B.E., Scholes, D., Young, B.E. & Voigt, L.F. (1991) Breast self-examination in relation to the occurrence of advanced breast cancer. *J. Natl Cancer Inst.*, **83**, 260–265

Newcomb, P.A., Olsen, S.J., Roberts, F.D., Storer, B.E. & Love, R.R. (1995) Assessing breast self-examination. *Prev. Med.*, **24**, 255–258

Ng, E.H., Ng, F.C., Tan, P.H., Low, S.C., Chiang, G., Tan, K.P., Seow, A., Emmanuel, S., Tan, C.H., Ho, G.H., Ng, L.T. & Wilde, C.C. (1998) Results of intermediate measures from a population-based, randomized trial of mammographic screening prevalence and detection of breast carcinoma among Asian women: The Singapore Breast Screening Project. *Cancer*, **82**, 1521–1528

Nguyen, M.Q., Nguyen, C.H. & Parkin, D.M. (1998) Cancer incidence in Ho Chi Minh City, Viet Nam, 1995–1996. *Int. J. Cancer*, **76**, 472–479

Nielsen, M., Jensen, J. & Andersen, J. (1984) Precancerous and cancerous breast lesions during lifetime and at autopsy: A study of 83 women. *Cancer*, **54**, 612–615

Nielsen, M., Thomsen, J.L., Primdahl, S., Dyreborg, U. & Andersen, J.A. (1987) Breast cancer and atypia among young and middle-aged women: A study of 110 medicolegal autopsies. *Br. J. Cancer*, **56**, 814–819

Nishizaki, T., Chew, K., Chu, L., Isola, J., Kallioniemi, A., Weidner, N., Waldman, F.M. (1997) Genetic alterations in lobular breast cancer by comparative genomic hybridization. *Int. J. Cancer*, **74**, 513–517.

Nixon, R., Prevost, T.C., Duffy, S.W., Tabár, L., Vitak, B. & Chen, H.H. (2000) Some random-effects models for the analysis of matched-cluster randomized trials: Application to the Swedish two-county trial of breast-cancer screening. *J. Epidemiol. Biostat.*, **5**, 349–358

Nolvadex Adjuvant Trial Organisation (1985) Controlled trial of tamoxifen as single adjuvant agent in management of early breast cancer. Analysis at six years by Nolvadex Adjuvant Trial Organisation. *Lancet*, **i**, 836–840

Nolvadex Adjuvant Trial Organisation (1988) Controlled trial of tamoxifen as a single adjuvant agent in the management of early breast cancer. 'Nolvadex' Adjuvant Trial Organisation. *Br. J. Cancer*, **57**, 608–611

Nyström, L. (2000) Assessment of population screening: The case of mammography. Thesis, Department of Public Health and Clinical Medicine, Umea University

Nyström, L., Rutqvist, L.E., Wall, S., Lindgren, A., Lindqvist, M., Ryden, S., Andersson, I., Bjurstam, N., Fagerberg, G. & Frisell, J. (1993) Breast cancer screening with mammography: Overview of Swedish randomised trials. *Lancet*, **341**, 973–978

Nyström, L., Larsson, L.G., Rutqvist, L.E., Lindgren, A., Lindqvist, M., Ryden, S., Andersson, I., Bjurstam, N., Fagerberg, G., Frisell, J. &. Tabàr, L. (1995) Determination of cause of death among breast cancer cases in the Swedish randomized mammography screening trials. A comparison between official statistics and validation by an end-point committee. *Acta Oncol.*, **34**, 145–152

Nyström, L., Larsson, L.G., Wall, S., Rutqvist, L.E., Andersson, I., Bjurstam, N., Fagerberg, G., Frisell, J. & Tabàr, L. (1996) An overview of the Swedish randomised mammography trials: Total mortality pattern and the representivity of the study cohorts. *J. Med. Screen.*, **3**, 85–87

Nyström, L., Andersson, I., Bjurstam, N., Frisell, J., Nordenskjold, B. & Rutqvist, L.E. (2002) Long-term effects of mammography screening: Updated overview of the Swedish randomised trials. *Lancet*, **359**, 909–919

O'Byrne, A., Kavanagh, A., Ugoni, A. & Diver, F. (2000) Predictors of non-attendance for second round mammography in an Australian mammographic screening programme. *J. Med. Screen.*, **7**, 190–194

O'Connor, A., Griffiths, C., Underwood, M. & Eldridge, S. (1998) Can postal prompts from general practitioners improve the uptake of breast screening? A randomised controlled trial in one East London general practice. *J. Med. Screen.*, **5**, 49–52

Ogawa, H., Tominaga, S., Yoshida, M., Kubo, K. & Takeuchi, S. (1987) Breast self-examination practice and clinical stage of breast cancer. *Jpn. J. Cancer Res.*, **78**, 447–452

Ohuchi, N., Yoshida, K., Kimura, M., Ouchi, A., Kamioki, S., Shiiba, K., Matoba, N., Kojima, S., Takahashi, K. & Matsuno, S. (1993) Improved detection rate of early breast cancer in mass screening combined with mammography. *Jpn. J. Cancer Res.*, **84**, 807–812

Ohuchi, N., Yoshida, K., Kimura, M., Ouchi, A., Shiiba, K., Ohnuki, K., Fukao, A., Abe, R., Matsuno, S. & Mori, S. (1995) Comparison of false negative rates among breast cancer screening modalities with or without mammography: Miyagi trial. *Jpn. J. Cancer Res.*, **86**, 501–506

Oliver-Vazquez, M., Sanhez-Ayebdez, M., Suarez-Perez, E. & Velez-Almodovar, H. (1999) Planning a breast cancer health promotion: Qualitative and quantitative data on Puerto Rican elderly women. *Promot. Educ.*, **6**, 16–19

Olivotto, I.A., Kan, L. & Coldman, A.J. (1998) Letter to the editor: False positive rate of screening mammography. *New Engl. J. Med.*, **339**, 560–564

Olivotto, I.A., Kan, L., d'Yachkova, Y., Burhenne, L.J., Hayes, M., Hislop, T.G., Worth, A.J., Basco, V.E. & King, S. (2000) Ten years of breast screening in the Screening Mammography Program of British Columbia, 1988–97. *J. Med. Screen.*, **7**, 152–159

Olsen, O. & Gotzsche, P.C. (2001) Cochrane review on screening for breast cancer with mammography. *Lancet*, **358**, 1340–1342

Olsen, J.H., Hahnemann, J.M., Börresen-Dale, A.L., Brondum-Nielsen, K., Hammarstrom, L., Kleinerman, R., Kääriäinen, H., Lönnqvist, T., Sankila, R., Seersholm, N., Tretli, S., Yuen, J., Boice, J.D., Jr & Tucker, M. (2001) Cancer in patients with ataxia-telangiectasia and in their relatives in the Nordic countries. *J. Natl Cancer Inst.*, **93**, 121–127

Olsson, P., Armelius, K., Nordahl, G., Lenner, P. & Westman, G. (1999) Women with false positive screening mammograms: How do they cope? *J. Med. Screen.*, **6**, 89–93

O'Malley, M.S. (1993) Cost–effectiveness of two nurse-led programs to teach breast self-examination. *Am. J. Prev. Med.*, **9**, 139–145

Ong, G. & Austoker, J. (1997) Recalling women for further investigation of breast screening: Women's experiences at the clinic and afterwards. *J. Public Health Med.*, **19**, 29–36

van Oortmarssen, G.J., Habbema, J.D., van der Maas, P.J., de Koning, H.J., Collette, H.J., Verbeek, A.L., Geerts, A.T. & Lubbe, K.T. (1990) A model for breast cancer screening. *Cancer*, **66**, 1601–1612

Örbo, A., Stalsberg, H. & Kunde, D. (1990) Topographic criteria in the diagnosis of tumor emboli in intramammary lymphatics. *Cancer*, **66**, 972–977

Ornstein, S., Garr, D., Jenkins, R., Rust, P. & Arnon, A. (1991) Computer-generated physician and patient reminders. Tools to improve population adherence to selected preventive services. *J. Fam. Pract.*, **32**, 82–90

O'Rourke, S., Galea, M.H., Morgan, D., Euhus, D., Pinder, S., Ellis, I.O., Elston, C.W. & Blamey, R.W. (1994) Local recurrence after simple mastectomy. *Br. J. Surg.*, **81**, 386–389

Orr, R.K. (1999) The impact of prophylactic node dissection on breast cancer survival—A Bayesian meta-analysis. *Ann. Surg. Oncol.*, **6**, 108–116

Orton, M., Fitzpatrick, R., Fuller, A., Mant, D., Mlynek, C. & Thorogood, M. (1991) Factors affecting women's response to an invitation to attend for a second breast cancer screening examination. *Br. J. Gen. Pract.*, **41**, 320–323

Osborne, C.K. (1998) Steroid hormone receptors in breast cancer management. *Breast Cancer Res. Treat.*, **51**, 227–238

Ota, J., Horino, T., Taguchi, T., Ishida, T., Izuo, M., Ogita, M., Abe, R., Watanabe, H., Morimoto, T., Itoh, S., Tashiro, H., Yoshida, K., Honda, K., Sasakawa, M., Enomoto, K., Kashiki, Y., Kido, C., Kuroishi, T. & Tominaga, S. (1989) Mass screening for breast cancer: Comparison of the clinical stages and prognosis of breast cancer detected by mass screening and in outpatient clinics. *Jpn. J. Cancer Res.*, **80**, 1028–1034

Overgaard, M., Hansen, P.S., Overgaard, J., Rose, C., Andersson, M., Bach, F., Kjaer, M., Gadeberg, C.C., Mouridsen,

H.T., Jensen, M.B. & Zedeler, K. (1997) Postoperative radiotherapy in high-risk premenopausal women with breast cancer who receive adjuvant chemotherapy. Danish Breast Cancer Cooperative Group 82b Trial. *New Engl.J. Med.*, **337**, 949–955

Owen, W.L., Hoge, A.F., Asal, N.R., Anderson, P.S., Jr, Owen, A.S. & Cucchiara, A.J. (1985) Self-examination of the breast: Use and effectiveness. *South. Med. J.*, **78**, 1170–1173

van Oyen, H. & Verellen, W. (1994) Breast cancer screening in the Flemish region, Belgium. *Eur. J. Cancer Prev.*, **3**, 7–12

Page, D.L., Dixon, J.M., Anderson, T.J., Lee, D. & Stewart, H.J. (1983) Invasive cribriform carcinoma of the breast. *Histopathology*, **7**, 525–536

Page, D.L., Anderson, T.J. & Sakamoto, G. (1987) *Diagnostic Histopathology of the Breast*, London, W.B. Saunders, pp. 193–235

Page, D.L., Kidd, T.E., Jr, Dupont, W.D., Simpson, J.F. & Rogers, L.W. (1991) Lobular neoplasia of the breast: Higher risk for subsequent invasive cancer predicted by more extensive disease. *Hum. Pathol.*, **22**, 1232–1239

Page, D.L., Dupont, W.D., Rogers, L.W., Jensen, R.A. & Schuyler, P.A. (1995) Continued local recurrence of carcinoma 15–25 years after a diagnosis of low grade ductal carcinoma in situ of the breast treated only by biopsy. *Cancer*, **76**, 1197–1200

PAHO (1998) *Health in the Americas 1998* (Scientific Publication No. 562), Washington DC

Palli, D., Rosselli del Turco, M., Buiatti, E., Carli, S., Ciatto, S., Toscani, L. & Maltoni, G. (1986) A case–control study of the efficacy of a non-randomized breast cancer screening program in Florence (Italy). *Int. J. Cancer*, **38**, 501–504

Palli, D., Rosselli del Turco, M., Buiatti, E., Ciatto, S., Crocetti, E. & Paci, E. (1989) Time interval since last test in a breast cancer screening programme: A case–control study in Italy. *J. Epidemiol. Community Health*, **43**, 241–248

Pamilo, M., Anttinen, I., Soiva, M., Roiha, M. & Suramo, I. (1990) Mammography screening—Reasons for recall and the influence of experience on recall in the Finnish system. *Clin. Radiol.*, **41**, 384–387

Pankow, J.S., Vachon, C.M., Kuni, C.C., King, R.A., Arnett, D.K., Grabrick, D.M., Rich, S.S., Anderson, V.E. & Sellers, T.A. (1997) Genetic analysis of mammographic breast density in adult women: Evidence of a gene effect. *J. Natl Cancer Inst.*, **89**, 549–556

Paquette, D., Snider, J., Bouchard, F., Olivotto, I., Bryant, H., Decker, K. & Doyle, G. (2000) Performance of screening mammography in organized programs in Canada in 1996. The database management subcommittee to the national committee for the Canadian breast cancer screening initiative. *Can. Med. Assoc. J.*, **163**, 1133–1138

Parkin, D.M. (2001) Global cancer statistics in the year 2000. *Lancet Oncol.*, **2**, 533–543

Parkin, D.M., Muir, C.S., Whelan, S.L., Gao, Y.T., Ferlay, J. & Powell, J., eds (1992) *Cancer Incidence in Five Continents, Volume VI* (IARC Scientific Publications No. 120), Lyon, IARCPress

Parkin, D.M., Whelan, S.L., Ferlay, J., Raymond, L. & Young, J., eds (1997) *Cancer Incidence in Five Continents, Volume VII* (IARC Scientific Publications No. 143), Lyon, IARCPress

Parkin, D.M., Pisani, P. & Bautista, A. (2001) Screening for cancer of the breast in the Philippines. In: *Biennial Report 2000–2001*, Lyon, IARCPress

Paskett, E.D., McMahon, K., Tatum, C., Velez, R., Shelton, B., Case, L.D., Wofford, J., Moran, W. & Wymer, A. (1998) Clinic-based interventions to promote breast and cervical cancer screening. *Prev. Med.*, **27**, 120–128

Paskett, E.D., Tatum, C.M., D'Agostino, R., Jr, Rushing, J., Velez, R., Michielutte, R. & Dignan, M. (1999) Community-based interventions to improve breast and cervical cancer screening: Results of the Forsyth County Cancer Screening (FoCaS) Project. *Cancer Epidemiol. Biomarkers Prev.*, **8**, 453–459

Patey, D.H. (1928) The position of histology in the prognosis of carcinoma of the breast. *Lancet*, **i**, 801–804

Pauli, R., Hammond, S., Cooke, J. & Ansell, J. (1996) Comparison of radiographer–radiologist double film reading with single reading in breast cancer screening. *J. Med. Screen.*, **2**, 18–22

Pedersen, L., Holck, S. & Schiodt, T. (1988) Medullary carcinoma of the breast. *Cancer Treat. Rev.*, **15**, 53–63

Peer, P.G., Verbeek, A.L., Straatman, H., Hendriks, J.H. & Holland, R. (1996) Age-specific sensitivities of mammographic screening for breast cancer. *Breast Cancer Res. Treat.*, **38**, 153–160

Peeters, P.H., Verbeek, A.L., Hendriks, J.H. & van Bon, M.J. (1989a) Screening for breast cancer in Nijmegen. Report of 6 screening rounds, 1975–1986. *Int. J. Cancer*, **43**, 226–230

Peeters, P.H., Verbeek, A.L., Straatman, H., Holland, R., Hendriks, J.H., Mravunac, M., Rothengatter, C., Dijk-Milatz, A. & Werre, J.M. (1989b) Evaluation of over-diagnosis of breast cancer in screening with mammography: Results of the Nijmegen programme. *Int. J. Epidemiol.*, **18**, 295–299

Pennypacker, H.S. & Pilgrim, C.A. (1993) Achieving competence in clinical breast examination. *Nurse Pract. Forum*, **4**, 85–90

Pennypacker, H.S., Bloom, H.S., Criswell, E.L., Neelakanten, P., Goldstein, M.K. & Stein, G.H. (1982) Toward an effective technology of instruction in breast self-examination. *Int. J. Mental Health*, **11**, 98–116

Pennypacker, H.S., Naylor, L., Sander, A.A. & Goldstein, M.K. (1999) Why can't we do better breast examinations? *Nurse Pract. Forum*, **10**, 122–128

Pereira, H., Pinder, S.E., Sibbering, D.M., Galea, M.H., Elston, C.W., Blamey, R.W., Robertson, J.F. & Ellis, I.O. (1995) Pathological prognostic factors in breast cancer. IV: Should you be a typer or a grader? A comparative study of two histological prognostic features in operable breast carcinoma. *Histopathology*, **27**, 219–226

Perou, C.M., Sorlie, T., Eisen, M.B., van de Rijn, M., Jeffrey, S.S., Rees, C.A., Pollack, J.R., Ross, D.T., Johnsen, H., Akslen, L.A., Fluge, O., Pergamenschikov, A., Williams, C., Zhu, S.X., Lonning, P.E., Borresen-Dale, A.L., Brown, P.O. & Botstein, D. (2000) Molecular portraits of human breast tumours. *Nature*, **406**, 747–752

Perry, N., Broeders, M., de Wolf, C., Törneberg, S. & Schouten, J., eds (2001) *European Guidelines of QA in Mammography Screening*, 3rd Ed., Brussels, Office for Official Publications of the European Communities

Philip, J., Harris, W.G., Flaherty, C., Joslin, C.A.F., Rustage, J.H. & Wijesinghe, D.P. (1984) Breast self-examination: Clinical results from a population-based prospective study. *Br. J. Cancer*, **50**, 7–12

Physician Insurers Association of America (1995) *Breast Cancer Study—June 1995*, Washington DC

Pilgrim, C., Lannon, C., Harris, R.P., Cogburn, W. & Fletcher, S.W. (1993) Improving clinical breast examination training in a medical school: A randomized controlled trial. *J. Gen. Intern. Med.*, **8**, 685–688

Pilnik, S. & Leis, H.P. (1978) Nipple discharge. In: Gallager, H.S., Leis, H.P., Snydermen, R.K. & Urban, J.A., eds, *The Breast*, St Louis, MO, Mosby Publishing

Pinder, K.L., Ramirez, A.J., Black, M.E., Richards, M.A., Gregory, W.M. & Rubens, R.D. (1993) Psychiatric disorder in patients with advanced breast cancer: Prevalence and associated factors. *Eur. J. Cancer*, **29A**, 524–527

Pinder, S.E., Ellis, I.O., Galea, M., O'Rouke, S., Blamey, R.W. & Elston, C.W. (1994) Pathological prognostic factors in breast cancer. III. Vascular invasion: Relationship with recurrence and survival in a large study with long-term follow-up. *Histopathology*, **24**, 41–47

Pinto, B.M. (1993) Training and maintenance of breast self-examination skills. *Am. J. Prev. Med.*, **9**, 353–358

Pisano, E.D., Earp, J., Schell, M., Vokaty, K. & Denham, A. (1998) Screening behavior of women after a false-positive mammogram. *Radiology*, **208**, 245–249

Poblano-Verastegui, O., Lopez-Carrillo, L., Clemenceau-Valdivia, J. & Lopez-Cervantes, M. (2000) The reproducibility of breast cancer diagnosis through mammography. A pilot study in Mexico. *Women Cancer J.*, **2**, 31–36

Poller, D., Silverstein, M.J., Galea, M., Locker, A.P., Elston, C.W., Blamey, R.W. & Ellis, I.O. (1994) Ductal carcinoma in situ of the breast: A proposal for a new simplified histological classification. *Modern Pathol.*, **7**, 257–262

Poplack, S.P., Tosteson, A.N., Grove, M.R., Wells, W.A. & Carney, P.A. (2000) Mammography in 53,803 women from the New Hampshire mammography network. *Radiology*, **217**, 832–840

Porter, P.L., El-Bastawissi, A.Y., Mandelson, M.T., Lin, M.G., Khalid, N., Watney, E.A., Cousens, L., White, D., Taplin, S. & White, E. (1999) Breast tumor characteristics as predictors of mammographic detection: Comparison of interval- and screen-detected cancers. *J. Natl Cancer Inst.*, **91**, 2020–2028

Potter, S., Mauldin, P. & Hill, H. (1996) Access to and participation in breast cancer screening: A review of recent literature. *Clin. Perform. Qual. Health Care*, **4**, 74–85

Prorok, P.C., Chamberlain, J., Day, N.E., Hakama, M. & Miller, A.B. (1984) UICC workshop on the evaluation of screening programmes for cancer. *Int. J. Cancer*, **34**, 1–4

Prorok, P.C., Kramer, B.S. & Gohagan, J.K. (1999) Screening theory and study design: The basics. In: Kramer, B.S., Gohagan, J.K. & Prorok, P.C., eds, *Cancer Screening: Theory and Practice*, New York, Marcel Dekker, pp. 29–53

Pruthi, S. (2001) Detection and evaluation of a palpable breast mass. *Mayo Clin. Proc.*, **76**, 641–647

Quinn, M., Allen, E., on behalf of the United Kingdom Association of Cancer Registries (1995) Changes in incidence of and mortality from breast cancer in England and Wales since introduction of screening. *Br. Med. J.*, **311**, 1391–1395

Quinn, M.J., Martinez-Garcia, C., Berrino, F. & the EUROCARE Working Group (1998) Variations in survival from breast cancer in Europe by age and country, 1978–1989. *Eur. J. Cancer*, **34**, 2204–2211

Qureshi, M., Thacker, H.L., Litaker, D.G. & Kippes, C. (2000) Differences in breast cancer screening rates: An issue of ethnicity or socioeconomics? *J. Women's Health Gender-based Med.*, **9**, 1025–1031

Rajakariar, R. & Walker, R.A. (1995) Pathological and biological features of mammographically detected invasive breast carcinomas. *Br. J. Cancer*, **71**, 150–154

Rapin, V., Contesso, G., Mouriesse, H., Bertin, F., Lacombe, M.J., Piekarski, J.D., Travagli, J.P., Gadenne, C. & Friedman, S. (1988) Medullary breast carcinoma. A reevaluation of 95 cases of breast cancer with inflammatory stroma. *Cancer*, **61**, 2503–2510

Rasbridge, S.A., Gillett, C.E., Sampson, S.A., Walsh, F.S. & Millis, R.R. (1993) Epithelial (E-) and placental (P-) cadherin cell adhesion molecule expression in breast carcinoma. *J. Pathol.*, **169**, 245–250

Rathore, S.S., McGreevey, J.D., III, Schulman, K.A. & Atkins, D. (2000) Mandated coverage for cancer-screening services: Whose guidelines do states follow? *Am. J. Prev. Med.*, **19**, 71–78

Recht, A., van Dongen, J.A., Fentiman, I.S., Holland, R. & Peterse, J.L. (1994) Third meeting of the DCIS Working Party of the EORTC (Fondazione Cini, Isola S. Giorgio, Venezia, 28 February 1994)—Conference report. *Eur. J. Cancer*, **30A**, 1895–1900

Retsky, M., Demicheli, R. & Hrushesky, W. (2001a) Premenopausal status accelerates relapse in node positive breast cancer: Hypothesis links angiogenesis, screening controversy. *Breast Cancer Res. J.* **65**, 217–224

Retsky, M., Demicheli, R. & Hrushesky, W. (2001b) Breast cancer screening for women aged 40–49 years. Screening may not be the benign process usually thought. *J. Natl Cancer Inst.*, **93**, 1572

Rezentes, P.S., De Almeida, A. & Barnes, G.T. (1999) Mammography grid performance. *Radiology*, **210**, 227–232

Richards, M.A., Braysher, S., Gregory, W.M. & Rubens, R.D. (1993) Advanced breast cancer: Use of resources and cost implications. *Br. J. Cancer*, **67**, 856–860

Richardson, W.W. (1956) Medullary carcinoma of the breast. A distinctive tumour type with a relatively good prognosis following radical mastectomy. *Br. J. Cancer*, **10**, 415–423

Richardson, J.L., Mondrus, G.T., Danley, K., Deapen, D. & Mack, T. (1996) Impact of a mailed intervention on annual mammography and physician breast examinations among women at high risk of breast cancer. *Cancer Epidemiol. Biomarkers Prev.*, **5**, 71–76

Rickard, M.T., Taylor, R.J., Fazli, M.A. & El Hassan, N. (1998) Interval breast cancers in an Australian mammographic screening program. *Med. J. Aust.*, **169**, 184–187

Ridolfi, R.L., Rosen, P.P., Port, A., Kinne, D. & Mike, V. (1977) Medullary carcinoma of the breast: A clinicopathologic study with 10 year follow-up. *Cancer*, **40**, 1365–1385

Rimer, B.K. & Bluman, L. (1997) The psychosocial consequences of mammography. *J. Natl Cancer Inst. Monogr.*, **22**, 131–138

Rimer, B.K. & Glassman, B. (1999) Is there a use for tailored print communications in cancer risk information? *J. Natl Cancer Inst. Monogr.*, **25**, 140–148

Rimer, B., Davis, S., Engstrom, P.F., Myers, R., Rosan, J., Fox, L. & McLaughlin, R. (1988) An examination of compliance and noncompliance in an HMO cancer screening program. *Prog. Clin. Biol. Res.*, **278**, 21–30

Rimer, B.K., Resch, N., King, E., Ross, E., Lerman, C., Boyce, A., Kessler, H. & Engstrom, P.F. (1992) Multistrategy health education program to increase mammography use among women ages 65 and older. *Public Health Rep.*, **107**, 369–380

Robbins, P., Pinder, S., de Klerk, N., Dawkins, H., Harvey, J., Sterrett, G., Ellis, I. & Elston, C. (1995) Histological grading of breast carcinomas: A study of inter-observer agreement. *Hum. Pathol.*, **26**, 873–879

Roberts, M.M., Alexander, F.E., Anderson, T.J., Chetty, U., Donnan, P.T., Forrest, P., Hepburn, W., Huggins, A., Kirkpatrick, A.E. & Lamb, J. (1990) Edinburgh trial of screening for breast cancer: Mortality at seven years. *Lancet*, **335**, 241–246

Roberts, C.S., Cox, C.E., Reintgen, D.S., Baile, W.F. & Gibertini, M. (1994) Influence of physician communication on newly diagnosed breast patients' psychologic adjustment and decision-making. *Cancer*, **74**, 336–341

Robles, S.C. & Galanis, E. (2002) Breast cancer in Latin America and the Caribbean. *Rev. Panam. Salud Publica* (in press)

Robra, B.P., Dierks, M.L., Frischbier, H.J. & Hoeffken, W. (1994) *The German Mammography Study—Results and Recommendations*, Hanover, Medizinische Hochschule Hannover

Rocha Alves, J.G., Cruz, D.B., Rodrigues, V.L., Goncalves, M.L. & Fernandes, E. (1994) Breast cancer screening in the central region of Portugal. *Eur. J. Cancer Prev.*, **3** (Suppl. 1), 49–53

Rodriguez-Cuevas, S., Macias, C.G., Franceschi, D. & Labastida, S. (2001) Breast carcinoma presents a decade earlier in Mexican women than in the United States or European countries. *Cancer*, **91**, 863–868

Rosai, J. (1991) Borderline epithelial lesions of the breast. *Am. J. Surg. Pathol.*, **15**, 209–221

Rosen, P.P. (1983) Tumor emboli in intra-mammary lymphatics in breast carcinoma: Pathologic criteria for diagnosis and clinical significance. *Pathol. Annu.*, **18**, 215–232

Rosen, P.P. (1991) *Breast Diseases,* Philadelphia, Lippincott, pp. 245–296

Rosen, P.P. (1997) *Rosen's Breast Pathology,* Philadelphia, Lippincott-Raven

Rosen, P.P., Saigo, P.E., Braun, D.W., Jr, Weathers, E. & DePalo, A. (1981) Predictors of recurrence in stage I (T1N0M0) breast carcinoma. *Ann. Surg.*, **193**, 15–25

Rosenberg, R.D., Yankaskas, B.C., Hunt, W.C., Ballard-Barbash, R., Urban, N., Ernster, V.L., Kerlikowske, K., Geller, B., Carney, P.A. & Taplin, S. (2000) Effect of variations in operational definitions on performance estimates for screening mammography. *Acad. Radiol.*, **7**, 1058–1068

Rosenman, K., Gardiner, J., Swanson, G., Mullan, P. & Zhu, Z. (1995) US farm women's participation in breast cancer screening practices. *Cancer*, **75**, 47–53

Roses, D.F., Bell, D.A., Flotte, T.J., Taylor, R., Ratech, H. & Dubin, N. (1982) Pathologic predictors of recurrence in stage 1 (T1N0M0) breast cancer. *Am. J. Clin. Pathol.*, **78**, 817–820

Rosvold, E.O., Hjartaker, A., Bjertness, E. & Lund, E. (2001) Breast self-examination and cervical cancer testing among Norwegian female physicians. A nation-wide comparative study. *Soc. Sci. Med.*, **52**, 249–258

Royal College of Pathologists http://www.rcpath.org/activities/publications/bcancer.html

Royal College of Radiologists (1997) Quality Assurance Guidelines for Radiologists (NHSBSP Publications No. 15), Sheffield, National Health Service Breast Screening Programme

Roylance, R., Gorman, P., Harris, W., Liebmann, R., Barnes, D., Hanby, A. & Sheer, D. (1999) Comparative genomic hybridization of breast tumors stratified by histological grade reveals new insights into the biological progression of breast cancer. *Cancer Res.*, **59**, 1433–1436

Rudolf, Z. (1994) Pilot study of breast cancer screening in six communes of Slovenia. In: Sankaranarayanan R., Wahrendorf J. & Demaret E., eds, *Directory of Ongoing Research in Cancer Epidemiology* (IARC Scientific Publications No. 130), Lyon, IARCPress

Ruffin, M.T., Gorenflo, D.W. & Woodman, B. (2000) Predictors of screening for breast, cervical, colorectal, and prostatic cancer among community-based primary care practices. *J. Am. Board Fam. Pract.*, **13**, 1–10

Russell, I.J., Hendricson, W.D. & Herbert, R.J. (1984) Effects of lecture information density on medical student achievement. *J. Med. Educ.*, **59**, 881–889

Rutledge, D.N., Barsevick, A., Knobf, M. & Bookbinder, M. (2001) Breast cancer detection: Knowledge, attitudes, and behaviors of women from Pennsylvania. *Oncol. Nurs. Forum*, **28**, 1032–1040

Saarenmaa, I., Salminen, T., Geiger, U., Holli, K., Isola, J., Kärkkäinen, A., Pakkanen, J., Piironen, A., Salo, A. & Hakama, M. (1999) The visibility of cancer on earlier mammograms in a population-based screening programme. *Eur. J. Cancer*, **35**, 1118–1122

Säbel, M. & Aichinger, H. (1996) Recent developments in breast imaging. *Phys. Med. Biol.*, **41**, 315–368

Säbel, M., Aichinger, U. & Schulz-Wendtland, R. (2001) [Radiation exposure in X-ray mammography]. *Fortschr. Rontgenstr.*, **173**, 79–91 (in German)

Sala, E., Warren, R., McCann, J., Duffy, S., Luben, R. & Day, N. (2000) High-risk mammographic parenchymal patterns, hormone replacement therapy and other risk factors: A case–control study. *Int. J. Epidemiol.*, **29**, 629–636

Salzmann, P., Kerlikowske, K. & Phillips, K. (1997) Cost-effectiveness of extending screening mammography guidelines to include women 40 to 49 years of age. *Ann. Intern. Med.*, **127**, 955–965

Sancho-Garnier, H. (1993) Evaluation of cancer screening programmes for breast cancer and uterine cervic in the EC. In: Frechia, G.N. & Theopilatoo, M., eds, *Health Service Research*, Amsterdam, IOS Press, pp. 403–419

Sankaranarayanan, R., Black, R.J. & Parkin, D.M. (1998) An overview of cancer survival in developing countries. In: Sankaranarayanan, R., Black, R.J., Swaminathan, R. & Parkin, D.M., eds, *Cancer Survival in Developing Countries* (IARC Scientific Publications No. 145), Lyon, IARCPress, pp. 135–173

dos Santos Silva, I. & Beral, V. (1997) Socioeconomic differences in reproductive behaviour. In: Kogevinas, M., Pearce, N., Susser, M. & Boffetta, P., eds, *Social Inequalities and Cancer* (IARC Scientific Publications No. 138), Lyon, IARCPress, pp. 285–308

Sarrazin, D., Le, M.G., Arriagada, R., Contesso, G., Fontaine, F., Spielmann, M., Rochard, F., Le Chevalier, T. & Lacour, J. (1989) Ten-year results of a randomized trial comparing a conservative treatment to mastectomy in early breast cancer. *Radiother. Oncol.*, **14**, 177–184

Sasco, A.J., Day, N.E. & Walter, S.D. (1986) Case–control studies for the evaluation of screening. *J. Chron. Dis.*, **39**, 399–405

Saunders, K.J., Pilgrim, C.A. & Pennypacker, H.S. (1986) Increased proficiency of search in breast self-examination. *Cancer*, **58**, 2531–2537

Scheuer, L., Kauff, N., Robson, M., Kelly, B., Barakat, R., Satagopan, J., Ellis, N., Hensley, M., Boyd, J., Borgen, P., Norton, L. & Offit, K. (2002) Outcome of preventive surgery and screening for breast and ovarian cancer in BRCA mutation carriers. *J. Clin. Oncol.*, **20**, 1260–1268

Schnitt, S.J. & Morrow, M. (1999) Lobular carcinoma in situ: Current concepts and controversies. *Semin. Diagn. Pathol.*, **16**, 209–223

Schnitt, S.J., Connolly, J.L., Tavassoli, F.A., Fechner, R.E., Kempson, R.L., Gelman, R. & Page, D.L. (1992) Interobserver reproducibility in the diagnosis of ductal proliferative breast lesions using standardized criteria. *Am. J. Surg. Pathol.*, **16**, 1133–1143

Schouten, L.J., de Rijke, J.M., Schlangen, J.T. & Verbeek, A.L. (1998) Evaluation of the effect of breast cancer screening by record linkage with the cancer registry, the Netherlands. *J. Med. Screen.*, **5**, 37–41

Schwartz, C.M., Woloshin, S., Sox, H.C., Fischholf, B. & Welch, H.G. (2000) US women's attitudes to false positive mammography results and detection of ductal carcinoma in situ: Cross-sectional survey. *Br. Med. J.*, **320**, 1635–1640

Scott, M.A., Lagios, M.D., Axelsson, K., Rogers, L.W., Anderson, T.J. & Page, D.L. (1997) Ductal carcinoma in situ of the breast: Reproducibility of histological subtype analysis. *Hum. Pathol.*, **28**, 967–973

Secretariat of Health (2000) [Project NOM-SSA-2000 for the Prevention, Diagnosis, Treatment, Control and Epidemiological Surveillance of Breast Cancer], Mexico City (in Spanish)

Segura, J.M., Castells, X., Casamitjana, M., Macia, F. & Ferrer, F. (2000) Utilization of screening mammography as a preventive practice piror to initiating a population-based breast cancer screening program. *J. Clin. Epidemiol.*, **53**, 595–603

Seidman, H., Gelb, S.K., Silverberg, E., LaVerda, N. & Lubera, J.A. (1987) Survival experience in the Breast Cancer Detection Demonstration Project. *CA Cancer ·l. Clin.*, **37**, 258–290

Seidman, J.D., Schnaper, L.A. & Aisner, S.C. (1995) Relationship of the size of the invasive component of the primary breast carcinoma to axillary lymph node metastasis. *Cancer*, **75**, 65–71

Semiglazov, V.F., Moiseyenko, V.M., Bavli, J.L., Migmanova, N.S., Seleznyov, N.K., Popova, R.T., Ivanova, O.A., Orlov, A.A., Chagunava, O.A., Barash, N.J., Matitzin, A.N., Dyatchenko, O.T., Kozhevnikov, S.Y., Alexandrova, G.I., Sanchakova, A.V. & Musayev, B.T. (1992) The role of breast self-examination in early breast cancer detection (Results of the 5-year USSR/WHO randomized study in Leningrad). *Eur. J. Epidemiol.*, **8**, 498–502

Semiglazov, V.F., Sagaidak, V.N., Moiseyenko, V.M. & Mikhailov, E.A. (1993) Study of the role of breast self-examination in the reduction of mortality from breast cancer. The Russian Federation/World Health Organization Study. *Eur. J. Cancer*, **29A**, 2039–2046

Semiglazov, V.F., Moiseenka, V.M., Manikhas, A.G., Protsenko, S.A., Kharikova, R.S., Seleznev, I.K., Popovu, R.T., Migmanova, N.S., Orlov, A.A., Borash, N.Y., Ivanova, O.A. & Ivanova, V.G. (1999) Interim results of a prospective randomized evaluation of self-examination for early detection of breast cancer (Russia/St Petersburg/WHO). *Vopr. Onkol.*, **45**, 265–271

Senie, R.T., Rosen, P.P., Lesser, M.L. & Kinne, D.W. (1981) Breast self-examination and medical examination related to breast cancer stage. *Am. J. Public Health*, **71**, 583–590

Senie, R.T., Lesser, M., Kinne, D.W. & Rosen, P.R. (1994) Method of tumour detection influences disease-free survival of women with breast carcinoma. *Cancer*, **73**, 1666–1672

Seow, A., Straughan, P.T., Ng, E.H., Emmanuel, S.C., Tan, C.H. & Lee, H.P. (1997) Factors determining acceptability of mammography in an Asian population: A study among women in Singapore. *Cancer Causes Control*, **8**, 771–779

Shapiro, S. (1994) Screening: Assessment of current studies. *Cancer*, **74**, 231–238

Shapiro, S. (1997) Periodic screening for breast cancer: The HIP randomized controlled trial. Health Insurance Plan. *J. Natl Cancer Inst. Monogr.*, **22**, 27–30

Shapiro, S., Strax, P. & Venet, L. (1966) Evaluation of periodic breast cancer screening with mammography. Methodology and early observations. *J. Am. Med. Assoc.*, **195**, 731–738

Shapiro, S., Strax, P. & Venet, L. (1967) Periodic breast cancer screening—The first two years of screening. *Arch. Environ. Health*, **15**, 547–553

Shapiro, S., Strax, P. & Venet, L. (1971) Periodic breast cancer screening in reducing mortality from breast cancer. *J. Am. Med. Assoc.*, **215**, 1777–1785

Shapiro, S., Venet, W., Strax, P., Venet, L. & Roeser, R. (1982) Ten- to fourteen-year effect of screening on breast cancer mortality. *J. Natl Cancer Inst.*, **69**, 349–355

Shapiro, S., Venet, W., Strax, P. & Venet, L. (1988a) *Periodic Screening for Breast Cancer: The Health Insurance Plan Project, 1963–1986, and Its Sequelae*, Baltimore, The Johns Hopkins University Press

Shapiro, S., Venet, W., Strax, P. & Venet, L. (1988b) Current results of the breast cancer screening randomized trial. The Health Insurance Plan (HIP) of Greater New York study. In: Day, N.E. & Miller, A.B., eds, *Screening for Breast Cancer*, Bern, Hans Huber, pp. 3–15

Shapiro, S., Coleman, E.A., Broeders, M., Codd, M., de Koning, H., Fracheboud, J., Moss, S., Paci, E., Stachenko, S. & Ballard-Barbash, R. (1998) Breast cancer screening programmes in 22 countries: Current policies, administration and guidelines. International Breast Cancer Screening Network (IBSN) and the European Network of Pilot Projects for Breast Cancer Screening. *Int. J. Epidemiol.*, **27**, 735–742

Sharp, D., Peters, T., Bartholomew, J. & Shaw, A. (1996) Breast screening: A randomised controlled trial in UK general practice of three interventions designed to increase uptake. *J. Epidemiol. Community Health*, **50**, 72–76

Sickles, E.A., Ominsky, S.H., Sollitto, R.A., Galvin, H.B. & Monticciolo, D.L. (1990) Medical audit of a rapid-throughput mammography screening practice: Methodology and results of 27,114 examinations. *Radiology*, **175**, 323–327

Silverstein, M.J., Poller, D.N., Waisman, J.R., Colburn, W.J., Barth, A., Gierson, E.D., Lewinsky, B., Gamagami, P. & Slamon, D.J. (1995) Prognostic classification of breast ductal carcinoma-in-situ. *Lancet*, **345**, 1154–1157

Silverstein, M.J., Lagios, M.D., Craig, P.H., Waisman, J.R., Lewinsky, B.S., Colburn, W.J. & Poller, D.N. (1996) A prognostic index for ductal carcinoma in situ of the breast. *Cancer*, **77**, 2267–2274

Sjonell, G. & Stahle, L. (1999) [Mammographic screening does not reduce breast cancer mortality]. *Lakartidningen*, **96**, 904–913 (in Swedish)

Slamon, D.J, Clark, G.M., Wong, S.G., Levin, W.J., Ullrich, A. & McGuire, W.L. (1987) Human breast cancer: Correlation of relapse and survival with amplification of the HER-2/neu oncogene. *Science*, **235**, 177–182

Slanetz, P.J., Giardino, A.A., McCarthy, K.A., Hall, D.A., Halpern, E.F., Moore, R.H. & Kopans, D.B. (1998) Previous breast biopsy for benign disease rarely complicates or alters interpretation on screening mammography. *Am. J. Roentgenol.*, **170**, 1539–1541

Slaytor, E. & Ward, J. (1998) How risks of breast cancer and benefits of screening are communicated to women: Analysis of 58 pamphlets. *Br. Med. J.*, **317**, 263–264

Sloane, J.P., Ellman, R., Anderson, T.J., Brown, C.L., Coyne, J., Dallimore, N.S., Davies, J.D., Eakins, D., Ellis, I.O., Elston, C.W., Humphreys, S., Lawrence, D., Lowe, J., McGee, J.O'D., Millis, R.R., Nottingham, J., Ryley, N., Scott, D.J., Sloan, J.M., Theaker, J., Trott, P.A., Wells, C.A. & Zakhour, H.D. (1994) Consistency of histopathological reporting of breast lesions detected by screening: Findings of the UK national external quality assessment (EQA) scheme. UK National Coordinating Group for Breast Screening

Pathology. *Eur. J. Cancer*, **30A**, 1414–1419

Sloane, J.P., Amendoeira, I., Apostolikas, N., Bellocq, J.P., Bianchi, S., Boecker, W., Bussolati, G., Coleman, D., Connolly, C.E., Eusebi, V., de Miguel, C., Dervan, P., Drijkoningen, R., Elston, C.W., Faverly, D., Gad, A., Jacquemier, J., Lacerda, M., Martinez-Penuela, J., Munt, C., Peterse, J.L., Rank, F., Sylvan, M., Tsakraklides, V. & Zafrani, B. (1999) Consistency achieved by 23 European pathologists from 12 countries in diagnosing breast disease and reporting prognostic features of carcinomas. European Commission Working Group on Breast Screening Pathology. *Virchows Arch.*, **434**, 3–10

Smith, E.M. & Burns, T.L. (1985) The effects of breast self-examination in a population-based cancer registry. *Cancer*, **55**, 432–437

Smith, E.M., Francis, A.M. & Polissar, L. (1980) The effect of breast self-exam practices and physician examinations on extent of disease at diagnosis. *Prev. Med.*, **9**, 409–417

Sneige, N., Lagios, M., Schwerting, R., Colburn, W., Atkinson, E., Weber, D., Sahin, A., Kemp, B., Hoque, A., Risin, S., Sabichi, A., Boone, C., Dhingra, K., Kelloff, G. & Lippman S. (1998) Interobserver reproducibility (IR) of the Lagios nuclear grading system for ductal carcinoma in situ (DCIS). *Modern Pathol.*, **11**, A28

Socialstyrelsen (1997) *Control of Mammography Equipment in the Southern Health Care Region. Sweden* (Art.No. 1997-00-31), Solna

Socialstyrelsen (1998) *Mammography Screening for Breast Cancer*, Solna

Solin, L.J., Yeh, I.T., Kurtz, J., Fourquet, A., Recht, A., Kuske, R., McCormick, B., Cross, M.A., Schultz, D.J., Amalric, R., et al. (1993) Ductal carcinoma in situ (intraductal carcinoma) of the breast treated with breast-conserving surgery and definitive irradiation. Correlation of pathologic parameters with outcome of treatment. *Cancer*, **71**, 2532–2542

Somkin, C., Hiatt, R., Hurley, L., Gruskin, E., Ackerson, L. & Larson, P. (1997) The effect of patient and provider reminders on mammography and Papanicolaou smear screening in a large health maintenance organization. *Arch. Intern. Med.*, **157**, 1658–1664

Sorlie, T., Perou, C.M., Tibshirani, R., Aas, T., Geisler, S., Johnsen, H., Hastie, T., Eisen, M.B., van de Rijn, M., Jeffrey, S.S., Thorsen, T., Quist, H., Matese, J.C., Brown, P.O., Botstein, D., Eystein, L.P. & Borresen-Dale, A.L. (2001) Gene expression patterns of breast carcinomas distinguish tumor subclasses with clinical implications. *Proc. Natl Acad. Sci. USA*, **98**, 10869–10874

Spencer, N.J., Evans, A.J., Galea, M., Sibbering, D.M., Yeoman, L.J., Pinder, S.E., Ellis, I.O., Elston, C.W., Blamey, R.W., Robertson, J.F., et al. (1994) Pathological–radiological correlations in benign lesions excised during a breast screening programme. *Clin. Radiol.*, **49**, 853–856

Stacey-Clear, A., McCarthy, K.A., Hall, D.A., Pile-Spellman, E., White, G., Hulka, C., Whitman, G.J., Mahoney, E. & Kopans, D.B. (1992) Breast cancer survival among women under age 50: Is mammography detrimental? *Lancet*, **340**, 991–994

Stanton, L., Villafana, T., Day, J.L. & Lightfoot, D.A. (1984) Dosage evaluation in mammography. *Radiology*, **150**, 577–584

Stockton, D., Davies, T., Day, N. & McCann, J. (1997) Retrospective study of reasons for improved survival in patients with breast cancer in East Anglia: Earlier diagnosis or better treatment? *Br. Med. J.*, **314**, 472–475

Stomper, P.C., Van Voorhis, B.J., Ravnikar, V.A. & Meyer, J.E. (1990) Mammographic changes associated with postmenopausal hormone replacement therapy: A longitudinal study. *Radiology*, **174**, 487–490

Stoner, T.J., Dowd, B., Carr, W.P., Maldonado, G., Church, T.R. & Mandel, J. (1998) Do vouchers improve breast cancer screening rates? Results from a randomized trial. *Health Serv. Res.*, **33**, 11–28

Stoutjesdijk, M.J., Boetes, C., Jager, G.J., Beex, L., Bult, P., Hendriks, J.H., Laheij, R.J., Massuger, L., van Die, L.E., Wobbes, T. & Barentsz, J.O. (2001) Magnetic resonance imaging and mammography in women with a hereditary risk of breast cancer. *J. Natl Cancer Inst.*, **93**, 1095–1102

Stratton, M.R., Collins, N., Lakhani, S.R. & Sloane, J.P. (1995) Loss of heterozygosity in ductal carcinoma in situ of the breast. *J. Pathol.*, **175**, 195–201

Strickland, C.J., Feigl, P., Upchurch, C., King, D.K., Pierce, H.I., Grevstad, P.K., Bearden, J.D., III, Dawson, M., Loewen,

W.C. & Meyskens, F.L., Jr (1997) Improving breast self-examination compliance: A Southwest Oncology Group randomized trial of three interventions. *Prev. Med.*, **26**, 320–332

Sudharsan, N.M., Ng, E.Y.-K. & Teh, S.L. (1999) Surface temperature distribution of a breast with/without tumor. *Int. J. Computer Meth. Biomech. Biomed. Eng.*, **2**, 187–189

Sutherland, H.J., Lockwood, G.A., Tritchler, D.L., Sem, F., Brooks, L. & Till, J.E. (1991) Communicating probabilistic information to cancer patients: Is there 'noise' on the line? *Soc. Sci. Med.*, **32**, 725–731

Sutton, S., Bickler, G., Sancho-Aldridge, J. & Saidi, G. (1994) Prospective study of predictors of attendance for breast screening in inner London. *J. Epidemiol. Community Health*, **48**, 65–73

Tabár, L. & Dean, P.B. (1982) Mammographic parenchymal patterns. Risk indicator for breast cancer? *J. Am. Med. Assoc.*, **247**, 185–189

Tabár, L., Fagerberg, C.J., Gad, A., Baldetorp, L., Holmberg, L.H., Grontoft, O., Ljungquist, U., Lundstrom, B., Manson, J.C. & Eklund, G. (1985) Reduction in mortality from breast cancer after mass screening with mammography. Randomised trial from the Breast Cancer Screening Working Group of the Swedish National Board of Health and Welfare. *Lancet*, **i**, 829–832

Tabár, L., Duffy, S.W. & Krusemo, U.B. (1987a) Detection method, tumour size and node metastases in breast cancers diagnosed during a trial of breast cancer screening. *Eur. J. Cancer Clin. Oncol.*, **23**, 959–962

Tabar, L., Faberberg, G., Day, N.E. & Holmberg, L. (1987b) What is the optimum interval between mammographic screening examinations? An analysis based on the latest results of the Swedish two-county breast cancer screening trial. *Br. J. Cancer*, **55**, 547–551

Tabár, L., Fagerberg, G., Duffy, S.W. & Day, N.E. (1989) The Swedish two county trial of mammographic screening for breast cancer: Recent results and calculation of benefit. *J. Epidemiol. Community Health*, **43**, 107–114

Tabár, L., Fagerberg, G., Duffy, S.W., Day, N.E., Gad, A. & Grontoft, O. (1992) Update of the Swedish two county program of mammographic screening for breast cancer. *Radiol. Clin. N. Am.*, **30**, 187–210

Tabár, L., Fagerberg, G., Chen, H.H., Duffy, S.W. & Gad, A. (1995) Screening for breast cancer in women aged under 50: Mode of detection, incidence, fatality and histology. *J. Med. Screen.*, **2**, 94–98

Tabár, L., Chen, H.H., Fagerberg, G., Duffy, S.W. & Smith, T.C. (1997) Recent results from the Swedish two-county trial: The effects of age, histologic type, and mode of detection on the efficacy of breast cancer screening. *Natl. Cancer Inst. Monogr.*, **22**, 43–47

Tabár, L., Duffy, S.W., Vitak, B., Chen, J.J. & Prevost, T.C. (1999) The natural history of breast carcinoma—What have we learned from screening? *Cancer*, **86**, 449–462

Tabár, L., Dean, P.B., Kaufman, C.S., Duffy, S.W. & Chen, H.H. (2000a) A new era in the diagnosis of breast cancer. *Surg. Oncol. Clin. N. Am.*, **9**, 233–277

Tabár, L., Vitak, B., Chen, H.H., Duffy, S.W., Yen, M.F., Chiang, C.F., Krusemo, U.B., Tot, T. & Smith, R.A. (2000b) The Swedish two-county trial twenty years later. Updated mortality results and new insights from long-term follow-up. *Radiol. Clin N. Am.*, **38**, 625–651

Tamburini, M., Massara, G., Bertario, L., Re, A. & Di Pietro, S. (1981) Usefulness of breast self-examination for an early detection of breast cancer. Results of a study on 500 breast cancer patients and 652 controls. *Tumori*, **67**, 219–224

Tan, P.H., Ho, J.T., Ng, E.H., Chiang, G.S., Low, S.C., Ng, F.C. & Bay, B.H. (2000) Pathologic–radiologic correlations in screen-detected ductal carcinoma in situ of the breast: Findings of the Singapore breast screening project. *Int. J. Cancer*, **90**, 231–236

Tanjasiri, S. & Sablan-Santos, L. (2001) Breast cancer screening among Chamorro women in southern California. *J. Women's Health Gender-based Med.*, **10**, 479–485

Taplin, S., Anderman, C., Grothaus, L., Curry, S. & Montano, D. (1994) Using physician correspondance and postcard reminders to promote mammography use. *Am. J. Public Health*, **84**, 571–574

Taplin, S.H., Mandelson, M.T., Anderman, C., White, E., Thompson, R.S., Timlin, D. & Wagner, E.H. (1997) Mammography diffusion and trends in late-stage breast cancer: Evaluating outcomes in a population. *Cancer Epidemiol. Biomarkers Prev.*, **6**, 625–631

Taplin, S.H., Barlow, W.E., Ludman, E., MacLehose, R., Meyer, D.M., Seger, D., Herta, D., Chin, C. & Curry, S. (2000) Testing reminder and motivational telephone calls to increase screening mammography: A randomized study. *J. Natl Cancer Inst.*, **92**, 233–242

Taplin, S.H., Rutter, C.M., Finder, C., Mandelson, M.T., Houn, F. & White, E. (2002) Screening mammography: Clinical image quality and the risk of interval breast cancer. *Am. J. Roentgenol.*, **178**, 797–803

Tarone, R.E. (1995) The excess of patients with advanced breast cancers in young women screened with mammography in the Canadian national breast screening study. *Cancer*, **75**, 997–1003

Tavassoli, F.A. & Stratton, M.R. (2002) Pathology and genetics of tumours of the breast and female genital organs. In: *WHO Classification of Tumours*, Lyon, IARCPress (in press)

Teh, W. & Wilson, A.R. (1998) The role of ultrasound in breast cancer screening. A consensus statement by the European Group for Breast Cancer Screening. *Eur. J. Cancer*, **34**, 449–450

Teppo, L., Pukkala, E. & Lehtonen, M. (1994) Data quality and quality control of a population-based cancer registry. Experience in Finland. *Acta Oncol.*, **33**, 365–369

Thilander-Klang, A.C. (1997) *Diagnostic Quality and Absorbed Dose in Mammography: Influence of X-ray Spectra and Breast Anatomy*, Thesis, Göteborg

Thilander-Klang, A.C., Ackerholm, P.H.R., Berlin, I.C., Bjurstam, I.C., Mattsson, S.L.J., Månsson, L.G., von Schéele, C. & Thunberg, S.J. (1997) Influence of anode–filter combinations on image quality and radiation dose in 965 women undergoing mammography. *Radiology*, **203**, 348–354

Thomas, L.R., Fox, S.A., Leake, B.G. & Roetzheim, R.G. (1996) The effects of health beliefs on screening mammography utilization among a diverse sample of older women. *Women Health*, **24**, 77–94

Thomas, D.B., Gao, D.L., Self, S.G., Allison, C.J., Tao, Y., Mahloch, J., Ray, R., Qin, Q., Presley, R. & Porter, P. (1997) Randomized trial of breast self-examination in Shanghai: Methodology and preliminary results. *J. Natl Cancer Inst.*, **89**, 355–365

Thomas, D.B., Gao, D.L., Ray, R.M., Wang, W.W., Allison, C.J., Chen, F.L., Porter, P., Hu, Y.W., Zhou, G.L., Pan, L.D., Li, W., Wu, C., Coriaty, Z., Evans, I., Lin, M.G., Stalsberg, H. & Self, S.G. (2002) Randomized trial of breast self-examination in Shanghai: Final results. *J. Natl Cancer Inst.*, **94** (in press)

Thompson, D.E., Mabuchi, K., Ron, E., Soda, M., Tokunaga, M., Ochikubo, S., Sugimoto, S., Ikeda, T., Terasaki, M., Izumi, S. &. Preston, D.L. (1994) Cancer incidence in atomic bomb survivors. Part II: Solid tumors, 1958–1987. *Radiat. Res.*, **137**, S17–S67

Thompson, R.S., Barlow, W.E., Taplin, S.H., Grothaus, L., Immanuel, V., Salazar, A. & Wagner, E.H. (1994) A population-based case–cohort evaluation of the efficacy of mammographic screening for breast cancer. *Am. J. Epidemiol.*, **140**, 889–901

Thurfjell, E.L. & Lindgren, J.A.A. (1994) Population-based mammography screening in Swedish clinical practice: Prevalence and incidence screening in Uppsala County. *Radiology*, **193**, 351–357

Thurfjell, E.L., Taube, A. & Tabár, L. (1994a) One-versus two-view mammographic screening. A prospective population based study. *Acta Radiol.*, **35**, 340–344

Thurfjell, E.L., Lernevall, K.A. & Taube, A.A.S. (1994b) Benefit of independent double reading in a population-based mammography screening program. *Radiology*, **191**, 241–244

Thurfjell, E.L., Holmberg, L.H. & Persson, I.R. (1997) Screening mammography: Sensitivity and specificity in relation to hormone replacement therapy. *Radiology*, **203**, 339–341

Tilanus-Linthorst, M.M., Bartels, C.C., Obdeijn, A.I. & Oudkerk, M. (2000a) Earlier detection of breast cancer by surveillance of women at familial risk. *Eur. J. Cancer*, **36**, 514–519

Tilanus-Linthorst, M.M., Obdeijn, I.M., Bartels, K.C., de Koning, H.J. & Oudkerk, M. (2000b) First experiences in screening women at high risk for breast cancer with MR imaging. *Breast Cancer Res. Treat.*, **63**, 53–60

Todd, J.H., Dowle, C., Williams, M.R., Elston, C.W., Ellis, I.O., Hinton, C.P., Blamey, R.W. & Haybittle, J.L. (1987) Confirmation of a prognostic index in primary breast cancer. *Br. J. Cancer*, **56**, 489–492

Tokunaga, M., Land, C.E., Tokuoka, S., Nishimori, I., Soda, M. & Akiba, S. (1994) Incidence of female breast cancer among atomic bomb survivors, 1950–1985. *Radiat. Res.*, **138**, 209–223

Törnberg, S., Carstensen, J., Hakulinen, T., Lenner, P., Hatschek, T. & Lundgren, B. (1994) Evaluation of the effect on breast cancer mortality of population based mammography screening programmes. *J. Med. Screen.*, **1**, 184–187

Tsongalis, G.J. & Ried, A., Jr (2001) HER2: The neu prognostic marker for breast cancer. *Crit. Rev. Clin. Lab. Sci.,* **38**, 167–182

Tsuda, H., Tani, Y., Hasegawa, T. & Fukutomi, T. (2001) Concordance in judgments among c-erbB-2 (HER2/neu) overexpression detected by two immunohistochemical tests and gene amplification detected by Southern blot hybridization in breast carcinoma. *Pathol. Int.*, **51**, 26–32

Turnbull, D., Irwig, L. & Adelson, P. (1991) A randomised trial of invitations to attend for screening mammography. *Aust. J. Public Health*, **15**, 33–36

Turnbull, D., Irwig, L., Simpson, J.M., Donnelly, N. & Mock, P. (1995) A prospective cohort study investigating psychosocial predictors of attendance at a mobile breast screening service. *Aust. J. Public Health*, **19**, 172–176

Turner, L., Swindell, R., Bell, W.G., Hartley, R.C., Tasker, J.H., Wilson, W.W., Alderson, M.R. & Leck, I.M. (1981) Radical versus modified radical mastectomy for breast cancer. *Ann. R. Coll. Surg.*, **63**, 239–243

Turner, K.M., Wilson, B. & Gilbert, F. (1994) Improving breast screening uptake: Persuading initial non-attenders to attend. *J. Med. Screen.*, **1**, 199–202

UICC (2002) *TNM Classification of Malignant Tumors*, 6th Ed., New York, Wiley

UK MRI Breast Screening Study Advisory Group (2000) Magnetic resonance imaging screening in women at genetic risk of breast cancer: Imaging and analysis protocol for the UK multicentre study. *Magn. Reson. Imaging*, **18**, 765–776

UK Trial of Early Detection of Breast Cancer Group (1988) First results on mortality reduction in the UK Trial of Early Detection of Breast Cancer. *Lancet*, **ii**, 411–416

UK Trial of Early Detection of Breast Cancer Group (1999) 16-year mortality from breast cancer in the UK Trial of Early Detection of Breast Cancer. *Lancet*, **353**, 1909–1914

UNSCEAR (1994) *Epidemiologic Studies of Radiation Carcinogenesis*, Annex A, New York

Urban, N., Anderson, G. & Peacock, S. (1994) Mammography screening: How important is cost as a barrier to use? *Am. J. Public Health*, **84**, 50–55

US Congress, Office of Technology Assessment (1987) *Breast Cancer Screening for Medicare Beneficiaries: Effectivness, Costs to Medicare and Medical Resources Required*, Washington DC, US Government Printing Office

US Preventive Task Force (1996) *Report of the US Preventive Services Task Force, Guide to Clinical Preventive Services*, 2nd Edition, Williams & Wilkins, Baltimore, pp. 73–88

Valdez, A., Banerjee, K., Ackerson, L., Fernandez, M., Otero-Sabogal, R. & Somkin, C.P. (2001) Correlates of breast cancer screening among low-income, low-education Latinas. *Prev. Med.*, **33**, 495–502

van't Veer, L.J., Dai, H., van de Vijver, M.J., He, Y.D., Hart, A.A., Mao, M., Peterse, H.L., van der, K.K., Marton, M.J., Witteveen, A.T., Schreiber, G.J., Kerkhoven, R.M., Roberts, C., Linsley, P.S., Bernards, R. & Friend, S.H. (2002) Gene expression profiling predicts clinical outcome of breast cancer. *Nature*, **415**, 530–536

Verbeek, A.L., Hendriks, J.H., Holland, R., Mravunac, M., Sturmans, F. & Day, N.E. (1984) Reduction of breast cancer mortality through mass screening with modern mammography. First results of the Nijmegen project, 1975–1981. *Lancet*, **1**, 1222–1224

Verbeek, A.L., Hendriks, J.H., Holland, R., Mravunac, M. & Sturmans, F. (1985) Mammographic screening and breast cancer mortality: Age-specific effects in Nijmegen Project, 1975–82. *Lancet*, **i**, 865–866

Verbeek, A.L.M., Straatmen,* H. & Hendriks, J.H.C.L. (1988) Sensitivity of mammography in Nijmegen women under age 50: Some trials with the Eddy model. In: Day, N.E. & Miller, A.B., eds, *Screening for Breast Cancer*, Toronto, Hans Huber, pp. 29–32

Verbeek, A.L.M., van den Ban, M.C. & Hendriks, J.H.C.L. (1991) A proposal for short-term quality control in breast cancer screening. *Br. J. Cancer*, **63**, 261–264

Vernon, S.W., Vogel, V., Halabi, S., Jackson, G., Lundy, R. & Peters, G. (1992) Breast cancer screening behaviors and attitudes in three racial/ethnic groups. *Cancer*, **69**, 165–174

Veronesi, U., Banfi, A., Salvadori, B., Luini, A., Saccozzi, R., Zucali, R., Marubini, E., del Vecchio, M., Boracchi, P., Marchini, S., Merson, M., Sacchini, V., Riboldi, G. & Santoro, G. (1990) Breast conservation is the treatment of choice in small breast cancer: Long-term results of a randomized trial. *Eur. J. Cancer*, **26**, 668–670

Veronesi, U., Galimberti, V., Zurrida, S. & et al. (1993a) Prognostic significance of number and level of axillary node metastases in breast cancer. *Breast*, **2**, 224–228

Veronesi, U., Luini, A., del Vecchio, M., Greco, M., Galimberti, V., Merson, M., Rilke, F., Sacchini, V., Saccozzi, R., Savio, T., Zucali, R., Zurrida, S. & Salvadori, B. (1993b) Radiotherapy after breast-preserving surgery in women with localized cancer of the breast. *New Engl. J. Med.*, **328**, 1587–1591

Veronesi, U., Maisonneuve, P., Costa, A., Sacchini, V., Maltoni, C., Robertson, C., Rotmensz, N. & Boyle, P. (1998) Prevention of breast cancer with tamoxifen: Preliminary findings from the Italian randomised trial among hysterectomised women. Italian Tamoxifen Prevention Study. *Lancet*, **352**, 93–97

Vincent, A.L., Bradham, D., Hoercherl, S. & McTague, D. (1995) Survey of clinical breast examinations and use of screening mammography in Florida. *South. Med. J.*, **88**, 731–736

Vleminckx, K., Vakaet, L., Jr, Mareel, M., Fiers, W. & van Roy, F. (1991) Genetic manipulation of E-cadherin expression by epithelial tumor cells reveals an invasion suppressor role. *Cell*, **66**, 107–119

de Waard, F., Collette, H.J., Rombach, J.J., Baanders-van Halewijn, E.A. & Honing, C. (1984a) The DOM project for the early detection of breast cancer, Utrecht, The Netherlands. *J. Chron. Dis.*, **37**, 1–44

de Waard, F., Rombach, J.J., Collette, H.J.A. & Slotboom, B. (1984b) Breast cancer risk associated with reproductive factors and breast parenchymal patterns. *J. Natl Cancer Inst.*, **72**, 1277–1282

de Waard, F., Kirkpatrick, A., Perry, N.M., Tornberg, S., Tubiana, M. & de Wolf, C. (1994) Breast cancer screening in the framework of the Europe against Cancer Programme. *Eur. J. Cancer Prev.*, **3**, 3–5

Wald, N.J., Murphy, P., Major, P., Parkes, C., Townsend, J. & Frost, C. (1995) UKCCCR multicentre randomised controlled trial of one and two view mammography in breast cancer screening. *Br. Med. J.*, **311**, 1189–1193

Waldman, F.M., Hwang, E.S., Etzell, J., Eng, C., Devries, S., Bennington, J. & Thor, A. (2001) Genomic alterations in tubular breast carcinomas. *Hum. Pathol.*, **32**, 222–226

Walker, L.G., Cordiner, C.M., Gilbert, F.G., Needham, G., Deans, H.E., Affleck, I.R., Hood, D.B., Mathieson, D., Ah-See, A.K. & Eremin, O. (1994) How distressing is attendance for routine breast screening? *Psych. Oncol.*, **3**, 299–304

Walter, S.D. & Day, N.E. (1983) Estimation of the duration of a pre-clinical disease state using screening data. *Am. J. Epidemiol.*, **118**, 865–886

Wang, H., Karesen, R., Hervik, A. & Thoresen, S.O. (2001) Mammography screening in Norway: Results from the first screening round in four counties and cost–effectiveness of a modeled nationwide screening. *Cancer Causes Control*, **12**, 39–45

Warner, E., Plewes, D.B., Shumak, R.S., Catzavelos, G.C., Di Prospero, L.S., Yaffe, M.J., Goel, V., Ramsay, E., Chart, P.L., Cole, D.E., Taylor, G.A., Cutrara, M., Samuels, T.H., Murphy, J.P., Murphy, J.M. & Narod, S.A. (2001) Comparison of breast magnetic resonance imaging, mammography, and ultrasound for surveillance of women at high risk for hereditary breast cancer. *J. Clin. Oncol.*, **19**, 3524–3531

Warren, R.M. & Duffy, S.W. (1995) Comparison of single reading with double reading of mammograms, and change in effectiveness with experience. *Br. J. Radiol.*, **68**, 958–962

Warren Burhenne, L.J., Wood, S.A., D'Orsi, C.J., Feig, S.A., Kopans, D.B., O'Shaughnessy, K.F., Sickles, E.A., Tabar, L., Vyborny, C.J. & Castellino, R.A. (2000) Potential contribution of computer-aided detection to the sensitivity of screening mammography. *Radiology*, **215**, 554–562

Waterhouse, J., Muir, C., Correa, P. & Powell, J., eds (1976) *Cancer Incidence in Five Continents, Volume III* (IARC Scientific Publications No. 15), Lyon, IARCPress

Waterhouse, J., Muir, C., Shanmugaratnam, K. & Powell, J., eds (1982) *Cancer Incidence in Five Continents, Volume IV* (IARC Scientific Publications No. 42), Lyon, IARCPress

Waterhouse, J., Mack, T., Powell, J. & Whelan, S., eds (1987) *Cancer Incidence in Five Continents, Volume V* (IARC Scientific Publications No. 88), Lyon, IARCPress

Weiss, N.S. (1983) Control definition in case–control studies of the efficacy of screening and diagnostic testing. *Am. J. Epidemiol.*, **118**, 457–460

Welch, H.G. & Black, W.C. (1997) Using autopsy series to estimate the disease 'reservoir' for ductal carcinoma in situ of the breast: How much more breast cancer can we find? *Ann. Intern. Med.*, **127**, 1023–1028

Welch, H.G. & Fisher, E.S. (1998) Diagnostic testing following screening mammography in the elderly. *J. Natl Cancer Inst.*, **90**, 1389–1392

Wellings, S.R., Jensen, H.M. & Marcum, R.G. (1975) An atlas of subgross pathology of the human breast with special reference to possible precancerous lesions. *J. Natl Cancer Inst.*, **55**, 231–273

Wellman, P.S., Dalton, E.P., Krag, D., Kern, K.A. & Howe, R.D. (2001) Tactile imaging of breast masses: First clinical report. *Arch. Surg*, **136**, 204–208

West, M., Blanchette, C., Dressman, H., Huang, E., Ishida, S., Spang, R., Zuzan, H., Olson, J.A., Jr., Marks, J.R. & Nevins, J.R. (2001) Predicting the clinical status of human breast cancer by using gene expression profiles. *Proc. Natl Acad. Sci. USA*, **98**, 11462–11467

Whelan, C., McLean, D. & Poulos, A. (1999) Investigation of thyroid dose due to mammography. *Australas. Radiol.*, **43**, 307–310

White, E., Velentgas, P., Mandelson, M.T., Lehman, C.D., Elmore, J.G., Porter, P., Yasui, Y. & Taplin, S.H. (1998) Variation in mammographic breast density by time in menstrual cycle among women aged 40–49 years. *J. Natl Cancer Inst.*, **90**, 906–910

Whitman, S., Ansell, D., Lacey, L., Chen, E.H., Ebie, N., Dell, J. & Phillips, C.W. (1991) Patterns of breast and cervical cancer screening at three public health centers in an inner-city urban area. *Am. J. Public Health*, **81**, 1651–1653

WHO Mortality Data Bank. Available at: http://www-depdb.iarc.fr/who/menu.htm

WHO (1999a) *Cancer Database for the Western Pacific Region: Essential Features and Data Analysis*, Manila, Regional Office for the Western Pacific

WHO (1999b) *1997–1999 World Health: Statistics Annual*, Geneva

Williams, K.L., Phillips, B.H., Jones, P.A., Beaman, S.A. & Fleming, P.J. (1990) Thermography in screening for breast cancer. *J. Epidemiol. Community Health*, **44**, 112–113

Williams, R., Boles, M. & Johnson, R. (1998) A patient-initiated system for preventive health care. A randomized trial in community-based primary care practices. *Arch. Fam. Med.*, **7**, 338–345

de Wolf, C.J.M. (2001) [Summary of EUREF programmes. Group of Epidemiologists of Latin Languages], Neuchatel (in French)

de Wolf, C.J.M. & Perry, N.M., eds (1996) *European Guidelines for Quality Assurance in Mammography Screening*, 2nd Ed., Europe Against Cancer Programme, Luxembourg, Commission of the European Communities

Worden, J.K., Solomon, L.J., Flynn, B.S., Costanza, M.C., Foster, R.S., Jr, Dorwaldt, A.L. & Weaver, S.O. (1990) A community-wide program in breast self-examination training and maintenance. *Prev. Med.*, **19**, 254–269

Workshop Group (1989) Reducing deaths from breast cancer in Canada. *Can. Med. Assoc. J.*, **141**, 199–201

Wrensch, M.R., Petrakis, N.L., Miike, R., King, E.B., Chew, K., Neuhaus, J., Lee, M.M. & Rhys, M. (2001) Breast cancer risk in women with abnormal cytology in nipple aspirates of breast fluid. *J. Natl Cancer Inst.*, **93**, 1791–1798

Wright, C.J. (1986) Breast cancer screening: A different look at the evidence. *Surgery*, **100**, 594–598

Wu, X., Gingold, E.L., Barnes, G.T. & Tucker, D.M. (1994) Normalized average glandular dose in molybdenum target–rhodium filter and rhodium target–rhodium filter mammography. *Radiology*, **193**, 83–89

Yamauchi, H., Stearns, V. & Hayes, D.F. (2001) When is a tumor marker ready for prime time? A case study of c-erbB-2 as a predictive factor in breast cancer. *J. Clin. Oncol.*, **19**, 2334–2356

Yanovitzky, I. & Blitz, C. (2000) Effect of media coverage and physician advice on utilization of breast cancer screening by women 40 years and older. *J. Health Communication*, **5**, 117–134

Yasuda, S., Ide, M., Fujii, H., Nakahara, T., Mochizuki, Y., Takahashi, W. & Shohtsu, A. (2000) Application of positron emission tomography imaging to cancer screening. *Br. J. Cancer*, **83**, 1607–1611

Yester, M.V., Barnes, G.T. & King, M.A. (1981) Experimental measurements of the scatter reduction obtained in mammography with a scanning multiple slit assembly. *Med. Phys.*, **8**, 158–162

Yokoe, T., Iino, Y., Maemura, M., Takei, H., Horiguchi, J., Matsumoto, H., Morishita, Y. & Koibuchi, Y. (1998) Efficacy of mammo-graphy for detecting early breast cancer in women under 50. *Anticancer Res.*, **18**, 4709–4711

Young, K.C. & Burch, A. (2000) Radiation doses received in the UK breast screening programme in 1997 and 1998. *Br. J. Radiol.*, **73**, 278–287

Young, K.C., Ramsdale, M.L. & Rust, A. (1996) Dose and image quality in mammography with an automatic beam quality system. *Br. J. Radiol.*, **69**, 555–562

Young, K.C., Wallis, M.G., Blanks, R.G. & Moss, S.M. (1997) Influence of number of views and mammographic film density on the detection of invasive cancers: Results from the NHS breast screening programme. *Br. J. Radiol.*, **70**, 482–488

Zambrana, R.E., Breen, N., Fox, S.A. & Gutierrez-Mohamed, M.L. (1999) Use of cancer screening practices by Hispanic women: Analyses by subgroup. *Prev. Med.*, **29**, 466–477

Zapka, J.G., Hosmer, D., Costanza, M.E., Harris, D.R. & Stoddard, A. (1992) Changes in mammography use: Economic, need, and service factors. *Am. J. Public Health*, **82**, 1345–1351

Zelen, M. & Feinleib, M. (1969) On the theory of screening for chronic diseases. *Biometrika*, **56**, 601–614

Ziegler, R.G., Hoover, R.N., Pike, M.C., Hildesheim, A., Nomura, A.M., West, D.W., Wu-Williams, A.H., Kolonel, L.N., Horn-Ross, P.L. & Rosenthal, J.F. (1993) Migration patterns and breast cancer risk in Asian–American women. *J. Natl Cancer Inst.*, **85**, 1819–1827

Zoetelief, J., Fitzgerald, M., Leitz, W. & Säbel, M. (1996) *European Protocol on Dosimetry in Mammography* (EUR 16263), Brussels, Commission of the European Communities

Zuur, C. & Broerse, J.J. (1985) Risk– and cost–benefit analyses of breast screening programs derived from absorbed dose measurements in The Netherlands. *Diagn. Imaging Clin. Med.*, **54**, 211–222

# Glossary

| | |
|---|---|
| **Background incidence rate:** | The breast cancer incidence rate expected in the absence of screening |
| **Invasive breast cancer detection rate:** | The number of histologically proven malignant lesions of the breast (invasive) detected at screening per 1000 women |
| **Total breast cancer detection rate:** | The number of histologically proven malignant lesions of the breast: in-situ (ductal only, not lobular) and invasive detected at screening per 1000 women |
| **Breast cancer incidence rate:** | The rate at which new cases of breast cancer occurs in a population. The numerator is the number of newly diagnosed cases of breast cancer that occurs in a defined period. The denominator is the population at risk of a diagnosis of breast cancer during this defined period, sometimes expressed in person-time. |
| **Breast cancer mortality rate:** | The rate at which deaths from breast cancer occur in a population. The numerator is the number of breast cancer deaths that occurs in a defined time period. The denominator is the population at risk of dying from breast cancer during this defined period, sometimes expressed as person–time. |
| **Breast cancer register:** | Recording of information on all new cases of and deaths from breast cancer occurring in a defined population |
| **Delay time:** | The time between when a cancer could be detected by screening and when it is actually detected |
| **Efficacy:** | The reduction in breast cancer mortality in randomized trials, under ideal conditions |
| **Effectiveness:** | The reduction in breast cancer mortality in screening practice, under real conditions |
| **Eligible population:** | The adjusted target population, i.e. the target population minus those women who are excluded according to screening policy on the basis of eligibility criteria other than age, sex and geographical location |
| **Further assessment:** | Additional diagnostic steps (either non-invasive or invasive) performed to clarify the nature of an abnormality detected at screening, either at the time of screening or on recall |
| **Interval cancer:** | A primary breast cancer diagnosed in a woman who had a result in a screening test, with or without further assessment, that was negative for malignancy, either:<br>• before the next invitation to screening was due or<br>• within a period equal to a screening interval for a woman who has reached the upper age limit for screening |

| | |
|---|---|
| **Interval cancer rate:** | The number of interval cancers diagnosed within a defined period since the last negative result in a screening examination per 1000 women with negative results |
| **Lead time:** | Period between when a cancer is found by screening and when it would be detected from clinical signs and symptoms (not directly observable) |
| **Length bias:** | The bias towards detection of cancers with longer sojourn times and therefore a better prognosis by screening |
| **Open biopsy:** | Surgical removal of (part of) a breast lesion |
| **Organized screening:** | Screening programmes organized at national or regional level, with an explicit policy, a team responsible for organization and for health care and a structure for quality assurance |
| **Opportunistic screening:** | Screening outside an organized or population-based screening programme, as a result of e.g. a recommendation made during a routine medical consultation, consultation for an unrelated condition, on the basis of a possibly increased risk for developing breast cancer (family history or other known risk factor) or by self-referral |
| **Overdiagnosis:** | Detection of breast cancers that might never have progressed to become symptomatic during a woman's life |
| **Participation rate:** | Number of women who have a screening test as a proportion of all women who are invited to attend for screening |
| **Population access:** | Proportion of the national population of elegible women who have access to a screening programme |
| **Positive predictive value:** | Proportion of all positive results at screening that lead to a diagnosis of cancer |
| **Recall:** | Physical recall of women to the screening unit, as a consequence of the screening examination, for:<br>• a repeat mammogram because of technical inadequacy of the screening mammogram (technical recall); or<br>• clarification of a perceived abnormality detected at screening, by performance of an additional procedure (recall for further assessment). |
| **Recall rate:** | The number of women recalled for further assessment as a proportion of all women who were screened |
| **Refined mortality:** | Mortality rate among women, excluding those in whom breast cancer was diagnosed before screening began |
| **Screening interval:** | Fixed interval between routine screenings decided upon in each programme, depending on screening policy |
| **Screening policy:** | Specific policy of a screening programme which dictates the targeted age and sex group, the geographical area, the screening interval (usually 2 or 3 years), etc. |

| | |
|---|---|
| **Screening test:** | Test applied to all women in a programme, consisting of a single or two-view mammogram with or without clinical examination |
| **Sensitivity:** | The proportion of truly diseased persons in the screened population who are identified as diseased by the screening test. The more general expression for 'sensitivity of the screening programme' refers to the ratio of true positives (breast cancers correctly identified at the screening examination) / true positives + false negatives (breast cancers not identified at the screening examination, detected as interval cases). |
| **Sojourn time:** | Detectable preclinical phase; time between that at which a tumour could be found by screening and that at which it would appear symptomatically (not directly observable) |
| **Specificity:** | Proportion of truly non-diseased persons in the screened population who are identified as non-diseased by the screening test (i.e. true negatives / true negatives + false positives) |
| **Target population:** | The age-eligible population for screening, e.g. all women offered screening according to the policy |

# Working Procedures

Prevention of cancer is one of the key objectives of IARC. Secondary prevention by early diagnosis and screening in non-symptomatic individuals is a fundamental component of any cancer control programme. The aim of secondary prevention is to reduce mortality and suffering from the disease. When screening is planned as part of a cancer control programme, only strategies proved to be effective should be proposed to the general population. Screening usually requires repeated interactions between 'healthy' individuals and health care providers, which can be inconvenient and costly. Furthermore, screening requires an ongoing commitment between the public and health care providers.

## Scope

Cochrane (1972) first discussed the concepts of efficacy and effectiveness in the context of health interventions. Efficacy was later defined by Last (1995) as "the extent to which a specific intervention, procedure or service produces a beneficial result under ideal circumstances". In contrast, the related term "effectiveness" is defined by the same author as "... a measure of the extent to which a specific intervention, procedure, regimen or service, when deployed in the field in routine circumstances, does what it is intended to do for a specific population." The distinction between efficacy as measured in experimental studies and the effectiveness of a mass population intervention is a crucial one for public health decision-making. In particular, the fact that the effectiveness of a screening procedure may be differ-

ent in different populations is often overlooked. A mass programme of screening must satisfy certain minimal requirements (e.g. acceptability, availability of relevant personnel, facilities for screening and access to pertinent health services) if it is to achieve the results that have been documented in randomized trials. The acceptance and use of screening services may vary from one population to another, implying that a given screening procedure is not universally effective. Even when a screening procedure is effective as a mass intervention, other outcomes such as harms and costs and the potential for other interventions to achieve equivalent benefits must be considered.

Efficacy is a necessary but not a sufficient basis for recommending screening. The efficacy of a screening procedure can be inferred if effectiveness can be proven. Screening has sometimes been implemented by a given procedure on the assumption that 'earlier is better', even when no evidence of efficacy was available. If such interventions result in a significant reduction in mortality that cannot otherwise be explained (by reduced incidence, due perhaps to primary prevention or better treatment), it can be inferred that the procedure is effective. However, uncontrolled interventions in which individuals are exposed to unknown risks and benefits should be avoided.

## Objectives

The objectives of the Working Group are:

(1) to evaluate the strength of the evidence for the efficacy of a screening procedure;
(2) to assess the effectiveness of defined screening interventions in defined populations;
(3) to assess the balance of benefit and harm in target populations; and
(4) to formulate recommendations for further research and for public health action.

The conclusions of the Working Group are published as a volume in the series of the IARC Handbooks of Cancer Prevention.

## Working groups

An international working group of experts is convened by the IARC. The tasks of the group are:

(1) to ascertain that all appropriate data have been retrieved;
(2) to select the data relevant for evaluation on the basis of scientific merit;
(3) to prepare accurate reviews of data to allow the reader to follow the reasoning of the working group;
(4) to evaluate the efficacy and effectiveness of the screening procedure;
(5) to summarize the potential adverse consequences of screening;
(6) to prepare recommendations for research and for public health action; and
(7) to prepare an overall evaluation of the screening procedure at the population level.

Approximately 13 months before a working group meets, the topics of the

Handbook are announced, and prospective participants are selected by IARC staff in consultation with other experts. Subsequently, relevant data are collected by the IARC from all available sources of published information. Working Group participants who contributed to the considerations and evaluations within a particular handbook are listed, with their addresses, at the beginning of each publication. Each participant serves as an independent scientist and not as a representative of any organization, government or industry. They are expected to put aside any stake they may have in a particular outcome and to evaluate the evidence objectively and with scientific rigour. Scientists nominated by national and international agencies, industrial associations and consumer and/or environmental organizations may be invited as observers. IARC staff members involved in the preparation of the handbook are listed.

About eight months before the meeting, the material collected is sent to meeting participants who are asked to prepare sections for the first drafts of the handbook. These drafts are then compiled by IARC staff and sent, before the meeting, to all participants of the working group for review.

### Data for handbooks
The handbooks do not necessarily cite all of the literature on the agent or strategy being evaluated. Only those data considered by the working group to be relevant to making the evaluation are included. Meeting abstracts and other reports that do not provide sufficient detail upon which to base an assessment of their quality are generally not considered.

With regard to reports of basic scientific research, epidemiological studies and clinical trials, only those that have been published or accepted for publication in the openly available scientific literature are reviewed by the working group. In certain instances, government agency reports that have undergone peer review and are widely available are considered. Exceptions may be made ad hoc to include unpublished reports that are in their final form and publicly available, if their inclusion is considered pertinent to making a final evaluation.

The available studies are summarized by the working group. In general, numerical findings are indicated as they appear in the original report; units are converted when necessary for easier comparison. The working group may conduct additional analyses of the published data and use them in their assessment of the evidence. These analyses are described in the handbook. Important aspects of a study, directly impinging on its interpretation, are brought to the attention of the reader.

## Evaluation of screening
The framework of a handbook on screening includes the following nine chapters:

## Chapter 1. Disease characteristics, global burden and rationale for screening

### Descriptive epidemiology
The purpose of this section is to document the importance of the disease in the context of the general health status of different populations. The worldwide burden of the cancer is described (mortality, incidence, prevalence and survival rates) and integrated with measures of the occurrence of cancers at other sites, of mortality from all causes and life expectancy. Expected trends in the absence of screening are a relevant component of this section.

### Natural history of the disease as relevant to screening
In this section, the natural history of the disease of interest and the relevance and potential of screening for early detection and for reducing mortality are described. Evolving concepts and principles pertinent to screening are also discussed.

There is now a wealth of evidence (both direct and indirect) to support the principle that screening and detection of certain cancers in appropriate target populations are associated with a lower probability of dying from the disease. The scheme (on the next page) illustrates the temporal framework commonly subscribed to in modern screening models

It should be noted that early diagnosis, due to greater awareness and improved access to appropriate medical services, has resulted in many countries in a reduction in diagnostic delay, probably reducing mortality. As a consequence, symptomatic cancers are frequently diagnosed and treated early after the onset of symptoms in many developed nations. In such instances, screening for the disease will improve outcomes (such as a reduction in mortality) only if treatment of the disease at an even earlier phase in its development provides additional benefit. The rapid evolution of molecular or genetic markers of pre-malignant conditions or individuals at 'high risk' has modified the concepts of 'disease onset' and 'lead time'. Hence, the model outlined above may require adaptation or development to allow for detection of pre-clinical conditions of undetermined significance (including serological and molecular markers and genetic predisposition), if they are relevant for screening for the cancer in question.

## Chapter 2. Screening tests
It is important to distinguish between screening tests and screening procedures, i.e. the test itself and the way in which it is administered. The two merit separate, detailed evaluation. Each of the screening tests to be considered is described. The ability of each test to detect cancer and to distinguish cancer from non-cancer conditions will be assessed as:

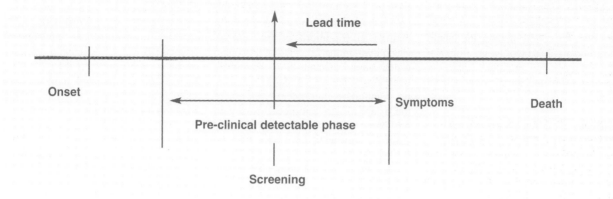

the validity of the test, expressed as its sensitivity and specificity under various conditions;

all known or potential side-effects; and

the cost of the test when implemented in mass screening programmes.

## Chapter 3. Delivery and uptake of screening

Information on how screening is delivered in different countries is reviewed in this section, with emphasis on the following aspects:

infrastructure for diagnosis and treatment: the nature of standard diagnostic procedures and treatment regimens and their availability to the target population;

extent of population coverage and participation rates;

equity, as defined by the extent to which access to the procedure (including diagnostic investigation and treatment) is ensured for all eligible individuals, irrespective of any personal characteristics;

informed decision and informed consent: the extent to which individual values are respected when information on potential benefit and harms is conveyed; and

behavioural and demographic considerations that affect participation in screening.

## Chapter 4. Efficacy of screening tests

In this section, evidence from experimental and observational studies is reviewed, and aspects of study design and analysis are critically discussed.

The handbooks are not intended to summarize all published studies. The working group considers the following aspects:

(1) the relevance of the study;
(2) the appropriateness of the design and analysis to the question being asked;
(3) the adequacy and completeness of the presentation of the data; and
(4) the degree to which chance, bias and confounding may have affected the results.

Studies that are judged to be inadequate or irrelevant to the evaluation are generally omitted. They may be mentioned briefly (i) when the information is considered to be a useful supplement to that in other reports, (ii) if they provide the only data available or (iii), in exceptional cases, if they have been widely perceived as being pertinent but are deemed otherwise by the Working Group. Their inclusion does not imply acceptance of the adequacy of the study design nor of the analysis and interpretation of the results, and their limitations are outlined.

The appropriate outcome(s) (mortality or incidence) of a given procedure, e.g. the detectable phase(s) of the natural history of the disease, are also defined. Aspects that are particularly important in evaluating experimental studies are: the selection of participants, the nature and adequacy of the randomization procedure, evidence that randomization achieved an adequate balance between the groups, the exclusion criteria used before and after randomization, compliance with the intervention in the screened group and 'contamination' with the intervention in the control group. Other considerations are the means by which the endpoint was determined and validated (either by screening or by other means of detection of the disease), the length and completeness of follow-up of the groups and the adequacy of the analysis.

Whenever possible, similar criteria should be used to evaluate non-experimental comparative studies.

In the Working Group's analysis of the efficacy of the screening procedure, a meta-analysis may be used, when applicable.

In evaluating case–control and cohort studies, particular attention is paid to the definition of cases, controls and exposure and, for cohort studies, the length and completeness of follow-up. Potential bias, especially selection bias, is carefully examined in all observational studies.

## Chapter 5. Effectiveness of population-based screening

The impact of the screening procedure when implemented in defined populations is examined in this section. Indicators used to monitor effectiveness, such as positive and negative predictive values, detection rate, rates of interval cancers and the number of tests performed, are reported. Time trends before and after implementation of screening as well as geographical comparisons of the occurrence of the disease and death from the disease in populations exposed and not exposed to screening are reviewed and interpreted. In doing this, the Working Group takes into account differences in screening procedures (e.g. frequency and the age of the target population) and of participation rates.

An integral component of this section is an evaluation of the benefits and harms of the screening procedure to the population. Reductions in mortality and/or incidence of invasive disease are fundamental measures of benefit. A reduction in the cumulative prevalence of advanced disease may be a useful predictor of a reduction in mortality from the disease. An additional benefit may be that more cases can be treated by less aggressive, less invasive procedures, thus improving the quality of life.

The spectrum of health care is dynamic, and a screening procedure should not be viewed in isolation. Greater awareness of the disease, brought about by publicity about screening that may result in early diagnosis, could be regarded as another benefit of a screening programme. This section should also consider the possibility that there might have been a change in treatment of the cancer, which even in the absence of screening would have resulted in a substantial decrease in mortality. As far as possible, an evaluation should be made of the extent to which improved treatment has been responsible for any changes seen in mortality from the specific disease.

Estimates of the rates of false-positive and false-negative findings in screened individuals and their consequences (false sense of security with false-negatives and false alarm with false-positives) are an integral part of this section. The rates of short- and long-term side-effects and the possibility of unnecessary treatment of borderline or indolent cases detected at screening are discussed. Management procedures for lesions detected at screening are reviewed. Psychological factors, such as anxiety induced by undergoing the test procedure, are also considered.

## Chapter 6. Cost-effectiveness of population-based screening

In this section, the cost-effectiveness of various modalities of test administration in various settings is considered. The discussion takes into account the costs per case detected and per death prevented.

## Chapter 7. Summary of data

In this section, the relevant data are summarized. Inadequate studies identified in the preceding text are generally not included.

## Chapter 8. Evaluation

### Evaluation of the efficacy of the screening procedure

An evaluation of the degree of evidence for the efficacy of a screening procedure is formulated according to the following definitions:

*Sufficient evidence of the efficacy of cancer-preventive activity* will apply when screening interventions by a defined procedure are consistently associated with a reduction in mortality from the cancer and/or a reduction in the incidence of invasive cancer, and chance and bias can be ruled out with reasonable confidence.

*Limited evidence of the efficacy of cancer-preventive activity* will apply when screening interventions by a defined procedure are associated with a reduction in mortality from the cancer and/or a reduction in the incidence of invasive cancer or a reduction in the incidence of clinically advanced cancer, but bias or confounding cannot be ruled out with reasonable confidence as alternative explanations for these associations.

*Inadequate evidence of the efficacy of cancer-preventive activity* will apply when data are lacking or when the available information is insufficient or too heterogeneous to allow an evaluation.

*Sufficient evidence that the screening procedure is not efficacious in cancer prevention* will apply when any of the following cases hold:

- the test does not result in earlier diagnosis than with standard tests already in use;
- the survival of cases detected at screening is no better than that of cases diagnosed routinely;
- the screening interventions are consistently associated with no reduction in mortality from the cancer, and bias can be ruled out with reasonable confidence.

In case of limited or inadequate evidence, the Working Group should highlight those aspects of the procedure for which information is lacking and which led to the uncertainty in evaluation. This will provide indications of research priorities.

## Overall evaluation

Finally, the body of evidence is considered as a whole, and summary statements are made about the cancer-preventive effects of the screening intervention in humans and other beneficial or adverse effects, as appropriate. The overall evaluation is usually in the form of a narrative. The data on the effectiveness of the screening intervention are summarized, including the factors that determine its success and failure under routine conditions. Finally, the balance between expected benefit and harm is described.

## Chapter 9. Recommendations

After its review of the data and its deliberations, the working group formulates recommendations, where applicable, for:

- further research and
- public health action.

## References

Cochrane, A.L. (1972) *Effectiveness and Efficiency: Random Reflections on Health Services*, Oxford: Nuffield Provincial Hospitals Trust

Last, J.M. (1995) *A Dictionary of Epidemiology*, Oxford: Oxford University Press

# Sources of figures

Figure 1   Ferlay *et al.* (2001)

Figure 2   Ferlay *et al.* (2001)

Figure 3   Descriptive Epidemiology Unit (International Agency for Research on Cancer) (DEP/IARC)

Figure 4   DEP (IARC)

Figure 5   DEP (IARC)

Figure 6   I. Ellis, Division of Histopathology, Nottingham City Hospital, UK

Figure 7   I. Ellis, Division of Histopathology, Nottingham City Hospital, UK

Figure 8   I. Ellis, Division of Histopathology, Nottingham City Hospital, UK

Figure 9   I. Ellis, Division of Histopathology, Nottingham City Hospital, UK

Figure 10   I. Ellis, Division of Histopathology, Nottingham City Hospital, UK

Figure 11   I. Ellis, Division of Histopathology, Nottingham City Hospital, UK

Figure 12   I. Ellis, Division of Histopathology, Nottingham City Hospital, UK

Figure 13   I. Ellis, Division of Histopathology, Nottingham City Hospital, UK

Figure 14   I. Ellis, Division of Histopathology, Nottingham City Hospital, UK

Figure 15   I. Ellis, Division of Histopathology, Nottingham City Hospital, UK,

Figure 16   I. Ellis, Division of Histopathology, Nottingham City Hospital, UK

Figure 17   I. Ellis, Division of Histopathology, Nottingham City Hospital, UK

Figure 18   I. Ellis, Division of Histopathology, Nottingham City Hospital, UK

Figure 19   Working Group

Figure 20   Working Group

Figure 21   Working Group

Figure 22   I. Andersson, Department of Diagnostic Radiology, Malmö, Sweden

Figure 23   I. Andersson, Department of Diagnostic Radiology, Malmö, Sweden

Figure 24   I. Andersson, Department of Diagnostic Radiology, Malmö, Sweden

Figure 25   Boyd *et al.* (2001)

Figure 26   I. Andersson, Department of Diagnostic Radiology, Malmö, Sweden

Figure 27   Working Group

Figure 28   Blackman *et al.* (1999)

Figure 29   Nyström *et al.* (2002)

Figure 30   Ford *et al.* (1998)

Figure 31   WHO (1999)

Figure 32   WHO (1999)

Figure 33   WHO WHO (1999)

Figure 34   WHO (1999)

Figure 35   Hakama *et al.* (1999)

Figure 36   Hakama *et al.* (1999)

Figure 37   Working Group

Figure 38   Working Group

Figure 39   Working Group

Figure 40   European Network of Cancer Registries (2001)

Figure 41   Working Group

Figure 42   S.H. Heywang-Köbrunner, Clinic of Radiology, Martin Luther University, Halle, Germany

Figure 43   National Cancer Institute (2001)

Figure 44   de Koning *et al.* (1991)

Figure 45   de Koning *et al.* (1991)

Figure 46   Boer *et al.* (1995)

---

Page 40   Clinical Breast Examination. JAMA (1999) 282, 1270–80 American Medical Association

Page 44   Breast Self examination. Sharon McLaren, University of Windsor, Canada

Page 46   Lancet Oncology, 3, p. 247 April 2002

Page 66   Access Arts Inc., Brisbane Powerhouse, Australia